PREDICTIVE TOXICOLOGY IN DRUG SAFETY

According to the Institute of Medicine and the U.S. Food and Drug Administration, "developing new scientific approaches to detecting, understanding, predicting, and preventing adverse events" was a critical path to the future of drug safety. This book brings together a collection of state-of-the-art chapters, written by experts in the drug safety field. It provides information on the present knowledge of drug side effects and their mitigation strategy during drug discovery, gives guidance for risk assessment, and promotes evidence-based toxicology. Each specific area of toxicology relevant for drug discovery is discussed in detail, including theory, experimental approaches, and data interpretation supported by comprehensive up-to-date references. Many chapters provide fascinating case studies, which are of general interest for those who have basic science training and are interested in how chemicals interact with the human body.

Dr. Jinghai J. Xu is currently Director of Knowledge Discovery and Knowledge Management at Merck & Company, Inc. Dr. Xu has won numerous awards, including the Central Research Achievement Award and Pfizer Global Research & Development Award. His most recently published book is *Drug Efficacy, Safety, and Biologics Discovery: Emerging Technologies and Tools* (2009).

Dr. Laszlo Urban is currently Executive Director and Global Head of Preclinical Safety Profiling at Novartis Institutes for Biomedical Research. Dr. Urban has been actively involved in organizations such as the European Neuropeptide Club, the Society for Biomolecular Sciences, and the International Association for the Study of Pain. His most recently published work is *Hit and Lead Profiling: Identification and Optimization of Drug-Like Molecules* (2009).

Predictive Toxicology in Drug Safety

Edited by

Jinghai J. Xu

Merck & Company, Inc.

Laszlo Urban

Novartis Institutes for Biomedical Research

CAMBRIDGE
UNIVERSITY PRESS

CAMBRIDGE UNIVERSITY PRESS
Cambridge, New York, Melbourne, Madrid, Cape Town, Singapore,
São Paulo, Delhi, Dubai, Tokyo, Mexico City

Cambridge University Press
32 Avenue of the Americas, New York, NY 10013-2473, USA

www.cambridge.org
Information on this title: www.cambridge.org/9780521763646

First published 2011

Printed in the United States of America

A catalog record for this publication is available from the British Library.

Library of Congress Cataloging in Publication data
Predictive toxicology in drug safety / [edited by] Jinghai J. Xu, Laszlo Urban.
p. ; cm.
Includes bibliographical references and index.
ISBN 978-0-521-76364-6 (hardback)
1. Drugs – Toxicity testing. I. Xu, Jinghai J. II. Urban, Laszlo, 1951–
[DNLM: 1. Drug Toxicity. 2. Drug Discovery. 3. Toxicity Tests. QV 600]
RA1238.P743 2011
615′.704–dc22 2010033857

ISBN 978-0-521-76364-6 Hardback

Contents

Contributors

Carl L. Alden D.V.M.
Millennium Pharmaceuticals
The Takeda Oncology Company
Cambridge, MA

Jiri Aubrecht Pharm.D., Ph.D.
Drug Safety Research and Development
Pfizer Global Research & Development
Groton, CT

Dejan Bojanic Ph.D.
Lead Finding Platform
Novartis Institutes for Biomedical Sciences
Cambridge, MA

Anita Büttner Ph.D.
University of Leipzig
Institute of Organic Chemistry
Leipzig, Germany

Glenn H. Cantor D.V.M., Ph.D.
Discovery Toxicology
Bristol-Myers Squibb
Princeton, NJ

Lucio G. Costa Ph.D.
Department of Environmental and Occupational Health Sciences
University of Washington
Seattle, WA

Thomas S. Davies Ph.D.
STA Preclinical Services LLC
Essex and Lyme, CT

Berengere Dumotier Ph.D.
Preclinical Safety
Novartis Pharma AG
Basel, Switzerland

David Gerhold Ph.D.
Department of Laboratory Sciences and Investigative Toxicology
Merck Research Laboratory
West Point, PA

Gennaro Giordano Ph.D.
Department of Environmental and Occupational Health Sciences
University of Washington
Seattle, WA

Bruce Gomes Ph.D.
Biotherapeutics Research and Development
Pfizer Inc.
Cambridge, MA

Sarah Gould Ph.D.
Non-Clinical Safety
Sanofi Pasteur
Marcy l'Etoile, France

Joaquin Guinea Ph.D.
ZF Biolabs
Madrid, Spain

Marina Guizzetti Ph.D.
Department of Environmental and Occupational Health Sciences
University of Washington
Seattle, WA

Ying Jiang Ph.D.
Department of Laboratory Sciences and Investigative Toxicology
Merck Research Laboratory
West Point, PA

Vivek J. Kadambi Ph.D.
Millennium Pharmaceuticals
The Takeda Oncology Company
Cambridge, MA

Amit S. Kalgutkar Ph.D.
Pharmacokinetics Dynamics and Metabolism Department
Pfizer Global Research & Development
Groton, CT

Nils Klüver Ph.D.
Helmholtz Centre for Environmental Research
Department of Bioanalytical Ecotoxicology
Leipzig, Germany

Frank Lee Ph.D.
Millennium Pharmaceuticals
The Takeda Oncology Company
Cambridge, MA

Lois D. Lehman-McKeeman Ph.D.
Discovery Toxicology
Bristol-Myers Squibb Company
Princeton, NJ

Albert P. Li Ph.D.
In Vitro ADMET Laboratories Inc.
Columbia, MD

Guohui Liu Ph.D.
Millennium Pharmaceuticals
The Takeda Oncology Company
Cambridge, MA

Bin Lu Ph.D.
Drug Safety Research and Development
Pfizer Global Research & Development
Groton, CT

Kapil Mayawala Ph.D.
Biotherapeutics Research and Development
Pfizer Inc.
Cambridge, MA

Timothy J. Maziasz Ph.D.
Millennium Pharmaceuticals
The Takeda Oncology Company
Cambridge, MA

Chester Ni Ph.D.
Computational Biology
University of Washington
Seattle, WA

Harry M. Olson D.V.M., Ph.D.
STA Preclinical Services LLC
Essex and Lyme, CT

Raymond Oomen Ph.D.
Discovery Bioinformatics
Sanofi Pasteur
Cambridge, MA

Monicah A. Otieno Ph.D.
Discovery Toxicology
Bristol-Myers Squibb Company
Princeton, NJ

Terence R. S. Ozolinš Ph.D.
Department of Pharmacology and Toxicology
Queen's University
Kingston, Canada

Shimoga Prakash Ph.D.
Millennium Pharmaceuticals
The Takeda Oncology Company
Cambridge, MA

Stefan Scholz Ph.D.
Helmholtz Centre for Environmental Research
Department of Bioanalytical Ecotoxicology
Leipzig, Germany

Lee Silverman D.V.M., Ph.D.
Millennium Pharmaceuticals
The Takeda Oncology Company
Cambridge, MA

Frank D. Sistare Ph.D.
Department of Laboratory Sciences and Investigative Toxicology
Merck Research Laboratory
West Point, PA

Martin Traebert Ph.D.
Preclinical Safety
Novartis Pharma AG
Basel, Switzerland

Laszlo Urban M.D., Ph.D.
Lead Finding Platform
Novartis Institutes for Biomedical Research
Cambridge, MA

Jörg Vollmer Ph.D.
Pfizer Oligonucleotides Therapeutics Unit
Coley Pharmaceutical GmbH
Düsseldorf, Germany

Jianling Wang Ph.D.
Metabolism and Pharmacokinetics
Novartis Institutes for Biomedical Research
Cambridge, MA

Susan Ward Ph.D.
Life Sciences Industries
Cambridge, MA

Jinghai J. Xu Ph.D.
Knowledge Discovery and Knowledge Management
Merck & Co., Inc.
Rahway, NJ

Li J. Yu Ph.D.
Drug Metabolism and Pharmacokinetics
Hoffmann–La Roche, Inc.
Nutley, NJ

Prologue

Predictive toxicology: a new chapter in drug safety evaluation

In 2007, the U.S. Food and Drug Administration (FDA) issued a report titled "The Future of Drug Safety – Promoting and Protecting the Health of the Public." In it, strengthening the science that supports drug safety evaluation was recognized as a critical path to improve drug safety assessment. In particular, "developing and qualifying techniques for predictive toxicology" was identified as one of the major unmet needs in advancing scientific approaches to detect, understand, predict, and prevent adverse events (http://www.fda.gov/).

With the cost of developing an FDA-approved medicine approaching $1 billion and time to develop a drug taking 10 to 15 years, late-stage failures or attritions pose a significant burden on the sustainability of the current pharmaceutical research and development (R&D) model. Because 90% of drug candidates that enter clinical development fail to reach the market, the root cause of rising R&D costs is a continuous investment in failure. By last account, clinical safety represents 20% and preclinical toxicology embodies 13% of failed development efforts. Together, drug safety reasons account for one-third of overall failure. Most of the current tools and models used for toxicology and human safety testing are decades old, including many that are recommended by the FDA. Better models, methodologies, and testing paradigms with demonstrated improvement in drug safety prediction than existing practices are clearly needed. Predictive toxicology, aimed at addressing this challenge using a combined knowledge and insight from all fields of science, is the central topic of this book.

This book is organized into two sections. The first section starts with a "current state" chapter on the predictivity of animal toxicology evaluation for human drug safety. This is followed by individual topics of toxicology, including genetic, cardiac, hepatic, drug–drug interactions, reactive metabolite, immune, neurologic, and developmental toxicology. The second section of the book emphasizes integrated approaches (integrated lead optimization, oncology drugs, mechanism-based toxicity), novel *in vivo* experimental models (zebrafish, genetically engineered models), emerging technologies (toxicogenomic pathway mining, safety biomarkers), and mathematical modeling approaches (PKPD modeling, biologics modeling). The book ends with a chapter on the safety evaluation of vaccines. Each chapter is authored by subject matter experts in that area. We are extremely grateful to all the contributing authors for sharing their knowledge and insight. It is our honor to experience their enthusiasm, professionalism, and collaboration from the beginning of this book project.

Even though there is a heavy emphasis on drug discovery and development, the predictive toxicology strategies and approaches described in this book should also be highly relevant and applicable to the fields of chemical, environmental, and other areas of toxicology where rational prediction of human safety risk becomes a fundamental duty for toxicologists. We hope that toxicologists in both practice and training will find this book thought-provoking and highly pertinent to the direction of toxicology in the twenty-first century.

Jinghai J. Xu, Ph.D.
Laszlo Urban, M.D., Ph.D.

PREDICTIVE TOXICOLOGY IN DRUG SAFETY

I SPECIFIC AREAS OF PREDICTIVE TOXICOLOGY

1 The human predictive value of combined animal toxicity testing

Current state and emerging approaches

Harry M. Olson and Thomas S. Davies

1.1 INTRODUCTION

Pharmaceutical development in the late twentieth and early twenty-first centuries has been a challenging enterprise. It is an expensive undertaking with a high degree of risk associated mainly with a high failure rate. A new chemical entity (NCE) that successfully completes the entire process of drug discovery and development reaching approval as a new therapeutic may accrue total development costs in excess of one billion dollars (U.S.).[1] Also, for the drugs that are successful, it typically takes 10 to 12 years from the initiation of research efforts to reach final marketing approval.[1] Experience in the past decade with the overall success/failure rate process – which now encompasses many new and emerging tools including early screening assays and *in silico* technologies, and the historical experience of "what works and doesn't work" – has so far not yielded the expected productivity improvements. Enigmatically, recent experience suggests that it is getting more difficult to identify successful lead molecules that lead to safe and effective therapeutics.

A high-level schematic overview of the current drug development process is shown in Figure 1.1. Candidate molecules entering preclinical development from the discovery process proceed through the stages of clinical development (Clinical Phases I, II, and III). During clinical development, safety (first) and efficacy are evaluated in consecutively larger groups of normal volunteers and patients. First-in-human (or FIH) studies number in the 10s of normal subjects or patients, and then the NCE is assessed in patients (100s in Phase 2, and 1,000s in Phase 3) with the disease of therapeutic interest. This overall "classical" approach is oriented mainly to small synthetic molecules, but it is applicable (with modifications) to other drug categories (e.g., biologicals and botanical products) as well.

The drug discovery phase preceding clinical drug development is when evaluation of many potential NCE molecules occurs and the numbers of promising structures is reduced and refined to a select handful of very promising candidates. The goal in discovery is to apply both pharmacology and toxicology screening processes relevant to the intended therapeutic indication and route of administration to identify candidate molecules with the most favorable efficacy

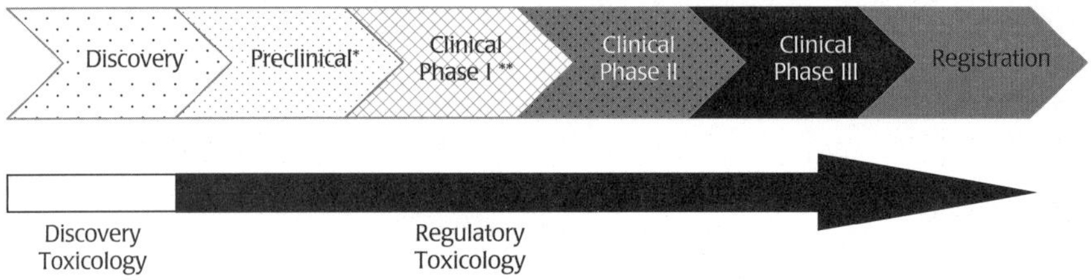

Clinical Phase	Objective	Subjects	No. Studied
Phase I	Safety, PK	Normal volunteers	10's
Phase II	Safety, Efficacy	Patients	100's
Phase III	Safety, Efficacy	Patients	1000's

Figure 1-1: Toxicology in drug development. Reprinted from *Regulatory Toxicology and Pharmacology*, vol. 32/1, Olson et al., "Concordance of the Toxicity of Pharmaceuticals in Humans and in Animals" 12, 2000, with permission from Elsevier.

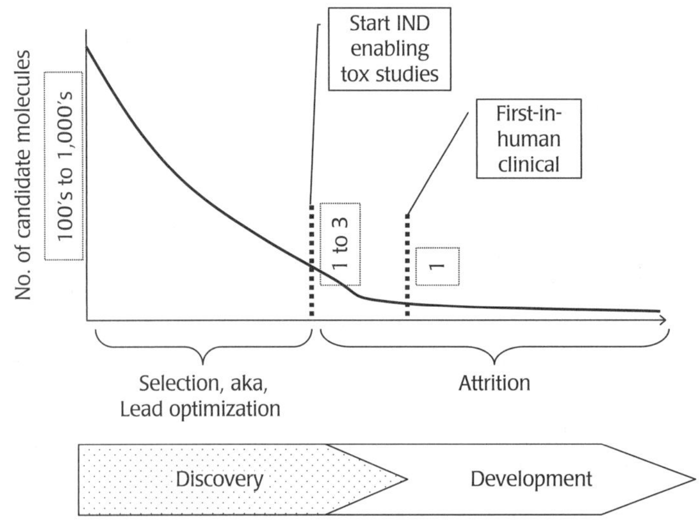

Figure 1-2: Selection and attrition in drug development. Reprinted from *Regulatory Toxicology and Pharmacology*, vol. 32/1, Olson et al., "Concordance of the Toxicity of Pharmaceuticals in Humans and in Animals" 12, 2000, with permission from Elsevier.

and safety attributes so that they can be considered for further development. This process is known as candidate selection (see Figure 1.2), or lead molecule optimization. The technologies and resources applied during candidate selection may include *in silico* methods (e.g., Quantitative Structure Activity Relationship [QSAR]), *in vitro* efficacy and safety screens, and also possibly some *in vivo* animal model assessment (e.g., pharmacokinetic and toxicology screening studies).[2,3]

1.1.1 Candidate selection and attrition – the inevitability of failure

As previously described, candidate selection is the approach in drug discovery that is expected to yield a small and select number of promising molecules for

Complex disease targets	Insufficient selectivity
Retention time in body too short or too long	Side effects
Adverse reactions	Unstable compound
Poor or low bioavailability	Competition (in marketplace)
Lack of adequate clinical effectiveness	Not practical to synthesize

Figure 1-3: Some common causes of attrition. Reprinted from *Regulatory Toxicology and Pharmacology*, vol. 32/1, Olson et al., "Concordance of the Toxicity of Pharmaceuticals in Humans and in Animals" 12, 2000, with permission from Elsevier.

the intended therapeutic indication (Figure 1.2). Many compounds or chemical classes during selection are evaluated in virtual or actual test systems. For toxicologists, this may include *in silico* assessment for structural alerts such as for genotoxic potential, cellular damage, or other potential toxic effects.[2,3] The next step in drug development of the selected lead molecule is attrition. Attrition is the loss of molecules or drug candidates that have entered the preclinical development or subsequent clinical development phases (Figure 1.2). A substantial number of development candidates fail because toxicity issues surfaced in preclinical Investigative New Drug Application (IND)-supporting studies (these compounds selected pre-FIH may never make it into Phase I clinical trials), in subsequent toxicology studies conducted during development, or as a result of significant clinical adverse events arising during development. Attrition can occur even after product registration and marketing, possibly resulting in withdrawal of the product from the market.

Some of the common reasons for attrition are shown in Figure 1.3; these include both toxicity-related findings and other deficiencies in drug candidates that can occur at any time during drug development. Indeed, attrition is about more than toxicity, which nonetheless does remain an important contributor to drug loss.[4] The other factors listed in Figure 1.3 should be kept in mind as key factors in this loss of NCE molecules during development. Unlike during the candidate selection phase, attrition is not a desirable outcome, but it is a normal and expected outcome of drug development. Historically (e.g., in large pharmaceutical company portfolios), attrition can reach or exceed a 90 percent failure rate of compounds identified as "promising" in the late discovery and early development phases. Overall, this may be considered as a kind of Darwinian "natural selection" process, to identify drugability shortcomings early and to focus available resources on the most promising candidates.

Optimally, drug developers want attrition to occur as early as possible, and in particular in the interval between start of the FIH- (or IND)-supporting studies and the end of the Phase II clinical trials (Figure 1.1). Later stage attrition (e.g., in Phase III clinical trials) can have a profound negative impact on drug development programs, timing, and costs.[1] The withdrawal of drugs from the marketplace due to toxicity or other issues can be discouraging and frustrating (or worse) to patients, drug manufacturers, and regulators.

The understanding of attrition occurring in drug development currently is more grounded historically to small, synthetic molecule development programs than to the more recent advent of biological therapeutics. While there is not yet the long history of experience with biologicals, some manufactured protein/polypeptides are typically "purpose designed" and configured as "humanized" to modulate or replace endogenous molecules, such as insulin, blood clotting factors, or other biomolecules. However, the early stage development of all ethical therapeutics – whether small molecules or biological therapeutics – must include preclinical toxicology evaluation in recognized and accepted (by regulatory authorities) *in vivo* test systems that are recognized as predictive of potential human toxicities or adverse effects.

1.1.2 *In silico, in vitro,* and *in vivo* – what approaches to use, and when?

The approach used to identify lead therapeutic molecules must be adaptable to – and take account of – the clinical program therapeutic goals, understand the attributes of the candidate molecule (both unique to the NCE and to the chemical class), and recognize the capabilities and limitations of any test systems used to characterize toxicity. As shown in Figure 1.4, the approach should begin with consideration of *in silico* approaches that may precede *in vitro* and *in vivo* studies.[2,3] Included here are access to the published literature, FOI (freedom-of-information) resources, and archival documentation including computer-based and searchable compound databases, which are important to review what is already known about potential target organ toxic effects for the chemical class. QSAR searchable artificial intelligence systems – a few are Internet accessible – can screen chemical structures and identify possible or "suspect" structural alerts. This information can be useful if applied judiciously to the process of optimizing lead molecule selection. Some *in silico* systems (MultiCASE) are useful to gather information sourced from historical databases and literature references. Many large pharmaceutical companies have systems that include data, summaries, and reports from internal investigative studies.

In vitro screening assays (Figure 1.4) are similarly useful to identify specific molecular characteristics such as receptor affinity, *ex vivo* cross-species comparative metabolite profile, compound metabolic stability, mutagenic potential or other specific attributes or liabilities.[2,3] In preclinical development preceding the Phase I clinical trial, there are specific regulatory requirements for *in vitro* studies conducted under Good Laboratory Practice (GLP) guidances,[3,4] including mutagenic potential in bacteria, structural chromosomal damage in mammalian cells, and also assessment of potassium channel inhibition in the human *Ether-à-go-go* Related Gene (hERG) test system.[2–4] Published data from investigative or regulatory *in vitro* systems may provide useful guidance of similar molecule characteristics. *In silico* and *in vitro* evaluations can contribute much to

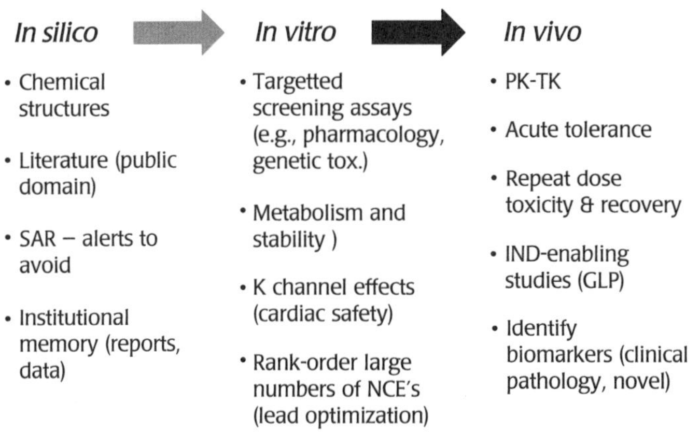

Figure 1-4: Strategic approach to *in vivo* study. Reprinted from *Regulatory Toxicology and Pharmacology*, vol. 32/1, Olson et al., "Concordance of the Toxicity of Pharmaceuticals in Humans and in Animals" 12, 2000, with permission from Elsevier.

the understanding of the molecular toxicity profile, including a preliminary estimate of the probability of success with the NCE development.[2] However, the results from *in vitro* systems have real limitations, and can't be used to reliably characterize the toxicity profile of a selected lead molecule as a therapeutic candidate. For this, the essential resource is *in vivo* toxicity testing.

The inclusion of laboratory animals in studies to assess the toxic potential of lead molecules as a basis for further clinical development is integral to the process of data-based decision making for drug development (Figure 1.4). As an outcome of the cause of death of seventy-six people from diethylene glycol poisoning, as a constituent of a sulphanilamide formulation (Elixir Sulfanilamide), came passage of the federal Food, Drug, and Cosmetic (FD&C) Act of 1938. With this legislation came – for the first time – the requirement of manufacturers of medicines to show that a drug was safe prior to marketing. This and other subsequent legislation mandated the key principles for testing and evaluating new drugs, including the mandate for *in vivo* animal toxicity testing.[5]

Mammalian test systems (notably rat, dog, and primate) are biochemically integrated, with metabolic capabilities for drug transformation and excretion, complex endocrine pathways and feedback loops, and internal organ systems and many clinical pathology biomarkers of toxic effects (e.g., elevated liver enzymes released from damaged hepatocytes or bone marrow toxicity revealed in hemogram changes) that mimic those in humans.[3,6] Therefore, these animal models – most typically one rodent and one nonrodent animal species – have been shown to provide an approximate integrated surrogate to assess possible in-life and target organ toxicity of the NCE. These preclinical studies are important to providing assurance of the safety profile prior to proceeding with studies in human volunteers or patients. Indeed, preclinical *in vivo* models are prime examples of *translation* of toxic effects to human risk assessment.[6] However, the outcome of toxicology studies performed in these test systems has not always predicted the identical outcomes in humans. But we have acquired much experience about the usefulness of these models to predict human toxicity, and also the limitations to identify certain types of clinical adverse effects.

In order to achieve the end-game of developing a marketable therapeutic, the requisite criteria are that the drug must be shown to be "pure, safe and effective" (Food, Drug and Cosmetic Act of 1938). Practice, experience, and updated regulatory guidance have provided guideposts for meeting each of these three criteria over the course of drug development. The remainder of this chapter will address the extent to which combined animal toxicity testing can help achieve an understanding of potential human toxicity, or adverse effects and what are the shortcomings that remain today.

1.2 MEANING AND VALUE OF PREDICTING HUMAN TOXICITY IN PHARMACEUTICAL DEVELOPMENT

Our attention in this chapter is to focus on contributions to reduce attrition by the pragmatic use of preclinical *in vivo* toxicity testing throughout drug development. This is provided by understanding the use, predictive value, and limitations of preclinical *in vivo* toxicology studies as they pertain to identifying possible human clinical toxicity, and how the safety data obtainable from these preclinical studies is being refined and continues to be improved.

Implicit in the title of this chapter, "The Human Predictive Value of Combined Animal Toxicity Testing," is the expectation *that there is predictive value* in preclinical animal toxicity testing. This is why these studies are done in pharmaceutical research and development, why toxicologists and clinical pharmacologists rely on the data and information from such studies, and, of course, why there are preclinical testing requirements mandated by regulatory authorities. Results from *in vivo* toxicity studies – both the toxicity and toxicokinetic data and their interpretation – are of direct use by clinical investigators to assess risk and benefit of a NCE exposure for patients, particularly in early phases of controlled clinical studies. Support for the predictive value of *in vivo* toxicity testing comes from long experience, historical precedence, published research and regulatory guidance, and requirements spanning many decades. The practice and requirements for animal toxicity design and testing (e.g., using the fewest number of animals needed to obtain a valid scientifically defensible outcome) have been incorporated into current preclinical toxicology study designs. With the availability of current methods to compare *in vitro* metabolism of compounds across species, and to measure plasma levels of parent drug and key (major) metabolites in animal toxicity studies (to compare with therapeutic plasma levels in clinical studies), it is possible to provide expected safety margin estimates for NCEs during development.[2,3]

1.3 *IN VIVO* TESTING STRATEGIES AND MODELS IN-USE FOR DRUG DEVELOPMENT

The background leading to today's preclinical regulatory study testing requirements has been described previously. Guidelines for testing of NCEs are provided in the M-3 Guidance[4] and other preclinical regulatory documents issued by review committees of the International Conferences on Harmonization (ICH). ICH was first convened in 1992 as a cooperative body to reduce duplicate testing of new medicines during the research and development phase. ICH guidance documents and revisions now provide a unified, standardized approach for toxicology testing, achieving greater harmonization of technical guidelines and study designs for product registration.

The main purpose of *in vivo* toxicity testing is to define the preclinical safety profile of the NCE. The safety profile doesn't mean that the drug candidate is absolutely safe in all respects or for all routes of dose administration, but instead that the safety profile of the prospective drug is known. This profile includes in-life effects and target organ toxicity endpoints in relationship to the schedule and route of intended dosing. The systemic drug exposure is reported also in animal toxicology studies. Therefore, "safe" means that the occurrence, incidence, severity, and reversibility of toxic effects and exposure to the NCE in the *in vivo* test system all contribute to determine how the NCE can be administered safely to human subjects. It is important to evaluate and understand the NCE dose-response relationship in studies that include lower doses near to the intended therapeutic exposure in patients, up to higher doses that test the tolerance (toxicology) limits. This dose-response concept was originated by Paracelsus (sixteenth-century "father of toxicology") who advised, "all substances may be poisons, *it is the dose that makes the poison*" (paraphrased, italics the author's).

Therefore, the safety profile of a NCE may include tolerance evaluation, clinical effects, blood or urine biomarkers that signal damage to target organs, and histopathology, which confirms the effect. Toxicokinetic measurements in these studies provide plasma exposure data on the parent compound and/or key metabolites that also occur in humans. During the past decade, the reversibility of toxicity effects is also often evaluated in the study design, by inclusion of a nondosing interval following the dosing phase. Based on this information *a safety margin* can be determined comparing the intended clinical plasma exposure with that in rodent and nonrodent studies to ensure the safety profile is consistent with the intended therapeutic indication. The main objective for drug registration (oncology therapeutics being an exception) is that the drug is expected to be safe under the conditions of intended human investigation and therapeutic use (by route and dose as prescribed).

1.3.1 Predictive value of animal testing

The rationale for laboratory animal testing is that the results from these studies are predictive of possible adverse effects in humans, and therefore can be used to manage the risk of subsequent human exposure. This is particularly true leading up to initial human trials – also called first-in-human studies – where there is no prior NCE clinical experience.

A very few investigations have been published to determine how predictive animal toxicity testing is related to human toxicities associated with investigative or marketed therapeutics.[7–13] The main aim of these studies was to understand how useful animal toxicity studies are to predict human clinical toxicity. Several of these studies have focused on cytotoxic anticancer therapeutics,[9–12] which have inherently narrow safety margins for tolerable toxicity since higher exposures may engender adverse effects in order to also achieve effective treatment of the disease. For anticancer therapeutics, the observed clinical toxicity in humans may be predicted for at the higher doses in the preclinical toxicity studies because of the very narrow safety margin. For the broader classes of pharmaceuticals (including but not limited to anticancer agents), the predictive value of preclinical animal toxicology studies is addressed by prediction of the clinical toxicity observed during clinical drug development trials (Figure 1.1). Two multinational pharmaceutical company surveys have been undertaken by the International Life Sciences Institute – Human and Environmental Sciences Institute (ILSI-HESI) organization to explore this aspect. The initial survey has been published,[7] and the second survey workshop was held in 2007 [HESI concordance of animal and human toxicity workshop, September 20–21, 2007, Washington, D.C.].

The multinational pharmaceutical company survey is the largest published survey of this kind, including a total of 150 compounds with 221 human toxicities (or adverse effects).[7] Some included drug candidates caused multiple clinical toxicities. In this survey, prediction of the human toxicity was the basis for evaluating whether animals were – or were not – effective to identify the corresponding target organ(s) human toxicity. Schein et al. examined the reported preclinical and human toxicities of twenty-five anticancer drugs in dog, primate, and human studies.[11] Owens reported toxicity findings of twenty-one anticancer drugs in rodent, dog, primate, and human studies,[9] and Freireich and colleagues reported toxicity findings of eighteen anticancer drugs in mouse, rat, hamster, dog, primate, and humans.[12]

The following summarizes the results and conclusions obtained from these published studies for the following organ systems:

Central nervous system (CNS). In a Japanese study of eighty-four drugs evaluated in general pharmacology studies, the reported capacity to predict adverse effects was mixed; however, it reported that changes in locomotor activity in rodents correlated with dizziness in humans.[13] In some studies, high doses in animals produced CNS-related effects (ataxia, convulsions) not observed in clinical trials.[7,14] The concordance in studies of general therapeutics[7] and anticancer therapeutics[9,11] was reported as moderate (predictive from 20 to 60 percent) as there was poor correlation with specific symptoms. Overall, nonrodent data were more predictive than rodent data for identifying adverse neurological effects in the clinic, and histopathologic evaluations were useful to detect serious neurotoxic effects.[15]

Cardiovascular. The overwhelming majority of concordance cases in these studies were reported in nonrodent species, specifically the dog and to a lesser extent the primate.[7,15] For general therapeutics the concordance rate was 80 percent,[7] and this was principally in pharmacology studies. The basis for evaluation includes safety pharmacology electrocardiographic effects and histopathologic toxicities. In these surveys, rodents were determined to have lesser utility because of the unsuitability of this model to evaluate cardiovascular function. Electrocardiographic (ECG) assessment in dogs – combined with *in vitro* assessment in hERG and Purkinje standardized test systems – is currently the regulatory standard to identify compounds presenting higher risk for human cardiac arrhythmias.[2,4]

Hematologic. There was a high concordance (91 percent) in both rodent and nonrodent species with human hematotoxic findings.[7,11,12] These cases are highly correlated with anticancer and antiinfective therapies. Current methods for identifying and evaluating bone marrow toxicity and coagulation effects in both preclinical toxicology and clinical studies are similar, providing the basis for consistent assessment and reliable cross-species and human comparison.

Gastrointestinal (GI). There was a high concordance (85 percent) of human GI toxicities with the animal findings most notably in nonrodent species.[7] This high concordance was particularly the case for anticancer, antiinfective, and antiinflammatory drug classes mediated by pharmacologic mechanisms. Similarly, safety pharmacology studies in a Japanese review of eighty-eight noncancer drugs showed a good correlation for rodent intestinal transport studies and clinical adverse effects (anorexia, constipation).[13] Other studies showed similar positive correlation outcomes across therapeutic classes, including anticancer drugs.[9,11,12,14] In particular the physiologic similarities of the dog and human gastrointestinal tracts may be useful and conducive in support of this high concordance.[16]

Hepatic. Hepatotoxicity remains a significant contributor to attrition in drug development portfolios of many pharmaceutical and biotech companies.[7] Recent surveys indicated that drug-induced liver damage accounts for over 50 percent of incidences of acute liver failure in the United States.[17] In the clinical and preclinical settings, measurement of liver enzymes in blood during NCE dose administration is the most reliable in-life method of detecting potential hepatotoxicity; liver histopathology is also important to confirm severity of effects in animal studies. One study reported a concordance of 80 percent in identifying hepatotoxicity from toxicity studies with known human hepatotoxicity.[18] Other studies assessing anticancer drugs reported good predictivity of hepatotoxic injury in humans with drugs, as evaluated by enzyme changes and liver histopathology.[9,11] In the large multinational industry survey, concordance was shown to be about 50 percent,[7] which was among the lower predictive markers. Possibly this is related to the occurrence of either: (a) subtle preclinical changes (i.e., minimal liver histopathologic changes or low-level increases in liver enzymes in only a few study animals) that fail to be recognized as hepatotoxic signals, or (b) occurrence of idiosyncratic hepatotoxicity with $< 1{:}10{,}000$

incidence in the population. In fact, idiosyncratic reactions are not uncommon and continue to have an impact on late-stage attrition of drugs in development or withdrawals from the marketplace.[15] For large pharmaceutical companies, the occurrence of liver enzyme changes in early drug development in rats is recognized as a common occurrence, generally related to propensity of this species to respond to metabolic inducers. NCEs that show evidence for liver effects and damage are usually presumed to be risky and are dropped in the early screening stages of drug development.

Renal. Renal toxicity – similar to hepatotoxicity – is assessed in preclinical toxicology studies by blood parameters (blood urea nitrogen [BUN], creatinine, electrolytes), urinalysis constituents, and histopathologic examination. Predictive results in studies with anticancer drugs were variable, with a tendency toward overprediction.[9,11] Concordance in the large multinational industry survey was about 70 percent.[7]

Pulmonary. The assessment of drug candidates on respiration is performed prior to FIH registration in either specific safety pharmacology respiratory studies – typically in rodents – or clinical evaluation of rodents and nonrodents in the postdose phase of conventional toxicology studies, and by histopathologic evaluation of lungs. Igarashi et al. reported that respiratory disturbances that occur clinically were not predicted by the safety pharmacology studies.[13] Both Schein and Fletcher reported a high degree of overprediction of respiratory effects in animal toxicity and safety pharmacology studies, compared to actual clinical adverse events.[11,14]

Endocrine. Endocrine changes may be identified by inclusion of specific hormone analyses (based on availability of bioanalytical methods for the species) in toxicology studies, or more typically by histopathologic evaluation of endocrine organs. Results from the multinational industry survey showed only moderate concordance (60 percent) from preclinical studies.[7] Fletcher reported that the findings from preclinical toxicology studies overpredicted effects in humans.[14]

Dermal. There are very few reported cases of skin reaction responses in the multinational industry survey,[7] and animal models in other surveys do not provide reliable predictive utility for these effects.[9,11,14] However, when they occur, dermal hypersensitivity-type reactions are a significant contributor to termination of drugs in various stages of development (Clinical Phases 2 and 3 in particular).[7,19]

Immunologic. The literature is replete with examples of xenobiotic (including therapeutics) immune effects in animal species, but except for hypersensitization few of these effects have been seen in human studies. In many cases immunologic endpoints in animal studies have not been evaluated for predictivity in humans. However, some specific individual species effects that are usefully compared to human immunologic effects (e.g., immune complex effects in rabbits, or immediate/delayed-type hypersensitivity in guinea pigs) have been reported.[20]

A workshop on Preclinical Evaluation of Peptides and Recombinant Proteins provided an integrated interpretation of preclinical toxicology data for several recombinant protein therapeutic molecules from studies in animals and humans.[21] A key conclusion of this analysis is that clinically relevant adverse effects can be obtained from well-designed preclinical toxicity studies. Examples of concordant effects with recombinant Hu interleukins include vascular leak syndrome (occurs in mouse, rat, primate) and hypotension (rabbit, primate). In the workshop discussion, it was noted that there may be quantitative differences in species sensitivity to clinical toxic effects. However, testing of the human protein in preclinical species – including species with and without the protein molecule receptor – may have value in identifying human-relevant toxicity. The importance of appropriate study design was emphasized, including species sensitivity, dose selection, and possible nonlinear dose response effects with biologicals, induction of an antibody response, and other factors.[21]

1.3.2 Predictive assessment of developmental and reproductive toxicology studies

Developmental and reproductive toxicology (DART) studies – usually conducted in the rat and rabbit – are performed during clinical development of synthetic and biological therapeutics.[4] The results of these studies may be included in the approved drug package insert with a category score to communicate risk. There is currently no published analysis of the predictive outcome of DART studies, nor are there any consistent reports of clinical teratogenic effects associated with exposure to drugs. However, a discussion of the significance and human risk assessment of preclinical teratogenic findings – at doses where maternal toxicity is or is not observed – is provided by Hood and Miller.[22]

1.4 LIMITATIONS OF *IN VIVO* TESTING IN DRUG DEVELOPMENT – EXAMPLE OF CARCINOGENICITY STUDIES

This section will focus on the current status and future trends of carcinogenicity testing in support of drug development. Even though the predictive value of the rodent bioassay remains controversial, the results of the rodent bioassay are currently required for approval of chronic use drugs in the United States and other countries. The safety and approval of drugs is based on a regulatory assessment of data from preclinical toxicology studies and clinical trials. The FDA Office of Pharmaceutical Science Web site states that toxicology studies are used to assess three broad categories of chemical toxicities that cannot be appropriately assessed in humans – genetic toxicity, reproductive and developmental toxicity, and carcinogenicity.[23] The default assumption is that positive effects in a rodent carcinogenicity study indicate that a drug candidate may have carcinogenic potential in humans. Thus, if no adequate human data are present, positive effects in a rodent carcinogenicity study become a basis for assessing the carcinogenic risk to humans. Results of carcinogenicity studies (and two other categories) are communicated by means of the drug label.

Historically, the regulatory requirements for the assessment of the carcinogenic potential of pharmaceuticals recommended the conduct of long-term carcinogenicity studies in two rodent species, usually the rat and the mouse. In the 1990s, the use of transgenic mice was introduced in an attempt to improve the process of hazard identification.[24] Deficiencies of the conventional bioassay are well known and include the following:[25,26]

- Approximately 50 percent of drugs tested yield positive results in bioassay.
- Bioassay often produces contradictory results – simultaneous tumor increases and decreases.
- Demonstrated lack of concordance of tumor sites in rodents and humans.
- Tumor type and/or incidence varies by species and strain/stock.
- Diet (calories) is a potential variable in carcinogenicity studies.
- Use of maximum tolerated dose (often not indicative of human exposure) is required.
- Bioassay is costly, time consuming, and resource intensive.

Interpretation and risk assessment of tumor findings in rodent bioassay would typically include evaluation of

- Adequacy of the study (dose selection, adequate survival)
- Type (rare vs. common), lethality, and time of onset of tumor
- Comparison of concurrent and historical control incidences of tumor type
- Dose response of tumor incidence data
- Presence/absence of preneoplastic lesions
- Occurrence of class effects for particular drug class
- Long-term tissue retention of drug
- The presence of a threshold (no-effect-level)
- Safety margin based on exposure multiples (mg/m^2 and/or AUC) at the no-effect-level
- Presence/absence of structural alerts and/or DNA reactivity
- Species/gender differences in tumor incidence, toxicokinetics (AUC), protein binding, and metabolism
- Molecular fingerprint of the tumor
- Need for mechanistic data, additional genotoxicity data, or transgenic mouse data

Drug candidate selected for full development are typically negative for genotoxic potential because of the recognized relationship between genotoxicity and tumor development. As a consequence of screening for lack of genotoxic potential, the majority of tumors identified in rodent bioassays conducted in support of pharmaceutical development occur by nongenotoxic (epigenetic) mechanisms, often at doses much higher than anticipated human exposure.

There is a general agreement concerning the need to improve risk assessment of bioassay data through the incorporation of more information on mechanism of action of tumor induction. Investigative studies to identify the mechanisms of action of rodent epigenetic carcinogens may clarify the relationship between

Table 1-1. Examples of tumor target organs and epigenetic mechanisms in rodents with little relevance for humans

Rodent target organ	Epigenetic mechanisms in rodents
Liver	Liver enzyme inducers that increase liver weight
	Inhibitors of TSH synthesis
Thyroid	Inhibitors of T_3-monodeiodinase (converts T_4 to T_3)
	Liver enzyme inducers (increase disposition of thyroid hormones)
Mesovarium	β-Adrenergic agonists
Mammary gland	Dopamine antagonists (increase prolactin)
Uterus	Dopamine agonists (decrease prolactin)
Stomach	Gastric acid antisecretory agents
Testis	5α-Reductase inhibitors
Pituitary, testis	LHRH-analogs
Pituitary, mammary gland Uterus	Estrogens
Blood	Immunosuppressants
Adrenal	Drugs that affect calcium absorption and homeostasis
	Drugs that affect catecholamine release from the adrenal medulla
Testis, ovary	Drugs that affect FSH or LH secretion
Urinary bladder	Carbonic anhydrase inhibitors
	Drugs that affect urinary pH

Source: Adapted from Monro.[27]

findings in rodents and likely effects in humans. Mechanistic data often lead to development of useful biomarkers. Numerous compounds induce tumors in rodents at doses and through mechanisms clearly not relevant to humans. Table 1.1 lists examples of epigenetic tumor formation in rodents with little relevance for human cancer risk.

A number of activities that hold promise for improvements in carcinogenic risk assessment of pharmaceuticals are underway. The Critical Path Institute, a nonprofit organization dedicated to implementing the FDA's Critical Path Initiative through collaborations between the FDA and industry, has recently established a Predictive Safety Testing Consortium (PSTC) of pharmaceutical companies.[28] One of several PSTC working groups, the Carcinogenicity Working Group, is evaluating the results of chronic rat studies as a predictor for 2-year rat carcinogenicity outcomes. The working group database contains approximately 240 chronic rat studies and matching carcinogenicity studies.[29] Preliminary analyses showed a strong sensitivity (87 percent) and negative predictivity (89 percent) of chronic study results for bioassay outcomes. Ultimately efforts like this may lead to improved predictivity, increased knowledge regarding human relevance of rodent tumors, revision of testing guidelines, reduced animal use, and reductions in time to market for new pharmaceuticals. Additional areas of research with potential promise for improvement in the current carcinogenicity risk assessment paradigm include predictive toxicogenomics and computational toxicology.[30,31]

1.5 REMAINING GAPS AND ADDITIONAL PERSPECTIVES ON PREDICTING HUMAN TOXICITY

The pragmatic application of toxicology data and interpretation from *in vivo* studies is of value to inform drug development stakeholders – including physicians, regulators, and the drug development sponsors – of potential human toxicity risks with an NCE and to facilitate safety risk management decision making (i.e., speed of dose escalation, identification of dose-limiting toxicity, making "go/no-go" project decisions). As shown previously, toxicity effects – including biomarkers identified with hematology, coagulation and clinical chemistry data or other novel urinary or blood biomarkers, and target tissue effects from macroscopic and histopathologic evaluation – are evaluated in the preclinical species.[2,3] This approach has continued to be effective over many decades in helping drug developers to manage and reduce the safety risks of repeated and long-term drug exposure in patients. The evidence of this is that controlled clinical trials have shown a long history and an overall excellent record of safety.

The predictive analysis of preclinical toxicology data has been shown previously in a quadrant model that takes account of the toxicity outcomes from preclinical studies and occurrence or nonoccurrence of adverse effects recorded in clinical trials (see Figure 1.5).[7] As shown in Figure 1.5, the "true positive" (upper left) and "true negative" (lower right) quadrants represent agreement ("concordance") between the clinical studies and the preclinical studies outcomes. That is, a clinical toxic effect in a target tissue was also identified – or predicted – in the preclinical model. This experience is important from the standpoint of placing reliance on whether toxicity signals observed in the test systems have shown reliable proficiency in identifying potential clinical toxicity. Conversely, does the absence of a toxic effect (perhaps characteristic of a chemical class) correctly predict that the clinical toxicity does not occur? Experience has shown that some unusual or rare (idiosyncratic) toxicities (e.g., liver) may not occur until after several years of marketing.

However we also know that the test systems are not infallible; they are subject to false positive outcomes (i.e., a false alert) or false negative outcomes (missing a human toxicity raises concern for all stakeholders). *False positive* outcomes may be the result of several factors, including occurrence of toxicity only at exaggerated dose levels (identifiable by determining safety margins based on comparative plasma exposure, or including biomarkers if available), or species-specific effects or toxic metabolites (as shown to not occur in humans). The consequence

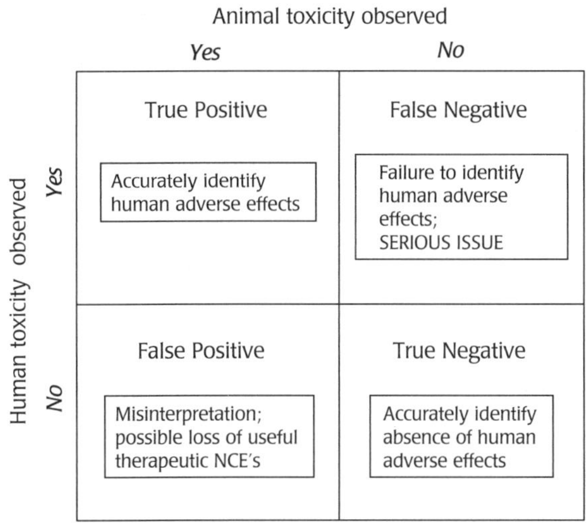

Figure 1-5: Quadrant analysis of clinical predictivity. Reprinted from *Regulatory Toxicology and Pharmacology*, vol. 32/1, Olson et al., "Concordance of the Toxicity of Pharmaceuticals in Humans and in Animals" 12, 2000, with permission from Elsevier.

of unrecognized false positive signals may be the attrition of a valuable human therapeutic as a consequence of misinterpretation of a nonrelevant preclinical effect. A *false negative* outcome as described earlier, carries the potential of a high safety risk impact on drug development. This depends directly on the incidence and severity of the human toxicity with the NCE and the clinical indication being treated. Ultimately, this becomes a risk–benefit decision by regulators and/or the sponsor. As shown previously, animal models do have limits in their ability to predict for some types of human toxicities including, for example, poor predictivity for dermal (rashes) and allergic or pseudoallergic adverse events.[7] These false negative outcomes and other examples of poor predictivity constitute a gap with current *in vivo* testing that will hopefully be addressed by emerging transgenic animal models, humanized *in vitro* test systems, *ex vivo* biomarkers, or some other novel approaches that are described in subsequent chapters.

Ongoing progress in identifying new blood, urine, or other biofluid markers of toxicity – potentially assessable in current animal models – also provides optimism that such refinements will expand the translational usefulness of these preclinical studies.[6,7] Recent examples of emerging or novel biomarkers that may become mainstream toxicity markers (as in research hospital clinical pathology assessments) are troponin markers for cardiac and skeletal muscle toxicity,[32] and kidney biomarkers to delineate specific regional toxic effects in the renal tubule/parenchyma.[33] Further development of these and similar assessable markers of toxicity will be pursued and usefully applied both preclinically and clinically.

In summary, combined animal toxicity testing, including toxic effects and signals recognized from safety pharmacology, clinical and histopathology, and toxicokinetics endpoints, provides a predictive and useful basis for human safety risk assessment in all phases of clinical development of new therapeutics. These test systems are essential to sustain the long track record of safety in clinical trials. The development of novel and robust biomarkers translatable from the preclinical to the clinical environments will help to provide toxicologists, clinicians, and regulators with reliable and appropriate risk management measures needed to address many potential safety concerns.

ACKNOWLEDGMENTS

The authors acknowledge the helpful input, comments, and perspective of the following contributors to the concepts included, and reviewers of this manuscript: William J. Dougherty, Ph.D., Thomas Monticello, DVM, Ph.D., and David Jacobsen-Kram, Ph.D.

REFERENCES

1. DiMasi JA, Hansen RW, Grabowski HG. The price of innovation: new estimates of drug development costs. *J Health Econ.* 2003;22:151–185.
2. Pritchard JF, Mille J-R, Reimer MLJ. Making better drugs: Decision gates in non-clinical drug development. *Nature Rev Drug Disc.* 2003;2:542–553.
3. Kramer JA, Sagartz JE, Morris DL. The application of discovery toxicology and pathology towards the design of safer pharmaceutical lead candidates. *Nature Rev Drug Disc.* 2007;6:636–649.
4. US FDA. M3(R2) Nonclinical safety studies for the conduct of human clinical trials and marketing authorization for pharmaceuticals, Revision 1, ICH Harmonized Tripartite Guideline, 2010.
5. Geiling EMK, Cannon, PR. Pathologic effects of elixir of sulphanilamide (diethylene glycol) poisoning. *JAMA.* 1938;111:919–926.
6. Mattes WB, Walker EG. Translational toxicology and the work of the predictive safety testing consortium. *Clin Pharmacol Ther.* 2009;85:327–330.
7. Olson HM, Betton G, Robinson D, et al. Concordance of the toxicity of pharmaceuticals in humans and in animals. *Reg Tox Pharma.* 2000;32:56–67.
8. Litchfield JT. Evaluation of the safety of new drugs by means of tests in animals. *Clin Pharmacol Ther.* 1962;3:665–672.
9. Owens AH. Predicting anticancer drug effects in man from laboratory animal studies. *J Chron Dis.* 1962;15:223–228.
10. Rozencweig M. Animal toxicology for early clinical trials with anticancer agents. *Cancer Clin Trials* 1981;4, 21–28.
11. Schein P, Davis RD, Carter S, et al. The evaluation of anticancer drugs in dogs and monkeys for the prediction of qualitative toxicities in man, *Clin Pharmacol Ther.* 1970;11,3–40.
12. Freireich EJ, Gehen EA, Rall DP, et al. Quantitative comparison of toxicity of anticancer agents in mouse, rat, hamster, dog, monkey and man. *Cancer Chemother Reports* 1966;50 219–244.
13. Igarashi T, Nakane S, Kitagawa, T. Predictability of clinical adverse reactions of drugs by general pharmacology studies. *J Toxicol Sci.* 1995;20:77–92.
14. Fletcher, AP. Drug safety tests and subsequent clinical experience. *J Royal Soc Med.* 1978;71:693–696.
15. Greaves P, Williams A, Eve M. First dose of potential new medicines to humans: How animals help. *Nature Rev Drug Disc.* 2004;3:226–236.

16. Dressman, JB. Comparison of canine and human gastrointestinal physiology. *Pharmacol Res.* 1986;3:123–131.
17. Lee, MW. Drug-induced hepatotoxicity. *N Engl J Med.* 2003;349:474–485.
18. Hayes, AW. Correlation of human hepatotoxicants with hepatic damage in animals. *Fund Appl Toxicol.* 1982;2:55–66.
19. Litchfield, JT. Forecasting drug effects in man from studies in laboratory animals. *JAMA*.1961;177:34–38.
20. Burrell R, Flaherty DK, Sauers LJ. *Toxicology of the Immune System – A Human Approach.* New York, NY: Van Nostrand Reinhold; 1992:228–232.
21. Hayes TJ. Interpretation of toxicological data from responsive and non-responsive species. In: *Preclinical Evaluation of Peptides and Recombinant Proteins.* Malmo, Sweden: Skogs Grafiska AB, A Sundwall, L Ekman, H-E Johansson – eds: 1990:15–18.
22. Hood RD, Miller DB. Maternally mediated effects on development. In: *Developmental and Reproductive Toxicology.* New York, NY: CRC Press; 2006:101–102.
23. FDA. Office of Pharmaceutical Science, Genetic Toxicity, Reproductive and Development Toxicity, and Carcinogenicity Database 2006. Retrieved from http://www.fda.gov/Cder/Offices/OPS_IO/. Accessed March 18, 2009.
24. ICH. Guideline S1B Testing for Carcinogenicity of Pharmaceuticals 1997.
25. Davies TS, Monro A. Marketed human pharmaceuticals reported to be tumorigenic in rodents. *J American College Toxicol.* 1995; 4:90–107.
26. Gold LS, Zeiger E,. Handbook of Carcinogenic Potency and Genotoxicity Databases. New York, NY: CRC Press; 1997. See also The Carcinogenic Potency Database. Retrieved from http://potency.berkeley.edu/index.html. Accessed March 18, 2009
27. Monro, A. Are Lifespan Rodent Carcinogenicity Studies Defensible for Pharmaceutical Agents. *Exp Toxic Pathol.* 1996; 48:155–166
28. Critical Path Institute. Predictive Safety Testing Consortium. 2008. Retrieved from http://www.c-path.org/pstc.cfm. Accessed March 18, 2009
29. Sistare F. An Analysis of Pharmaceutical Experience with Decades of Rat Carcinogenicity Testing: Should We Modify Current Testing Guidelines for Assessing Pharmaceutical Carcinogenicity Risk? Annual Congress for the 30th Spring Meeting of the British Toxicology Society 2009; 22–25 March 2009, University of Warwick, UK. Abstract S002.
30. Predictive Safety Testing Consortium (PSTC). Carcinogenicity Working Group. Interlaboratory evaluation of genomic signatures for predicting carcinogenicity in the rat. *Toxicol Sci.* 2008;103:28–34.
31. MatthewsEJ, Kruhlak NL, Cimino MC, et al. An analysis of genetic toxicity, reproductive and developmental toxicity, and carcinogenicity data: II. Identification of genotoxicants, reprotoxicants, and carcinogens using in silico methods. *Regul Tox Pharm.* 2006;44:97–110.
32. Wallace KB, Hausner E, Herman E, et al. Serum troponins as biomarkers of drug-induced cardiac toxicity. *Tox Path.* 2004;32:106–121.
33. Rached E, Hoffmann D, Blumbach K, et al. Evaluation of putative biomarkers of nephrotoxicity after exposure to Ochratoxin A in vivo and in vitro. *Toxicol Sci.* 2008;103:371–381.

2 Screening approaches for genetic toxicity

Jiri Aubrecht and Jinghai J. Xu

2.1 INTRODUCTION

Assessing human cancer risk associated with exposure to chemicals is an essential component of the safety assessment paradigm for drugs, cosmetics, and industrial chemicals. The current testing paradigm mainly relies on *in vitro* genotoxicity testing followed by 2-year carcinogenicity bioassays in mice and rats. Because of the technical complexity, high costs, and animal usage associated with 2-year bioassays, the genetic toxicology battery has been designed to be highly sensitive in predicting chemical carcinogenicity.[1,2] In fact, the genotoxicity testing is used as a surrogate for carcinogenicity testing and is required for initiation of clinical trials[3] and for most industrial chemicals. Since the beginning of genotoxicity testing in the early 1970s, many different test systems have been developed and used. Since no single test is capable of detecting all genotoxic agents, present routine genotoxicity evaluation of pharmaceutical compounds incorporates a standard battery of *in vitro* and *in vivo* assays.[4] These tests include (a) bacterial reverse-mutation tests, (b) *in vitro* tests for chromosomal damage (cytogenetic assays and *in vitro* mouse lymphoma thymidine kinase assay), and (c) an *in vivo* test for chromosomal damage (micronucleus test). To further enhance human genotoxic risk assessment, the international ICH working group together with other scientific groups have also suggested additional tests such as the measurement of DNA adducts, DNA strand breaks, DNA repair, and recombination to complement the standard battery in certain cases.[5]

Recent progress in molecular biology, genomics, and bioinformatics has revolutionized drug discovery research. The current discovery process utilizes high-throughput pharmacologically based screens for the identification of lead compounds. Since standard genetic toxicology assays originated in the 1970s and are still being employed, it is expected that their throughput will not satisfy future needs. To facilitate testing, the standard assays must be re-engineered or replaced to both accommodate the increased numbers of compounds submitted to testing and to provide more mechanistically based outcomes to enhance human genotoxic risk assessment.

The goal of genetic toxicity screening assays is to predict the outcome of the assays required by regulatory agencies (Figure 2.1.). Considering cost and uncertain

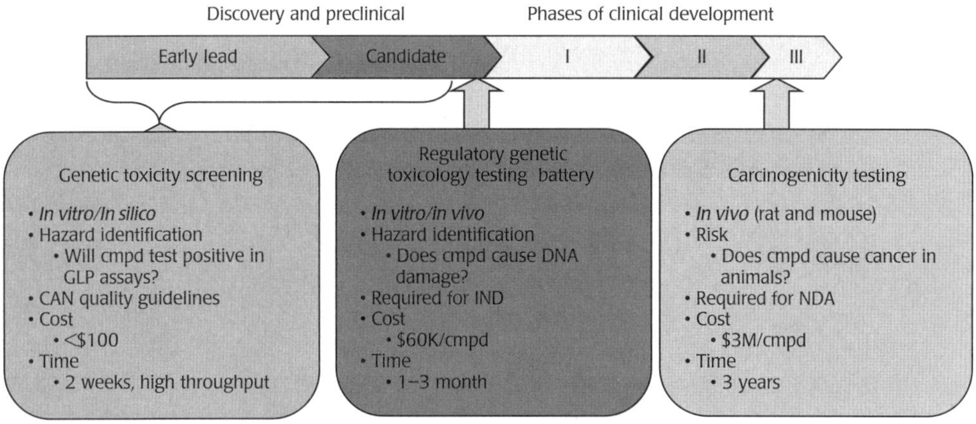

Figure 2-1: Integration of genetic toxicity screening into safety assessment paradigm. Genetic toxicity screening is used as a surrogate for carcinogenicity assessment and is required for investigational new drug (IND) submissions. The goal of genetic toxicity screening assays is to predict the outcome of the assays required by regulatory agencies. Considering cost and uncertain drug development options associated with positive results in a regulatory genetic toxicology testing battery, the application of genetic toxicity screening at early stages of drug development for selecting clean chemical series and compounds is essential.

drug development options associated with positive results in the regulatory genetic toxicology testing battery, the application of genetic toxicity screening at early stages of drug development for selecting clean chemical series and compounds is essential. There are three major themes providing foundation for the development of screening assays. The compound's potential to produce point mutations (mutagenicity) is assessed mostly via miniaturized *Salmonella* assay platforms. Typically, these assays utilize the same endpoint as the regulatory assay and provide reliable data. Because of mainly practical reasons, the screening assays for chromosome damage (clastogenicity) utilize alternative, more automation friendly endpoints such as micronuclei and Comets (DNA breakage) instead of microscopic evaluation of chromosome aberrations, which regulatory agencies typically require for evaluation of chromosome damage. Since compounds producing chromosome damage are not uncommon in drug development pipelines and regulatory assays are laborious and time consuming, those screening assays are quite valuable for evaluation of chemical series and selection of drug candidates. The third theme applied to developing mainly high-throughput assays is genotoxic stress response (also called SOS response) in bacteria. Genotoxic stress triggers a variety of biological responses including the transcriptional activation of genes regulating cell survival. This idea led to the development of promoter–reporter construct-based platforms (biosensors) for detecting genotoxicity in bacteria, yeast, and mammalian cells (reviewed in Reference 6). Since genotoxic stress response provides a fingerprint corresponding to the mechanisms of action of tested chemical, arrays of tester strains have been developed where each tester strain or cell line carries a promoter–reporter construct (biosensor) capable of detecting induction of a single stress response pathway. An array of such biosensors covering multiple genotoxic stress-associated pathways provides even more complex insight into genotoxic mechanisms (reviewed in Reference 6).

2.2 SCREENING APPROACHES FOR MUTAGENICITY

The analysis of mutations in specific bacterial marker genes serves as indicators of mutagenicity. The *Salmonella* (Ames) assay has been developed to measure reversions of specific auxotrophic bacterial mutations in *Salmonella typhimurium*.[7] The *Salmonella* test has been validated in studies using several hundred chemicals and remains the required mutagenicity test by regulatory agencies.[8] However, the standard *Salmonella* test protocol is laborious, time consuming, and requires a large amount of test article. Because of the high concordance of positive *Salmonella* test results with rodent carcinogenicity, the positive findings in this assay typically lead to discontinuation of development. Therefore, the application of screening assay platforms capable of detecting bacterial mutagens in the regulatory *Salmonella* assay is important. To increase the throughput of the *Salmonella* assay, several modifications and alternative approaches have been developed.

Spiral modification of *Salmonella* assay[9] was developed to eliminate the need for serial dilutions and multiple plates. The sample delivery by a spiral plater allows fixed as well as variable dilution depositions onto the agar plate. As a result, this system permits testing over a wide range of concentrations on a single agar plate using about 35–50 mg of test article. Although the introduction of the Spiral assay has significantly enhanced compound screening, the requirement for agar plates and limited potential for full automation restricts its future application.

Gradient plate assay (GPA) also utilizes the concentration gradient of tested compounds in the agar plates.[10] The concentration gradient is established by a plating technique without the need for special instrumentation. In addition, each gradient plate allows simultaneous testing of multiple *Salmonella* tester strains. The GPA platform also eliminates the need for serial dilutions and multiple plates. However, the assay produces rather qualitative mutagenicity assessment, and its potential for full automation is limited.

To increase the throughput a **Miniscreen assay** platform has been developed. In principle, the Miniscreen is a scaled down version of the standard AMES assay.[11] Since the assay is performed in multiwell plates, only 20 mg of test article is needed. However, Miniscreen does not eliminate the serial dilution steps and is not suitable for automation. In addition, it is also rather difficult to obtain quantitative data for mutagenicity assessment.

On the other hand, a **Mutascreen assay** platform is a fully automated instrument for mutagenicity assessment[12]. It is suitable for experiments involving all bacterial tester strains. Its major advantages are streamlined protocol and elimination of agar plates. The assay exploits the turbidity measurements of liquid bacterial cultures for the detection of bacterial growth. Small volumes of cultures are treated in multiwell plates, and the turbidity in each well is monitored intermittently over a 24-h period by using a vertical pathway photometer.

The analysis of growth kinetics allows calculations of mutation frequencies and assessment of overall toxicity of tested compounds. Although this assay provides streamlined protocol and can be fully automated, the turbidimetric measurements of cell density are not highly sensitive or accurate.

In contrast to Mutascreen, the **AmesII assay** utilizes fluctuation analysis for calculation of reversion frequency. Besides the standard *Salmonella* tester strain TA98, the AmesII assay also includes new strains each designed to revert by only one specific base pair substitution mutation.[13] Thus, when mixed, all six base pair substitutions can be represented in one culture.

The concept of a biosensor yielded the establishment of bacterial mutagenicity assays that employ bioluminescent or biofluorescent gene products. The *lux* genes permit cells to emit light due to bioluminescence that can be easily detected using a luminometer. The bioluminescence test[14] and its commercialized version (**Mutatox assay**) uses dark mutants of luminous bacteria *Vibrio fischeri* and determines the ability of various genotoxic agents to restore the luminescence by inducing mutations.[15] The increase of light emission in treated liquid culture over the control is indicative of mutagenicity. This assay has potential for full automation.

A special TA98 *Salmonella* tester strain carrying *luxAB* genes under the control of constitutive promoter is used in a bioluminescence *Salmonella* assay platform.[16] The authors have shown that the light emission corresponds to the number of living cells in culture (biomass). The mutagenicity is evaluated as an increase of revertant biomass using a microluminometer. Since only viable cells are capable of light emission, this technique also permits easy evaluation of overall toxicity of tested chemical. This elegant approach eliminates the need for multiple agar plates and reduces laborious pipetting steps. In addition it can be easily automated and miniaturized.

Biofluorescence is utilized in a green fluorescent protein (GFP)-based *E. coli* mutation assay.[17] In this system, the *E. coli* tester strains carrying the GFP form of *Aequorea victoria* jellyfish serve as mutation biosensors. In the reversion system, the treatment of bacteria carrying a specific frameshift mutation in the GFP gene with genotoxic agents yields fluorescent colonies indicating that reversion to the wild type has occurred. In the forward system, the wild type GFP is under the control of arabinose P_{BAD} promoter. Mutations in the control region that derepress the promoter result in the expression of GFP and biofluorescence.

Recently, we have reported the development of the **bioluminescent reverse mutation assay** in *Salmonella* as a fully automated higher-throughput platform applicable for the screening of large sets of test compounds[18] (Figure 2.2). The bioluminescent *Salmonella* assay utilizes genetically engineered standard Ames *Salmonella* tester strains TA98 and TA100 expressing the *lux* (CDABE) operon from *Xenorhabdus luminescens*. The assay employs bioluminescence as a sensor of changes in bacterial metabolism associated with starvation, hence effectively identifying colonies of histidine-independent revertant cells. In this assay, the cells are treated in agar medium on a multiwell plate. The cells that acquired the reverse mutation and thus can function in the absence of histidine form small

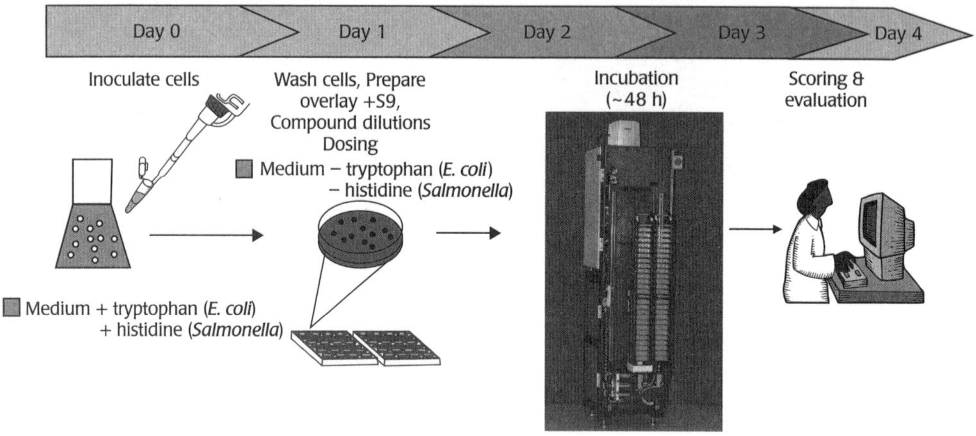

Figure 2-2: Bioluminescent *Salmonella* assay workflow. The luminescent histidine-dependent cells are exposed to tested compounds in agar overlay containing only traces of histidine in multiwell-plate format. The reverse-mutation events restore endogenous histidine synthesis resulting in luminescent colonies of histidine-independent cells that can be visualized via CCD camera. The fully automated instrument in conjunction with automated image analysis of plates enables the analysis of 100 plates in one run.

luminescent colonies. These colonies can be easily detected and counted via a sensitive charge-coupled device (CCD) camera, which captures the luminescent image of an entire multiwell plate at once. The digitized image is then analyzed using an automated image analysis algorithm. Since the image analysis algorithm actually counts the number of revertant colonies, it avoids the common mistakes associated with gross luminescent measurements that cannot distinguish the difference between lots of small colonies and fewer but larger colonies. The bioluminescent *Salmonella* assay coupled with the automated image analysis algorithm provides an economical, higher-throughput tool for assessment of mutagenicity with high concordance to outcomes in the current Ames standard plate incorporation method[18] and provides reliable data across multiple laboratories.[19]

2.3 SCREENING APPROACHES FOR CLASTOGENICITY

The incidence of chromosome damage findings among lead compounds in drug discovery is quite common (approximately 30 percent of drug candidates testing positive). Although the impact of the positive findings is not as severe as in case of positive mutagenicity findings, the application of screening tools capable of providing data in sufficient throughput in early drug discovery is essential to avoid delays in drug development or potential attrition of the drug candidate.

***In vitro* micronucleus (IVMN, or MN) assay** detects extra-nuclear chromatin present in the cell's cytoplasm arisen after cell division as a consequence of chromosome (DNA) breakage (clastogenicity) or lagging chromosome (aneugenicity). The lagging chromosome is caused by the compound's interference

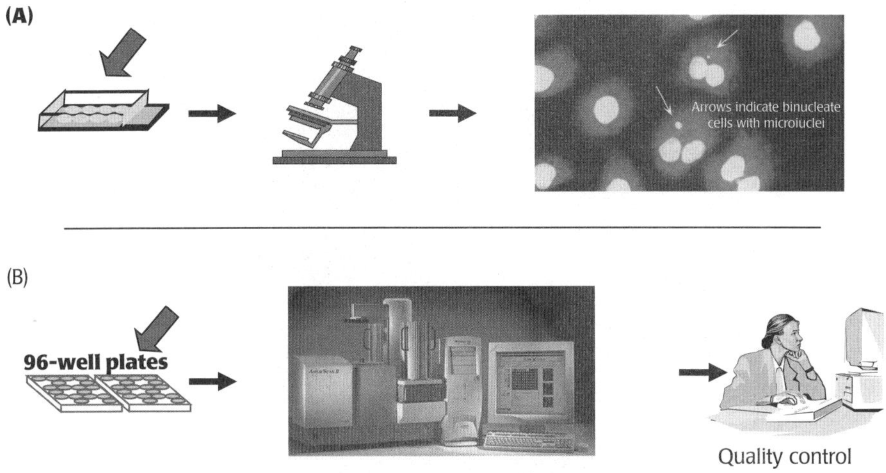

Figure 2-3: Comparison of manual (microscopic) and automated image analysis-based *in vitro* micronucleus assay platforms. **(A)** The cells are treated on chambered microscopic slides. Visual microscopic analysis of micronuclei is performed after fixation and staining with DNA-specific dye via fluorescent microscope. Since the microscopic analysis is laborious and time consuming, the throughput is limited to four to six compounds per week. **(B)** The automated image analysis–based platforms typically utilize 96-well plates for the treatment of cells. After fixation, the cells are stained with DNA-specific dye, and images of nuclei and micronuclei are acquired using high-throughput scanner technology. Application of sophisticated image analysis algorithms enables fast detection of micronuclei. The assay operator then typically performs only quality control of the data. The automated platform provides opportunity for testing typically 100–200 compounds per week.

with the spindle apparatus or cellular signaling pathways. The mode of micronucleus formation can be investigated via use of kinetochore antibody staining to identify micronuclei containing centromeric DNA indicating the whole chromosome[20]. The MN assay can be conducted in most proliferating cell lines but is typically performed in Chinese hamster ovary (CHO), Chinese hamster lung (CHL), human lymphocytes or mouse lymphoma cells L5178Y. The cells are exposed to the test compound in the presence and absence of liver S9 homogenate, and the incidence of micronuclei of the compound-treated sample is compared with the vehicle-treated controls. The positive response is characterized as a dose-dependent increase of incidence of micronuclei.

The advantage of the MN assay is its relative simplicity and low compound requirement. It is possible to provide data with 20–30 mg of test compound. The presence and incidence of micronuclei is typically examined and enumerated microscopically. However, the laborious and time-consuming microscopic analysis severely limits assay throughput and its application as a screening tool in drug discovery. Thus, alternative methods for detection of micronuclei have been developed[21–23] (Figure 2.3). One approach exploits image analysis algorithms. The advantage of image analysis is the ability to use the 96-well format and high-throughput microscopic scanning instrument such as the ArrayScan (by Cellomics, now Thermo Fisher). A variety of algorithms have been developed for the enumeration of micronuclei.[24–26] In our laboratory, we have developed

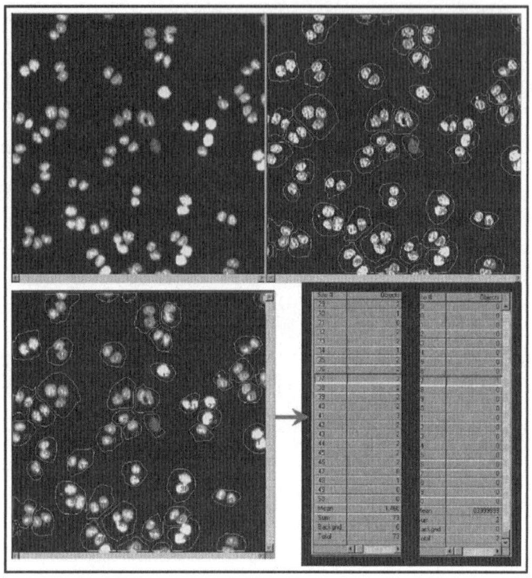

Figure 2-4: Automated image analysis of the *in vitro* micronucleus assay. *See color plates.*

a fully automated approach relying on an image analysis algorithm. The cells are treated in 96-well plates using standard laboratory automation methods and stained with the DNA-specific dye Hoechst 33342. This dye stains main nuclei and micronuclei with sufficiently high signal-to-background ratio to allow automated identification of these target objects. The cells are counterstained with acridine orange, a dye that stains RNA and proteins in cytoplasm. Then the plates are scanned using ArrayScan with a setting of 20× magnification and an XF93 filter. The 20× magnification allows image capture from a larger field of view compared to the traditionally used 40× or 60×, while maintaining sufficient resolution to detect micronuclei. The ArrayScan captures the nuclei/micronuclei and cytoplasm images in separate wavelength or channels, and saves all the images and their associated meta-data. These images are then analyzed using an image analysis algorithm. In the first step, raw image of the acridine orange channel is used to "identify" cell outlines (e.g., as in Figure 2.4a). This step converts the acridine orange image into a binary map, where the extracellular space becomes "0" and intracellular space becomes "1." Next, the acridine orange image undergoes a series of image "dialation" and "erosion" steps in order to automatically segment adjacent and contacting cells into individual cells. The segmented "cell outline" is then combined with the raw nuclei image from the Hoechst channel (e.g., as in Figure 2.4b). The algorithm automatically "identifies" main nuclei within a cell, according to predefined ranges of size and shape (e.g., Figure 2.4b). Following that, the algorithm further "searches" for micronuclei according to the following criteria: (1) having a size that is less than a third the size of the main nucleus, (2) being located within the cell outline, (3) not touching the main nucleus, (4) having no more than two micronuclei within the same cell, and (5) having a round or close-to-round shape. If a cell possesses more than two micronuclei, the algorithm reports them as such (which can be an indication of nuclear fragmentation, e.g., due to apoptosis). After the micronuclei are found (e.g., as in Figure 2.4c), the algorithm automatically compiles cell-by-cell data (e.g., as in Figure 2.4d), as well as well-level statistics including micronuclei incidence. The whole system including plate handling, automated image acquisition, and data calculation is capable of providing data for 100–150 compounds per week.

An alternative approach for automating MN assay relies on flow cytometry.[27,28] In principle, the flow cytometer is used for detecting nuclei and small micronuclei after they were released from cells by cell lysis. The limiting factor for application of flow cytometry for detection of micronuclei is its difficulty to differentiate micronuclei from apoptotic and genotoxic events. Therefore, a fluorescent dye is covalently linked by photoactivation to chromatin of apoptotic and dying cells prior to lysing the cell membranes. This results in true micronuclei being labeled with a DNA dye and apoptotic or chromatin fragments from dying cells being stained with both the DNA and covalently linked dye. The flow cytometric analysis provides an elegant method enabling simultaneous detection of micronuclei and cell cycle analysis.

***In vitro* comet assay** provides a sensitive tool for detection of DNA breakage in individual cells. In addition, the comet assay can detect DNA lesions that can be converted to DNA strand breaks. Typically, the comet assay is conducted in CHO, CHL, human lymphocytes, or mouse lymphoma cells LY-1457. Briefly, the cells are treated with tested compounds in presence or absence of exogenous S9 rat liver homogenate and then resuspended into single-cell suspension in agarose gel on microscope slides. After the slides are prepared, the cell membrane is lysed, and the nuclei are exposed to alkaline electroporesis.[29,30] During this procedure, long strands of chromosomal DNA denaturate, and low molecular weight DNA fragments that arose as a consequence of DNA damage migrate toward positive electrode when an electrical field is applied, forming a comet-like pattern. Thus, the nucleus of undamaged DNA appears to be round, whereas the nucleus with damaged DNA forms a trailing comet tail. The advantage of this assay is a relatively small compound requirement (10 mg) and the potential for full automation of the comet analysis. The disadvantage of this assay platform is the unknown role of cytotoxicity in comet formation that might contribute to false positive results in comparison with the clastogenicity assay accepted by regulatory agencies.

The DEL (deletion) recombination assay detects the incidence of intrachromosomal recombination events between two truncated alleles of HIS3 gene arranged as a head to tail repeat in *Saccharomyces cerevisiae*.[31,32] The recombination events produce deletions of the intervening sequence resulting in restoration of the functional HIS3 allele. Briefly, the yeast cells are treated with tested compound in presence and absence of S9 rat liver homogenate. The HIS3-proficient cells can be easily detected as yeast colonies arisen in histidine-free medium. The positive signal in this assay is considered as a dose-dependent increase of HIS3-proficient colonies when compared to vehicle-treated controls. Earlier mechanistic studies have shown that double-strand breaks in DNA cause increased DEL recombination frequency.[33,34] Since the DNA deletions detected by the DEL assay represent one kind of chromosome aberration, the DEL assay data correlate with other chromosome aberration assays.[35,36] The deletion recombination is also sensitive to other DNA lesions including DNA adduction, oxidative stress, and so on. In fact, the DEL assay is capable of differentiating direct (DNA reactive) from indirect (DNA nonreactive) mechanisms of genotoxicity based on the shape of the dose response curve. Direct-acting compounds display a linear dose response, whereas indirect-acting compounds display a threshold response, only at cytotoxic concentrations.[37] Since the DEL assay detects clastogenic as well as mutagenic compounds,[38] this test has a potential to reduce the screening battery into a single test replacing the separately run mutagenicity and clastogenicity assays[39]. In addition, the assay has potential to provide insights into mechanisms of genotoxicity (i.e., DNA reactive vs. DNA nonreactive).

Tumor cells frequently contain genome rearrangements such as deletions, transversions, and translocations. In fact, an elevated frequency of recombination and genome rearrangements is found in cells from human patients suffering from cancer-prone diseases such as ataxia telangiectasia, Li-Fraumeni syndrome, Blooms syndrome and Werners syndrome, Cockayne's syndrome, Fanconi's anaemia, Lynch syndromes I and II, Wiscott-Aldrich syndrome, and xeroderma pigmentosum (extensively reviewed in Reference 40). These data indicate that a high frequency of genetic rearrangements may be a causative factor in tumor development and thus provide mechanistic relevance for the DEL assay as a tool for detection of carcinogens. In fact, the DEL assay is inducible by carcinogens with varying mechanisms of genotoxicity.[41] Application of the DEL assay in drug development as a screening tool is limited by the permeability of the yeast cell wall for larger lipophilic compounds. Thus, a clear direction for future assay improvement, namely development of a permeable yeast tester strain, has been identified.[36] The application of improved tester strain is expected to increase the sensitivity of the assay, and it is crucial for future large-scale validation of the DEL assay as a clastogenicity screen. Nevertheless, the high degree of concordance with the IVMN and other assays for clastogenicity, the consistency of results, amenability to automation, and economical nature of the DEL assay makes it an excellent candidate for use as a genotoxicity assay for screening of new compounds.

2.4 STRESS (SOS) RESPONSE-BASED SCREENING ASSAYS

Early studies in mammalian cells using ionizing radiation and prototypical DNA-damaging compounds have identified genes that are induced by DNA damage.[42–44] These genes have been shown to play major roles in basic cellular processes such as cell cycle and growth arrest, cellular signaling and apoptosis (see review in Reference 45). The discovery of these genes has lead to the idea that genotoxicity can be identified by monitoring the expression of stress responsive genes. In bacteria, the transcriptional activation of the SOS response, measured using promoter–reporter constructs (biosensors) was exploited for detecting genotoxicity of chemicals (Table 2.1, Figure 2.5).[46–51] Similarly in the

Table 2-1. Selected bacterial biosensor-based assays used for detecting genotoxicity

Assay	Promoter	Reporter gene(s)	Stressors detected	Host	Reference #
SOS chromotest	sfiA	lacZ, alkaline phosphatase	Benzofurans, naphtafurans, fungal toxins, MMC, NCS, MMS, EMS, DMS, DES, b-propiolactone, propane sultone, DMN, DEN, MNNG, B[a]P, 4NQO, DMSO, NaCl, Caffeine, Aspirin	*E. coli*	50
Umu-test	umu	lacZ	DNA-damaging agents (radiation or chemical)	*S. typhimurium*	48
Rec-lac test	recA	lacZ	DNA-damaging agents (radiation or chemical), 4NQO, MMC, MNNG, nalidixic acid, DMS, H_2O_2, formaldehyde, UV radiation, tert-butyl hydroperoxide, cumene hydroperoxide, and streptonigrin	*E. coli*	47
SOS-lux test	cda, recA	luxCDABFE	DNA-damaging agents (radiation or chemical), MMC, MNNG, nalidixic acid, DMS, H_2O_2, formaldehyde, UV and gamma irradiation	*E. coli*	49
VITOTOX	recN	luxCDABE	PAHs	Bacterial (*E. coli*, *S. typhimurium*)	60
GreenScreen	rad54	gfp	DNA-damaging agents	*S. cerevisiae*	52
GreenScreenHC	GADD45	gfp	DNA-damaging agents	Human TK6	65

Notes: 4NQO: 4-nitroquinoline-N-oxide; AP: Alkaline phosphatase; B[a]P: Benzo[a]pyrene; cda: Cytidine deaminase; DEN: Diethylnitrosamine; DES: Diethyl sulfate; DMN: Dimethylnitrosamine; DMS: Dimethyl sulfate; DMSO: Dimethyl sulfoxide; EMS: Ethyl methanesulfonate; GFP: Green fluorescent protein; H202: Hydrogen peroxide; lacZ: β-galactosidase; lux: Luciferase; MMC: Mitomycin C; MMS: Methylmethanesulfonate; MNNG: N-methyl-N-nitro-N-nitroso guanidine; NaCl: Sodium chloride; NCS: Neocarsinostatin; PAHs: Polyaromatic hydrocarbons; rad 54: Radiation sensitive (or related); rec: Recombination protein; sfiA: Cell division inhibitor; umu: Mutagenesis by UV and mutagens. Reprinted with permission from Pharmacogenomics 2005;6(4):419–428.

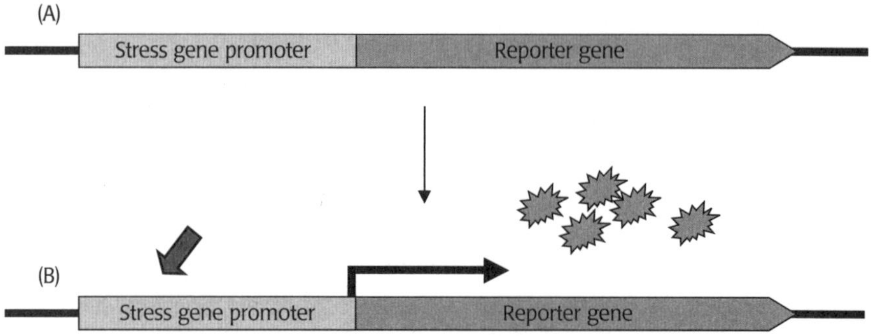

Figure 2-5: Principle of biosensor-based assay platforms. **(A)** A promoter-reporter construct consisting of stress gene promoter and appropriate reporter such as green fluorescent protein or luciferase (biosensor) is integrated into the genome of cells used for detection of genotoxicity. In case of bacterial assays the promoter–reporter construct may reside on an episomal plasmid. **(B)** The treatment of biosensor-carrying cells with genotoxic agents activates the otherwise silent stress promoter and initiate reporter gene transcription and production of reporter protein. The resulting fluorescence or luminescence is detected via high-throughput detectors. Since these assay platforms can be performed in high-density plates, the throughput can reach 1,000 compounds per week.

yeast, RAD54 promoter activity[52,53] has been utilized to detect genotoxic stress. Recently, the development of GreenScreen GC and GreenScreen HC has been reported.[52,65] Those assays utilize GFP as reporter for RAD54 in *Saccharomyces* and GADD45 in human TK6 cells. However, monitoring transcriptional activity of a single gene provides only limited characterization of the cellular stresses. Accordingly, arrays of biosensors consisting of bacterial strains with promoter–reporter constructs sensitive to various stresses were developed and used to study the mechanisms of action of unknown toxicants (Table 2.2). The major advantage of this approach relies on relatively easy adaptation of biosensor assay platforms to high-throughput screening that is suitable for testing hundreds of compounds.

Since the activation of stress genes expression is a mechanistically different endpoint than structural or numerical chromosome damage or point mutations, the concordance of data from biosensor-based assays with traditional assay platforms detecting chromosome damage or mutagenicity is not perfect. For instance, monitoring mRNA levels of GADD45 in HepG2 cells was utilized as a screen for genotoxicity to test chemicals from combinatorial libraries in drug discovery.[54] Although, a correlation between chemical structure and up-regulation of GADD45 mRNA levels was apparent, the change in GADD45 transcript did not correlate with the ability of test compounds to produce mutations in a standard *Salmonella* reverse-mutation test.[54] Furthermore, monitoring p53 protein levels after treatment with chemicals was also proposed as a tool for identifying potential genotoxic carcinogens.[55,56] However, although the p53 pathway or the induction of GADD45 can be activated by a wide spectrum of DNA-damaging agents, other stresses such as hypoxia, nutrient, starvation, alteration of the ubiquitin pathway, or ribonucleotide depletion have also been shown to affect the p53 pathway and/or the GADD45 gene levels.[44,57–59] Despite these stresses, applying a

Table 2-2. Examples of arrays of biosensors utilized to evaluate toxic mechanisms

Assay	Promoter	Reporter genes	Stressors detected	Host	Reference #
	micF, lon, fabA, lac, katG, uspA, micF	luxCDABE	sodium azide, 4-nitrophenol, phenol, 3,5-DCP, proflavine hemi sulfate, $NiSO_4$, CTAB, fluoranthene, $PbCl_2$, $HgCl_2$, $CdCl_2$, H_2O_2, KH_2AsO_4, $ZnCl_2$, 2,4-DNP, PCP, 2,4,5-T, 2,4,6-TCP, 2,4-D, benzidine, methyl viologen, parathion, malthion, SDS, propiconazole	Bacterial (*E. coli*)	46
Pro-tox (C)	katG, micF, osmY, uspA, recA, zwf, umuDC, merR, ada, dinD, soi28, nfo	lacZ	(DNA damage) trivalent chromium	Bacterial (*E. coli*)	61
Cat-tox (L)	cyp1A1, gstYa, hmtIIA, Fos, xhf, hsp70, gadd153, gadd45, grp78, xre, NF-κBRE, gre, p53RE, RARE	CAT	DNA-damaging agents (vanadocene complexes, cisplatin, 3-MC, PMA, RA, MMS, heavy metals, arsenic)	Mammalian (human liver cells)	62, 63
Cat-tox (D)	DNA polβ, p53, gadd153, gadd45, cfos, tPARE, tPA	CAT	DNA-damaging agents (UV irradiation, MMS, EMS, MNNG, DMN, MMC, actinomycin D, Hydroxyurea)	Mammalian (human colon cells)	64

Notes: 2,4,5-T: 2,4,5-trichlorophenoxy acetic acid; 2,4,6-TCP: 2,4,6-trichlorophenol; 2,4-D: 2,4-dichlorophenoxy-acetic acid; 2,4-DNP: 2,4-dinitro phenol; 3-MC: 3-methylcholanthrene; 3,5-DCP: 3,5-dichlorophenol; ada: Transcriptional adaptor; CAT: Chloramphenicol acetyltransferase; CdCl2: Cadmiumchloride; PCP: Pentachloro phenol; CTAB: Cetyl trimethyl ammonium bromide; CYP: Cytochrome P450; dinD: DNA-damage-inducible protein; DMN: Dimethylnitrosamine; DNA polb: DNA polymerase b; EMS: Ethyl methanesulfonate; fabA: β-hydroxydecanoyl thioester dehydrase; Fos: Protooncogeneprotein; GADD: Growth arrest and DNA-damage-inducible; gre: glutocorticoid response element; grp78: Glucose-regulated proteinprecursor; gstYa: Glutathione S-transferase Ya chain; H202: Hydrogen peroxide; HgCl2: Mercury chloride; hmtIIA: Heavy metal tolerance protein; hsp70: Heat shock protein 70; katG: catalase-peroxidase protein G; KH2AsO4: Potassium arsenate; lacZ: β-galactosidase; lux: luciferase; merR: Bacterial regulatory protein; micF: small RNA/regulatory antisense RNA; MMC: Mitomycin C; MMS: Methylmethanesulfonate; MNNG: N-methyl-Nnitro-N-nitroso guanidine; NF-kBRE: Nuclear factor κB response element; nfo: Endonuclease IV; NiSO4: Nickel sulfate; osmY: Osmotically inducibleprotein Y; p53RE: Tumor suppressor p53 regulatory element; PbCl2: Lead chloride; PMA: Phorbol 12-myristate 13-acetate; RA: Retinoic acid; RARE: Retinoic acid response element; rec: Recombination protein; SDS: Sodium dodecyl sulfate; soi28: Superoxide inducible gene; tPA: Tissueplasminogen activator; tPARE: Tissue plasminogen activator response element; uspA: Universal stress protein A; xhf: Collagenase; xre: Phage-related transcriptional regulator; ZnCl2: Zinc chloride; zwf: Glucose-6-phosphate dehydrogenase. Reprinted with permission from Pharmacogenomics 2005;6(4):419–428.

biosensor-based approach could be quite useful for prioritizing chemical series in early drug discovery where positive results in the biosensor assay provide a measure of risk for genotoxic liability.

2.5 CONCLUSIONS

Because of the technical complexity, high costs, and animal usage associated with the 2-year carcinogenicity testing in laboratory animals, the *in vitro* genetic toxicology battery has been designed to be highly sensitive in predicting chemical carcinogenicity. The genotoxicity testing is used as a surrogate for carcinogenicity testing and is required for initiation of clinical trials and for most industrial chemicals. Positive data in regulatory-approved genotoxicity assays result in delays and often the discontinuing of development for drug candidates. Recent progress in molecular biology, genomics, and bioinformatics has revolutionized drug discovery research. The current drug discovery process utilizes high-throughput pharmacologically based screens for the identification of lead compounds. Since the standard genotoxicity assays are laborious and time consuming, their throughput cannot satisfy either current or future needs of drug discovery. The development, validation, and application of higher-throughput genetic toxicity screening technologies is essential for identifying safer lead compounds and drug candidates. The field of genotoxicity screening will continue to progress toward higher accuracy, greater efficiency, less compound usage, and enhanced capacity to provide insights in structure–activity relationship and mechanistic understanding. Ultimately, this will lead to reduced usage of laboratory animals, while maintaining a high degree of protection against carcinogenicity in human beings.

REFERENCES

1. Kirkland D, Aardema M, Henderson L, et al. Evaluation of the ability of a battery of three in vitro genotoxicity tests to discriminate rodent carcinogens and non-carcinogens: I. Sensitivity, specificity and relative predictivity. *Mutat Res.* 2005;584(1–2):1–256.
2. Kirkland D, Aardema M, Muller L, et al. Evaluation of the ability of a battery of three in vitro genotoxicity tests to discriminate rodent carcinogens and non-carcinogens: II. Further analysis of mammalian cell results, relative predictivity and tumour profiles. *Mutat Res.* 2006;608(1):29–42.
3. Jacobs A, Jacobson-Kram D. Human carcinogenic risk evaluation, Part III: Assessing cancer hazard and risk in human drug development. *Toxicol Sci.* 2004;81(2):260–262.
4. Muller L, Kikuchi Y, Probst G, et al. ICH-harmonised guidances on genotoxicity testing of pharmaceuticals: evolution, reasoning and impact. *Mutat Res.* 1999;436(3):195–225.
5. Thybaud V, Aardema M, Clements J, et al. Strategy for genotoxicity testing: Hazard identification and risk assessment in relation to in vitro testing. *Mutat Res.* 2007;627(1):41–58.
6. Aubrecht J, Caba E. Gene expression profile analysis: An emerging approach to investigate mechanisms of genotoxicity. *Pharmacogenomics.* 2005;6(4):419–428.

7. Ames BN, Durston WE, Yamasaki E, et al. Carcinogens are mutagens: A simple test system combining liver homogenates for activation and bacteria for detection. *Proc Natl Acad Sci USA*. 1973;70(8):2281–2285.
8. Muller A, Boitier E, Hu T, et al. Laboratory variability does not preclude identification of biological functions impacted by hydroxyurea. *Environ Mol Mutagen*. 2005;46(4):221–235.
9. Houk VS, Schalkowsky S, Claxton LD. Development and validation of the spiral Salmonella assay: An automated approach to bacterial mutagenicity testing. *Mutat Res*. 1989;223(1):49–64.
10. Rexroat MA, Oberly TJ, Bewsey BJ, et al. The gradient plate assay: A modified Ames assay used as a prescreen for the identification of bacterial mutagens. *Mutat Res*. 1995;341(3):185–192.
11. Brooks TM. The use of a streamlined bacterial mutagenicity assay, the MINISCREEN. *Mutagenesis*. 1995;10(5):447–448.
12. Falck K, Partanen P, Sorsa M, et al. Mutascreen, an automated bacterial mutagenicity assay. *Mutat Res*. 1985;150(1–2):119–125.
13. Gee P, Maron DM, Ames BN. Detection and classification of mutagens: A set of base-specific *Salmonella* tester strains. *Proc Natl Acad Sci USA*. 1994;91(24):11606–11610.
14. Ulitzur S. Bioluminescence test for genotoxic agents. *Methods Enzymol*. 1986;133:264–274.
15. Sun TS, Stahr HM. Evaluation and application of a bioluminescent bacterial genotoxicity test. *J AOAC Int*. 1993;76(4):893–898.
16. Cote C, Blaise C, Delisle CE, et al. A miniaturized Ames mutagenicity assay employing bioluminescent strains of *Salmonella typhimurium*. *Mutat Res*. 1995;345(3–4):137–146.
17. Cariello NF, Narayanan S, Kwanyuen P, et al. A novel bacterial reversion and forward mutation assay based on green fluorescent protein. *Mutat Res*. 1998;414(1–3):95–105.
18. Aubrecht J, Osowski JJ, Persaud P, et al. Bioluminescent *Salmonella* reverse mutation assay: A screen for detecting mutagenicity with high throughput attributes. *Mutagenesis*. 2007;22(5):335–342.
19. Ackerman J, Sharma R, Hitchcock J, et al. Inter-laboratory evaluation of the bioluminescent Salmonella reverse mutation assay using 10 model chemicals. *Mutagenesis*. 2009;24(5):433–438.
20. Parry EM, Parry JM, Corso C, et al. Detection and characterization of mechanisms of action of aneugenic chemicals. *Mutagenesis*. 2002;17(6):509–521.
21. Bryce SM, Bemis JC, Avlasevich SL, et al. In vitro micronucleus assay scored by flow cytometry provides a comprehensive evaluation of cytogenetic damage and cytotoxicity. *Mutat Res*. 2007;630(1–2):78–91.
22. Frieauff W, Potter-Locher F, Cordier A, et al. Automatic analysis of the in vitro micronucleus test on V79 cells. *Mutat Res*. 1998;413(1):57–68.
23. Smolewski P, Ruan Q, Vellon L, et al. Micronuclei assay by laser scanning cytometry. *Cytometry*. 2001;45(1):19–26.
24. Decordier I, Papine A, Plas G, et al. Automated image analysis of cytokinesis-blocked micronuclei: An adapted protocol and a validated scoring procedure for biomonitoring. *Mutagenesis*. 2009;24(1):85–93.
25. Diaz D, Scott A, Carmichael P, et al. Evaluation of an automated in vitro micronucleus assay in CHO-K1 cells. *Mutat Res*. 2007;630(1–2):1–13.
26. Varga D, Johannes T, Jainta S, et al. An automated scoring procedure for the micronucleus test by image analysis. *Mutagenesis*. 2004;19(5):391–397.
27. Bryce SM, Avlasevich SL, Bemis JC, et al. Interlaboratory evaluation of a flow cytometric, high content in vitro micronucleus assay. *Mutat Res*. 2008;650(2):181–195.

28. Avlasevich SL, Bryce SM, Cairns SE, et al. In vitro micronucleus scoring by flow cytometry: Differential staining of micronuclei versus apoptotic and necrotic chromatin enhances assay reliability. *Environ Mol Mutagen*. 2006;47(1):56–66.
29. Hartmann A, Schumacher M, Plappert-Helbig U, et al. Use of the alkaline in vivo Comet assay for mechanistic genotoxicity investigations. *Mutagenesis*. 2004;19(1): 51–59.
30. Kiskinis E, Suter W, Hartmann A. High throughput Comet assay using 96-well plates. *Mutagenesis*. 2002;17(1):37–43.
31. Schiestl RH. Nonmutagenic carcinogens induce intrachromosomal recombination in yeast. *Nature*. 1989;337(6204):285–288.
32. Carls N, Schiestl RH. Evaluation of the yeast DEL assay with 10 compounds selected by the International Program on Chemical Safety for the evaluation of short-term tests for carcinogens. *Mutat Res*. 1994;320(4):293–303.
33. Galli A, Schiestl RH. Effects of DNA double-strand and single-strand breaks on intrachromosomal recombination events in cell-cycle-arrested yeast cells. *Genetics*. Jul 1998;149(3):1235–1250.
34. Galli A, Schiestl RH. Hydroxyurea induces recombination in dividing but not in G1 or G2 cell cycle arrested yeast cells. *Mutat Res*. 1996;354(1):69–75.
35. Kirpnick Z, Homiski M, Rubitski E, et al. Yeast DEL assay detects clastogens. *Mutat Res*. 2005;582(1–2):116–134.
36. Sobol Z, Engel ME, Rubitski E, et al. Genotoxicity profiles of common alkyl halides and esters with alkylating activity. *Mutat Res*. 2007;633(2):80–94.
37. Galli A, Schiestl RH. *Salmonella* test positive and negative carcinogens show different effects on intrachromosomal recombination in G2 cell cycle arrested yeast cells. *Carcinogenesis*. 1995;16(3):659–663.
38. Galli A, Schiestl RH. Cell division transforms mutagenic lesions into deletion-recombinagenic lesions in yeast cells. *Mutat Res*. 1999;429(1):13–26.
39. Ku WW, Aubrecht J, Mauthe RJ, et al. Genetic Toxicity Assessment: Employing the Best Science for Human Safety Evaluation Part VII: Why Not Start with a Single Test: A Transformational Alternative to Genotoxicity Hazard and Risk Assessment. *Toxicol Sci*. 2007;99(1):20–25.
40. Bishop AJ, Schiestl RH. Homologous Recombination and Its Role in Carcinogenesis. *J Biomed Biotechnol*. 2002;2(2):75–85.
41. Hontzeas N, Hafer K, Schiestl RH. Development of a microtiter plate version of the yeast DEL assay amenable to high-throughput toxicity screening of chemical libraries. *Mutat Res*. 2007;634(1–2):228–234.
42. Fornace AJ, Jr., Alamo I, Jr., Hollander MC. DNA damage-inducible transcripts in mammalian cells. *Proc Natl Acad Sci USA*. 1988;85(23):8800–8804.
43. Holbrook NJ, Fornace AJ, Jr. Response to adversity: molecular control of gene activation following genotoxic stress. *New Biol*. 1991;3(9):825–833.
44. Amundson SA, Myers TG, Fornace AJ, Jr. Roles for p53 in growth arrest and apoptosis: putting on the brakes after genotoxic stress. *Oncogene*. 1998;17(25):3287–3299.
45. Smith ML, Fornace AJ, Jr. Mammalian DNA damage-inducible genes associated with growth arrest and apoptosis. *Mutat Res*. 1996;340(2–3):109–124.
46. Ben-Israel O, Ben-Israel H, Ulitzur S. Identification and quantification of toxic chemicals by use of Escherichia coli carrying lux genes fused to stress promoters. *Appl Environ Microbiol*. 1998;64(11):4346–4352.
47. Nunoshiba T, Nishioka H. 'Rec-lac test' for detecting SOS-inducing activity of environmental genotoxic substance. *Mutat Res*. 1991;254(1):71–77.
48. Oda Y, Nakamura S, Oki I, et al. Evaluation of the new system (umu-test) for the detection of environmental mutagens and carcinogens. *Mutat Res*. 1985;147(5):219–229.
49. Ptitsyn LR, Horneck G, Komova O, et al. A biosensor for environmental genotoxin screening based on an SOS lux assay in recombinant *Escherichia coli* cells. *Appl Environ Microbiol*. 1997;63(11):4377–4384.

50. Quillardet P, Huisman O, D'Ari R, et al. The SOS chromotest: Direct assay of the expression of gene sfiA as a measure of genotoxicity of chemicals. *Biochimie.* 1982;64(8–9):797–801.
51. Vollmer AC. Genotoxic sensors. *Methods Mol Biol.* 1998;102:145–151.
52. Cahill PA, Knight AW, Billinton N, et al. The GreenScreen genotoxicity assay: A screening validation programme. *Mutagenesis.* 2004;19(2):105–119.
53. Lichtenberg-Frate H, Schmitt M, Gellert G, et al. A yeast-based method for the detection of cyto and genotoxicity. *Toxicol In Vitro.* 2003;17(5–6):709–716.
54. Todd MD, Lin X, Stankowski LF, Jr., et al. Toxicity screening of a combinatorial library: Correlation of cytotoxicity and gene induction to compound structure. *J Biomol Screen.* 1999;4(5):259–268.
55. Duerksen-Hughes PJ, Yang J, Ozcan O. p53 induction as a genotoxic test for twenty-five chemicals undergoing in vivo carcinogenicity testing. *Environ Health Perspect.* 1999;107(10):805–812.
56. Yang J, Duerksen-Hughes P. A new approach to identifying genotoxic carcinogens: p53 induction as an indicator of genotoxic damage. *Carcinogenesis.* 1998;19(6):1117–1125.
57. Ko LJ, Prives C. p53: Puzzle and paradigm. *Genes Dev.* 1996;10(9):1054–1072.
58. Linke SP, Clarkin KC, Di Leonardo A, et al. A reversible, p53-dependent G0/G1 cell cycle arrest induced by ribonucleotide depletion in the absence of detectable DNA damage. *Genes Dev.* 1996;10(8):934–947.
59. Lopes UG, Erhardt P, Yao R, et al. p53-dependent induction of apoptosis by proteasome inhibitors. *J Biol Chem.* 1997;272(20):12893–12896.
60. van der Lelie D, Regniers L, Borremans B, et al. The VITOTOX test, an SOS bioluminescence Salmonella typhimurium test to measure genotoxicity kinetics. *Mutat Res.* 1997;389(2–3):279–290.
61. Plaper A, Jenko-Brinovec S, Premzl A, et al. Genotoxicity of trivalent chromium in bacterial cells. Possible effects on DNA topology. *Chem Res Toxicol.* 2002;15(7):943–949.
62. Aubrecht J, Narla RK, Ghosh P, et al. Molecular genotoxicity profiles of apoptosis-inducing vanadocene complexes. *Toxicol Appl Pharmacol.* 1999;154(3):228–235.
63. Todd MD, Lee MJ, Williams JL, et al. The CAT-Tox (L) assay: A sensitive and specific measure of stress-induced transcription in transformed human liver cells. *Fundam Appl Toxicol.* 1995;28(1):118–128.
64. Beard SE, Capaldi SR, Gee P. Stress responses to DNA damaging agents in the human colon carcinoma cell line, RKO. *Mutat Res.* 1996;371(1–2):1–13.
65. Hastwell PW, Chai LL, Roberts KJ, et al. High-specificity and high-sensitivity genotoxicity assessment in a human cell line: Validation of the GreenScreen HC GADD45a-GFP genotoxicity assay. *Mutat Res.* 2006;607(2):160–175.

3 Cardiac safety

Martin Traebert and Berengere Dumotier

3.1 INTRODUCTION: THE STATUS OF THE PROBLEM

Over the last two decades, several medicines were withdrawn from the market because their use in patients has been discovered to be associated with the development of a very specific potentially life-threatening polymorphic ventricular tachycardia, Torsade de pointes (TdP).[1] In approximately 20 percent of the cases, TdP can develop into ventricular fibrillation and lead to sudden death. The recently finalized ICH S7B guideline defines the prolongation of the QT interval (measure of time between Q and T waves in the electrocardiogram) on the surface electrocardiogram as an appropriate biomarker for predicting the torsadogenic risk of a given compound. However, a growing body of evidence suggests that the QT interval prolongation is an incomplete biomarker of a drug's torsadogenic potential.[2] The generation of TdP is triggered more by dynamic combination of multiple predisposing factors and components and favored by myocardial substrate rather than by a single electrophysiological event. Following recommendations of the respective guideline, the pharmaceutical industry has intensively implemented methodologies to assess the potential risk of QT prolongation and TdP in man. The key task of each cardiac safety testing strategy requires a case-by-case analysis; how to find the best combination of different test capabilities considering their strengths and limitations to detect the liability of a chemical structure to induce lethal arrhythmia of very low clinical incidence. This chapter will provide a brief overview on the current methodologies and considerations that are useful in predicting QT prolongation in man and/or a torsadogenic liability.

3.2 THE REGULATORY SITUATION

National and international health authorities have acknowledged the cardiovascular risk during drug development by providing stringent guidelines for cardiotoxicity testing. Nonclinical cardiotoxicity (as well as clinical) assessments are therefore key requirements in pharmaceutical frameworks. In addition to the evaluation of cardiotoxicity based on toxicological and pathological endpoints, cardiac safety pharmacology is the paramount subject of a few important

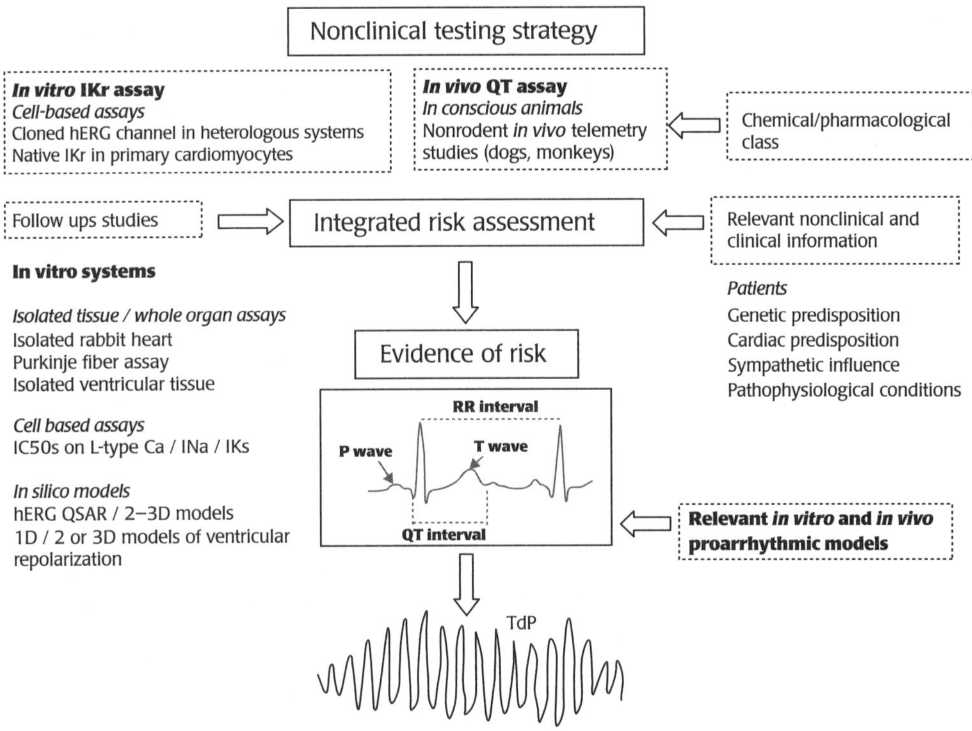

Figure 3-1: Integrated risk assessment strategy. Reprinted from *Cell Biology and Toxicology*, vol. 23, issue 4, Dumotier et al. "Preclinical cardio-safety assessment of torsadogeic risk and alternative methods to animal experimentation: The inseparable twins," Jan. 1, 2007, with permission from Elsevier.

guidelines. It appears that public health authorities now expect all new chemical entities to be tested in cardiac electrophysiological studies.[3]

In 1997, the Committee for Proprietary Medicinal Products (CPMP) of the European Union issued a "points to consider" document[4] on the assessment of the potential for QT interval prolongation by noncardiovascular medicinal products. The CPMP document was followed by the Canadian draft in 2001, the Health Canada/USA draft in 2002, and the International Conference on Harmonization on preclinical guidelines (ICH) S7A (*in vivo*)[5] and S7B (*in vitro*).[6]

All medicines that have been related to the occurrence of TdP in patients display moderate to high affinity for the most important ion current highly expressed in the ventricle, that is, the rapidly activating component of the delayed rectifier K+ current I_{Kr} whose alpha subunit is encoded by the **h**uman *Ether-à-go-go* **R**elated **G**ene(hERG). Even a small I_{Kr} inhibition can cause a slowing of the final repolarization phase of the ventricular action potential, which can translate into a prolongation of the QT interval in the surface electrocardiogram.[7] Therefore, drug safety testing presently considers drug-related hERG blockage and QT prolongation as predictors of TdP. Nonclinical evaluation of the potential of a drug to induce delayed ventricular repolarization is addressed in detail in the ICH S7B guideline, recommending a testing strategy (Figure 3.1) based on electrophysiology studies *in vitro* as well as *in vivo*.[6] The

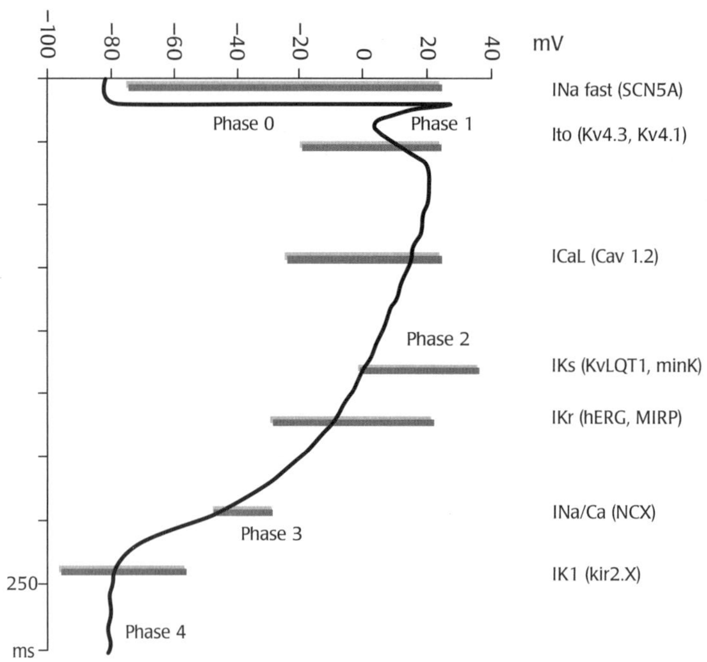

Figure 3-2: Contribution of main ion currents (and respective genes) to time course of membrane potential changes constituting the cardiac action potential. Horizontal gray bars indicate the voltage range ion current participation in the different depolarization/repolarization phases.

in vitro studies evaluate drug effects on channels (mainly hERG channels) expressed in heterologous systems and native I_{Kr} in primary cardiomyocytes as well as effects at the tissue level (e.g., repolarization assays on papillary muscle or on Purkinje fibers) or at the organ level (e.g., retrogradely perfused "Langendorff" isolated hearts). Nonrodent *in vivo* telemetry studies in conscious animals (dogs, monkeys, guinea pigs) are recommended to specifically evaluate drug effects on parameters such as the QT interval of the ECG, blood pressure, heart rate, PR interval (measure of time between P and R waves in the electrocardiogram), and QRS duration of the ECG.

3.3 ION CHANNELS INVOLVED IN CARDIAC ACTION POTENTIAL AND PACEMAKER ACTIVITY

The cardiac action potential can be divided into five phases, numbered 0–4. These phases result from the subsequent or parallel activity of ion channels (Figure 3.2) and/or transporters. Initially, the cell is polarized to near the electrochemical potential for potassium ions because of high K+ conductance at rest. A rapid depolarization is initiated by the activation of the fast inward Na+ current (phase 0). This depolarization is followed by a brief partial repolarization mainly resulting from the activation of the transient outward current (I_{to}) and the inactivation of the sodium current (phase 1). The plateau phase of the action potential is the result of a fine balance between the net calcium influx via L-type Ca2+ channels and Na–Ca exchanger activity, the late inward sodium current and the K+ efflux via different potassium channels (phase 2). In the last part of the action potential (phase 3), two major physiological and pharmacological different outward potassium currents (see next paragraph) play in concert to terminate the plateau phase and initiate a relatively fast final repolarization.[8] This last step restores the original resting potential of the myocyte near –85 mV (phase 4).

The first ion channel identified to be involved in the congenital type 2 long QT syndrome (LQT2) was the hERG channel. This ion channel has been demonstrated to be responsible for the drug-induced LQTS.[9] The hERG channel is a voltage-gated potassium channel, which mediates the rapid component of the delayed rectifier outward potassium current, I_{Kr}.[10] The slow component of the delayed rectifier outward potassium current is the I_{Ks} current, mainly constituted by the KvLQT1/mink protein complex.[11] The subsequent finding that several mutations in the gene encoding I_{Ks} were involved in a different form of congenital LQTS (LQT1)[12] raised the possibility that a loss of function of this channel induced by pharmacological inhibition of this current might also contribute to acquired LQTS. However, even though the role of I_{Ks} in repolarization of human ventricular myocytes has been questioned,[13] it cannot yet be ruled out.

In the myocardium, automaticity is the ability of the cardiac muscle to depolarize spontaneously (i.e., without external electrical stimulation from the autonomic nervous system). This spontaneous depolarization is due to the plasma membrane within the heart that has reduced permeability to potassium (K+) but still allows passive transfer of calcium ions, allowing a net charge to build. Automaticity is most often demonstrated in the sinoatrial (SA) node, the so-called pacemaker cells. Abnormalities in automaticity result in rhythm changes. The mechanism of automaticity involves the pacemaker channels of the HCN (Hyperpolarization-activated, Cyclic Nucleotide-gated) family[14] (e.g., I_f, "funny" current). These poorly selective cation channels conduct more current as the membrane potential becomes more negative, or hyperpolarized. They conduct both potassium and sodium ions. The activity of these channels in the SA node cells causes the membrane potential to slowly become more positive (depolarized) until, eventually, calcium channels are activated and an action potential is initiated.

3.4 HETEROGENEITY OF REPOLARIZATION AND DISPERSION

Some studies conducted over the past two decades have provided evidence that the ventricular myocardium may comprise three electrophysiological and functionally distinct cell types in some species: epicardial, M, and endocardial cells.[15] Ventricular epicardial, but not endocardial, cells generally display a prominent phase 1 because of a large 4-aminopyridine-sensitive transient outward current (Ito), giving the action potential a notched configuration. Differences in the magnitude of the action potential notch and corresponding differences in Ito have also been described between the right ventricular (RV) and left ventricular (LV) epicardium.[16] This distinction is thought to form the basis for why Brugada syndrome, a congenital (channelopathy) form of sudden death, is an RV disease (reference).

An important feature of the M cells is the ability of its action potential duration (APD) to exceed epicardial or endocardial APD in response to a slowing of rate or in response to agents that prolong APD. Similar to Purkinje fibers, M cells show a prominent APD prolongation and develop early after depolarizations (EAD) in response to hERG (I_{Kr}) blockers, whereas the epicardium and endocardium do not.[17] Cells with the characteristics of M cells have been described in canine, guinea pig, and swine ventricles, but so far they cannot be demonstrated in rabbit heart,[18] and there is still no absolute evidence of their presence in human heart when recorded in patients[19] despite few studies reporting the presence of the M cells *in vitro* in human ventricular slices[20].

The transmural increase in APD from the epicardium to the endocardium is relatively gradual, except between the epicardium and subepicardium, where there is often a sharp increase in APD. In summary the degree of electrotonic coupling, together with the intrinsic differences in APD, determines the extent to which transmural dispersion of repolarization (TDR) is present in the ventricular myocardium.

The ionic features that distinguish the M cells also sensitize them to a variety of pharmacological agents. Agents that block I_{Kr} or I_{Ks} or increase I_{Ca} or late I_{Na} generally produce a much greater prolongation of the APD of the M cells than of epicardial or endocardial cells, leading to amplification of TDR. Amplification of transmural heterogeneities normally present in the early and late phases of the action potential and can lead to the development of a variety of arrhythmias, including long QT, Brugada, and short QT syndromes, as well as catecholaminergic ventricular tachyarrhythmias (VT).[21]

A delay of the ventricular transmural repolarization is an important component to define the proarrhythmic potential of a drug. The milder the delay of transmural repolarization is, the lower the likelihood of developing proarrhythmic events is.

3.5 PREDICTIVITY OF AVAILABLE CARDIOSAFETY ASSAYS

3.5.1 *In silico* predictions

The early prediction of hERG K(+) channel affinity of drug candidates is becoming increasingly important in the drug discovery process. Both structure-based and ligand-based approaches have been undertaken to shed more light on the molecular basis of drug-channel interactions[22]. Drug binding to a receptor or ion channel is based on certain structural requirements. The affinity of new chemical entities to a target can be theoretically predicted based on the three-dimensional structure of the molecule when the structure of binding domains of the targets is well known. Unfortunately, there is no crystal structure model available for the hERG channel so far, which makes a reliable quantitative-structure-activity relationship (QSAR) approach based on docking simulations at the channel currently impossible. At present there are only a few structure-activity approaches that try to find structural similarities between hERG-blocking agents.[23–26] Compounds with a tri-alkylated nitrogen like halofantrine and lumefantrine, which undergo protonation in aqueous solution or cellular environment, display inhibitory effects on hERG and other voltage-gated K+ channels. One of the hypotheses suggests that quaternary ammonium ions block the channel pore by interacting with the four tyrosine residues at the extracellular entryway.[23] In addition, inhibitory effects on the hERG channel may also be influenced by the molecular mass/charge ratio and by the adjacent moieties of the tri-alkylated nitrogen. An aromatic ring in proximity to the alkylated nitrogen showing a strong field effect could effectively shield the quaternary ammonium ion and therefore decrease the affinity for hERG K+ channels. Increased potency in blocking I_{Kr} has been suggested when the length of the alkyl side chain attached to the nitrogen is increased.[25] As combinatory chemistry made huge advances over the past years, the chemical structure of a lead compound can be modified in order to avoid cardiotoxic side effects. This step is often performed as early as possible in discovery, and when it comes to hERG, it is frequently used as a prefilter when new chemical structures are to be synthesized. One disadvantage is that *in silico* prediction of hERG inhibitory potency of new molecular entities is hampered by the existence of overlapping binding sites in the central cavity of the channel for different hERG channel blockers.[22]

Different computational hERG models have been developed. These include classification methods, homology models (3D protein sequence) and 2D/3D QSAR models. Different factors may strongly influence the promiscuity of the hERG channel: (a) the presence of intralumind Phe and Tyr at positions 652 and 656, (b) the large size of the hERG channel cavity (approx. 12 Å), (c) well-tolerated variation in hERG pharmacophore because of the formation of multiple binding sites by intraluminal aromatic rings. Pearlstein[27] and colleagues developed a CoMSiA model based on internal patch clamp data for 28 compounds, including several sertindole analogs. The model proposed two major ways of reducing the hERG inhibition, that is, (a) decreasing the positive charge on the central nitrogen or (b) increasing the steric bulk on the hydrophobic end of the molecule.

Interestingly, a recent study compared two of the most common and powerful tools used to address a number of biological topics,[28] that is, comparative molecular field analysis (CoMFA) methodology and grid-independent descriptors (GRIND)-based 3D-QSAR model. Results indicated that both models give good and comparable predictions of the hERG potassium channel blocking activity; however, these models mainly differ in the treatment of the molecule hydrophobicity. The authors suggest using both methods, if feasible, or at least to first identify the main features of the interaction (polar or hydrophobic) and the lipophilicity and flexibility of the compound. Indeed, in case of hydrophobicity would be relevant for the interaction, the use of the GRIND-based model would request a close inspection of the information due to DRY probe. In case of the use of the CoMFA model, one should keep in mind that some crucial region of interaction may not be present on the contour maps before designing new molecules.

The predictivity of hERG *in silico* tools depends on the number of hERG-blocking structures, which are the fundament of each database. A molecule with an unknown hERG toxicophore may not be classified as an hERG blocker. In addition, the predictivity strongly depends on the amount of data compiled in the library and on the variability of the data that can be influenced by experimental settings (i.e., voltage protocols, cell lines, solutions, temperature) across laboratories. In this respect, pharmaceutical companies try to develop their own internal libraries and *in silico* models in the aim to use this tool for decision making as soon as possible in drug development. The *in silico* approaches, will in all cases, benefit from the fast development of (very) high-throughput technologies generating huge amount of data finally (a) improving the quality/homogeneity of the libraries and (b) helping in validating new *in silico* approaches or concepts.

In silico prediction of cardiac toxicity at tissue or organ level requires complex models simulating ion channel block–induced changes of cardiac repolarization, refractoriness, and conduction. The contribution varies significantly between species and different models are needed for dog, rabbit, and human. The predictivity of such models will correlate to the number and quality of data that are fed into the model. Examples of such data are ion channel type, density and kinetics, and incorporation of exchangers and transporters present in the cardiac muscle. Ideally, the three-dimensional structure, including fiber orientation, should also be incorporated. The fully developed model may then be utilized for investigations of the outcome of perturbation of ion channel function, which mimics disease conditions and drug effects. These *in silico* studies will then complement experimental studies and could work as a first preliminary step in evaluating drug-induced cardiotoxicity.

3.5.2 Considerations on the hERG assay

I_{Kr} is a voltage- and time-dependent outward (repolarizing) current that is activated upon depolarization and plays a prominent role in the final repolarization in ventricular tissue.[9] In humans, I_{Kr} is encoded by the hERG gene and is typically referred to as the hERG current. Numerous studies have demonstrated that the hERG block may delay repolarization and prolong the QT interval on the ECG. For most drugs, blocking hERG current results from drug binding within the channel pore after gaining access from the cytoplasmic pool.[29] Virtually all drugs associated with TdP block I_{Kr}/hERG current,[30] but the converse relationship is not always true. It is now relatively easy to study drug effects on the hERG channel by simple radio-ligand binding assays or functionally by measuring the hERG current using voltage clamp techniques such as manual patch clamp or automated planar patch techniques applied to heterologous expression systems. One caveat is that binding assays usually work with crude membrane preparations,whereas the electrophysiological assays are performed with intact cells. Thus, drugs that do not pass the membrane barrier may be overestimated in the radio-ligand binding assay because most of the important hERG-blocking sides are located on the intracellular side of the hERG channel pore. In electrophysiology, an hERG channel block is usually evaluated based on changes in the amplitude of the deactivating tail current measured upon repolarization. Block potency is typically compared based on IC_{50} values derived from fitting concentration–response curves; Hill coefficients for derived fits and confidence intervals should also be provided. Testing an accepted positive control should be included as should the analytical determination of the bath concentrations; the later is crucial to prevent underestimating block potency resulting from c reduced bath concentrations (resulting, for example, from drug absorption to tubing, aggregation). Experimental conditions like temperature or different voltage clamp protocols may affect IC_{50} determinations. Even though comparable IC_{50} values are attained using such varied conditions with most drugs, a few compounds provide substantially different values.[31] More recent studies have underlined the importance of the stimulation rate on the hERG current block[32]. Modulation of the block by stimulation rate likely relates to unique kinetics of drug binding and unbinding to the channel. For insoluble compounds, the hERG assay is typically conducted with concentrations to the limit of solubility. For drugs shown to accumulate in the myocardium, it may be difficult to directly translate an hERG block measured in simple CHO or HEK293 cell expression systems to electrophysiological effects *in vivo*. IC_{50} values for an hERG block are typically compared to predicted (or actual) clinical C_{max} values in order to characterize safety margins for QT prolongation. Redfern et al.[33] have proposed that an IC_{50} value for an hERG block 30-fold greater than the maximal calculated unbound effective therapeutic plasma concentration (ETPC-unbound) provides a reasonable, balanced compromise for delineating torsadogenic risk and calculating safety margins. Safety margins based on IC_{20} values are most likely more variable because they are obtained in the nonlinear part of the concentration–response relationship.

More importantly, the calculated safety margin is not chiseled in stone and should reflect the pharmacokinetic profile of the drug, the patient population, and its potential predisposing factors to arrhythmias, the severity of the disease, the age of the target population and the competitive landscape to name a few.

Apart from the hERG channel electrophysiology, the hERG channel cell biology has recently become increasingly important. Several mutations in hERG were identified to produce trafficking-deficient channels that are retained in the endoplasmic reticulum (ER), and either not expressed at the cell membrane,or expressed but misfolded so that it is nonfunctional. Surface expression of certain mutations (i.e., hERG G601S) can be restored by specific I_{Kr} channel blockers. For instance, the chaperones Hsp70 and Hsp90, cytosolic proteins, can interact transiently with wild type hERG. Inhibition of Hsp90 prevents maturation and reduces hERG/I_{Kr} currents by reducing the number of hERG channels expressed in the cell surface.[34] A well-known example is arsenic trioxyde, which interferes with the formation of hERG/chaperone complexes and inhibits hERG maturation causing a decreased hERG whole cell current, a prolonged action potential, and ECG abnormalities.[35] These trafficking effects have been observed also for other drugs (e.g., pentamidine)[36] but are easily missed when applying short-term *in vitro* electrophysiological experiments because their effects on ventricular repolarization develop in a time period > 10 h.

3.5.3 Repolarization assays

It is increasingly evident that not all the hERG blockers are proarrhythmic. Indeed, even a potent blockade of the hERG channel *in vitro* does not necessarily lead to a QT prolongation in man. For example, the calcium channel blocker verapamil does not lead to QT interval prolongation despite an IC_{50} on hERG in the low micromolar range. The reason for this apparent discrepancy is simply that the myocardial action potential configuration is the net result of the concerted activity of numerous ion channels, and effects on a given channel can be masked by the activities of other competing channels.[37] Thus, measuring effects on the myocardial action potential allows one to assess the physiological relevance of any activity on hERG channels that may be present assuming the system used for testing the drug liability for cardiac ion channels is highly sensitive.[38] It is increasingly recognized that the performance of hERG channel assay together with action potential recording may provide an early risk assessment with a better correlation to the *in vivo* and clinical setting than with just one of these assays alone[60]. Drug effects on the myocardial action potential are typically measured *in vitro* in myocardial tissue such as Purkinje fibers,[39] papillary muscles, ventricular wedge preparation, or the isolated heart model.[40] The focus of all these approaches is to assess the APD measured as the time required to a given percentage of repolarization (e.g., APD90 or the duration at 90 percent repolarization) and changes in AP morphologies, such as triangulation. In addition, some of these models can respond to hERG-blocking drugs with EADs thought to be the cellular event for triggering arrhythmia. The use of the myocardial wedge preparation (a three-dimensional piece of the ventricle) also addresses the important issue of potential transmural differences in drug-induced effects on repolarization,[15] an aspect that cannot be addressed by using isolated tissue such as Purkinje fibers or papillary muscles.

Studies in isolated Purkinje fibers can detect compound induced effects on the action potential configuration and potential EADs. For hERG-dependent effects on the APD, not only APD90 but also the slowing of repolarization as measured by triangulation (APD90-APD30; 30 percent of repolarization) are increasingly being reported. Most compounds known to block hERG-mediated potassium current induce triangulation in this model. The model is capable of detecting both prolongation and shortening of the action potential, and it should not be forgotten that other drug-induced effects on electrophysiological function can be detected, including effects on sodium (e.g., effects on the rate of depolarization) and calcium currents (e.g., effects on the plateau phase of the action potential). In comparison to the papillary muscle or the monophasic action potential in the intact heart, the effects of the drugs prolonging APD are considerably larger. Whereas this is not necessarily a disadvantage, the model has been viewed as possibly being too sensitive for drug-induced effects on repolarization. It must be stressed, however, that most hERG-blocking drugs do lead to an action potential prolongation in this model, especially in dogs and rabbits, and that exceptions are rare. Also, potent hERG-blocking compounds that do not prolong the QT interval and are not proarrhythmic (such as verapamil) do not prolong the action potential in this model. Purkinje fibers from the dog or rabbit have been used typically[41] and are considered as the most appropriate models. Studies in isolated rabbit Purkinje fibers have also been utilized to assess the risk of QT interval prolongation by drugs.[42]

Another commonly used model for assessing myocardial action potential uses the guinea pig papillary muscle. It has an appropriate size since the papillary muscle from larger species may be compromised by ischemia in the middle of the muscle during the experiment. In contrast to the Purkinje fiber, the papillary muscle is a strong contractile tissue, thus allowing the measurement of contractile force,[43] together with the action potential configuration. Since effects on the inotropic state of the myocardium can also affect the action potential, this is a useful secondary measurement to interpret possible drug effects.

3.5.4 Arterially perfused wedge left ventricular preparations

The M cell is a unique myocardial cell type found in the deeper layers of the ventricular wall.[15] These cells respond more sensitively to agents that block hERG channels and, as such, contribute to possible drug-induced transmural heterogeneity of ventricular repolarization and thereby the proarrhythmic potential. The arterially perfused left ventricular myocardial wedge preparation is designed to allow the study of transmural differences in drug action on the action potential and may therefore provide a better assessment of possible proarrhythmic potential of a test article. A similar system has been adapted to the rabbit ventricle, where the presence of M cells could not be recorded. In rabbit species, transmural dispersion is, therefore, described as the difference in duration between the epicardium and the endocardium, believed in rabbits to display similar sensitivity to drug effects than the M cells in dogs. A transmural electrocardiogram is recorded using extracellular silver chloride electrodes placed near the epicardial and endocardial surfaces of the preparation. Transmembrane action potentials were simultaneously recorded from the epicardial, endocardial, and mid-myocardium using three separate intracellular floating microelectrodes. The evaluation is based on the measurement of the QT interval of the electrocardiogram, together with the action potential configuration measured using the transmurally located electrodes. The APD of the M cells is expected to be longer than either endocardial or epicardial cells. The rate dependency of a given drug effect is also amplified in the M cells and may importantly contribute to the proarrhythmic potential of a drug. The measurement of a transmural electrocardiogram (ECG) together with local action potentials from across the ventricular wall of the dog provides one of the most sophisticated *in vitro* approaches for determining drug-induced effects on repolarization, as well as having implications on its proarrhythmic potential. Its main disadvantage is the experimental complexity that makes it accessible only in specialized laboratories and requires extensive training to master the technical preparation.

3.5.5 Isolated heart systems

Studies similar to those described using myocardial tissue *in vitro* can be conducted by using the entire isolated heart. One measures an external monophasic action potential, as opposed to an intracellular myocardial action potential.[40] Hearts are typically perfused retrogradely from the aorta in variations of the so-called Langendorff preparation. The isolated perfused rabbit heart has become a useful model to study proarrhythmia induced by class III antiarrhythmic drugs.[44] Hondeghem developed an automatically analyzed isolated rabbit heart technology that measures several proarrhythmic parameters known as TRIaD (i.e., Triangulation, Reverse use-dependence, Instability, and Dispersion).[45] The model was extensively validated in a blinded way by several pharmaceutical companies. So far, none of the torsadogenic drugs has been demonstrated to be safe in this model.

3.5.6 Measurement of the concentration of test article in *in vitro* systems

The results from studies designed to assess potential drug effects on hERG channels or on the action potential *in vitro* are used as an early risk assessment for clinically relevant effects on the QT interval duration and even proarrhythmic activity. The use of these data for the estimation of safety margins necessitates an accurate measurement of the drug concentrations present in the test system. The perfusion baths used are typically protein free, and one needs to consider potential protein binding of a compound when comparing to the *in vivo* situation. At early stages of drug research, these data may not be available; however, these can have a substantial impact on the risk assessment since the safety margins are determined with unbound drug fraction.[33] Furthermore, compounds may adhere to glass or plastic used in the experimental setups or may undergo rapid degradation in the test solutions with the possibility that the intended drug concentrations are not reached, particularly at lower concentrations.[46] Drug solubility in aqueous solutions at pH 7.4 can also limit the concentrations being tested.

3.5.7 Nonrodent *in vivo* telemetry

According to the ICH S7B guideline, an *in vivo* QT assay is included as one of the most important component of the general testing strategy. Intact animal models are believed to be very informative for extrapolations to the clinical situation because they enable evaluation of metabolites and estimation of safety margins. The use of conscious unrestrained animals with a telemetry device that transmits wirelessly the recorded ECG data has great advantages for eliminating the influences of anesthetic and restraint-induced stress since these factors may alter the sensitivity of the models to detect an effect on QT interval. The beagle dog is a popular species for evaluating the effects on ECG and heart rate; and the conscious dog model, which allows monitoring of blood pressure, heart rate, and ECG, has been widely used as a primary test system for the *in vivo* QT assay.[47] Although the use of nonhuman primates[48] is increasing due to a variety of development factors (limited compound requirements, canine toxicity, biotechnology products), the animals usually show a large interindividual variability with regard to their ECG response.

The conscious dog model either with invasive or noninvasive telemetry (jacket telemetry) is most commonly advocated for toxicology or safety pharmacology studies (especially for good laboratory practice (GLP)-compliant studies).[49] In a typical GLP telemetry dog study, the dog receives single ascending doses with ECG monitoring that lasts for 24 h after dosing. Individual PK is difficult to obtain because telemetered dogs do not usually have implanted catheters, and blood sampling is likely to disrupt the cardiovascular or ECG measurements for a significant period of time.

The anesthetized dog model provides tremendous control over measurement of cardiovascular parameters[50] in combination with the possibility to measure pharmacokinetics (PK) relationships. This latter point is extremely important because without an individual PK relationship, comparisons to reported clinical outcomes and determinations of therapeutic indices generally cannot be reliably estimated from experiments with relatively few animals. In addition, higher drug exposure can be achieved in case the test compound induces nausea or vomiting, which is a frequent side effect of drugs with oncology indications. ECG interval changes and even APDs can be precisely recorded through direct measures either at sinus rate or during pacing to alleviate the need for corrections of the QT interval. The caveat with this model is that normal autonomic nervous system-mediated events will be blunted by anesthetics or overridden completely if pacing is used. It is also possible that anesthetics may interfere with the cardiac repolarization and sensitize the model for proarrhythmia.

For most species it has been shown that the duration of the QT interval is inversely related to the heart rate.[51] Thus, any changes in the raw QT interval must be carefully interpreted and corrected for this physiological variation to isolate the drug-induced component from the QT interval modulation. Since the QT interval has a rate-dependent nature, various mathematical formulae were developed to adjust this variable for values obtained at different heart rates resulting in a "corrected" QT interval (i.e., QTc). The scientific debate about the appropriate QT correction formula is still ongoing, but frequently, the Bazett's formula, Fridericia's formula and Van de Water et al.'s formula are used. In addition, several individual correction factors were published by different laboratories.[52–54] Usually a QTc increase by more than 10 percent or of statistical significance is regarded as a positive *in vivo* QT signal.

Independent of the selected experimental approach, various aspects of a study can optimize the quality of the ECG data collected. Animals should be calm and acclimatized to the procedure, and the restraint approaches and the placement of the ECG leads should be consistent. The environment should be quiet and electronically shielded, and on the days of ECG recordings there should be no disturbances (e.g., blood sampling). A sufficient pretest period (e.g., one day) is necessary to provide data for individual correction factors.

As for any other model, the question of whether the dog is a good model for predicting effects in humans must be taken into context with the differences in physiology. The normal conscious dog responds much as humans do with respect to the QT–RR interval relationship and has proven to be a good predictor of response based on pharmacokinetic/pharmacodynamic (PK/PD) relationship. The dog also has a much more profound sinus arrhythmia than humans, which is beneficial when using the beat-to-beat technique for comparison of QT intervals at comparable heart rate (RR) intervals. Because of this species-specific sinus arrhythmia, the dog must necessarily cope with sudden heart rate accelerations and decelerations that could trigger arrhythmias through impaired hysteresis of the QT interval. In summary, the preceding data validates the dog as a highly useful model for predicting ECG outcomes in humans.

3.6 INTEGRATED CARDIAC RISK ASSESSMENT

In the drug development process, an integrated cardiosafety assessment is necessary before entering the clinical phase to evaluate the molecule's potential QT liability and its proarrhythmic risk. A strict adherence to the ICH S7 guidelines will result in a narrow cardiovascular assessment that does not address all potentially important aspects of cardiovascular function. Data from all available *in vitro* and *in vivo* assays have to be considered. Since none of the assays is predictive enough when considered alone, the cardiosafety package should contain at least an *in vitro* hERG channel study combined with *in vivo* ECG studies. Although actually considered as "mechanistic studies," the results from repolarization assays may be very important in case of positive findings. The results of each preclinical assay must be judged on the calculation of a therapeutic index or safety margin (i.e., the concentration of the undesired effect divided by the concentration of the desired effect). The concentration of the undesired effect is reflected by an IC_{50} value (e.g., hERG channel 50 percent inhibition), and the concentration of the desired effect is expressed ideally as the free therapeutic plasma concentration in man (or an estimated value). If in early phases of drug development the estimation of potential therapeutic concentration is difficult, it can be replaced by pharmacological receptor binding (Kd) data or by EC_{50} or IC_{50} values from different robust pharmacological *in vitro* target (e.g., cell-based) assays. In the case of highly plasma protein bound compounds, "corrected" IC_{50} reflecting calculated (equivalent) total plasma drug concentrations are sometimes provided. However, it should be recognized that plasma protein binding varies with species, is not necessarily linear across drug concentrations, and represents only one factor that determines drug distribution to the myocardium. Controversy exists in regards to "correcting" for plasma protein binding with *in vitro* studies. Some drugs have been shown to accumulate in cardiac tissues and cardiac tissue/plasma. In principle, similar calculations can be performed for inhibitory values of drugs on other cardiac ion channels like sodium and calcium.

An hERG IC_{50} value ≤ 1 μ*M* or $\leq 30 \times$ free therapeutic plasma concentration is regarded as a strong positive signal by the health authorities.[33,55] In *in vivo* animal studies, a given QT_c interval prolongation exceeding 10 percent or reaching statistical significance is regarded as a positive signal. In clinical trials, a maximum group means QT_c prolongation ≥ 5 ms is a regarded as a positive finding.[55]

A nonscientific but important driver is the availability of drug substance as these assays have a major step in terms of compound requirement from low milligram quantities to hundreds of milligrams or even gram amounts in *in vivo* models. One should recognize that potential hemodynamic activity (changes in arterial blood pressure, heart rate) can be addressed easily in small animal models including the rat and guinea pig. These studies may be done later during lead optimization when candidate selection and prioritization is initiated.

The electrophysiological mechanisms that underlie the development of TdP are complex and influenced by a wide variety of factors that are not completely understood. Nevertheless, it seems clear that a delay in the ventricular repolarization process reflected by a QT interval prolongation is not the sole determinant of a torsadogenic effect of a drug. Thus, the use of preclinical cardiac electrophysiology data to predict the potential of a drug to cause TdP requires a comprehensive and integrated approach in which the risk for TdP of a given drug includes characterization of the drug effects on different cardiac ion channels (including kinetics of block) from the cellular to the whole organism level.

However, there is a growing body of evidence that a deeper evaluation is requested for drug torsadogenicity.[56–58] Dispersion of repolarization and beat-to-beat variability are key factors in torsadogenic effects. There is actually a strong need to develop robust and scientifically validated models that use these two parameters so that they can be used routinely to screen compounds in the early phase of development. Indeed, beat-to-beat variability and dispersion of repolarization may also indicate potential risk for other types of lethal arrhythmias such as ventricular fibrillation related to conduction disturbances. Nevertheless, the pharmaceutical industry would gain in confidence by detecting, in early preclinical phase of development, not only lethal arrhythmias related to delayed repolarization (TdP) but also those where a shortening of the cardiac wavelength may precipitate ventricular fibrillation by the sole effect of the drug.

Although TdP episodes result from a complex electrophysiological mechanism, QT interval prolongation and I_{Kr} block are still regarded as surrogate markers for TdP-like arrhythmia.

In the end, there is no cookbook to perform a tasty integrated safety assessment because each drug combined with the mode of action and indication is unique in its features. Good pharmacological science should drive the individual tailor-made solutions.

Integrating a safety pharmacological assessment into drug discovery and development has become essential to fulfill new regulatory requirements, but more importantly this assessment provides important data for the selection of drug candidates. As mentioned from the onset, only doing GLP safety pharmacology studies on drugs prior to phase I clinical trials will mean that data are available too late for lead optimization and the drug candidate selection process. Thus, a thorough cardiovascular safety pharmacological assessment should consider additional aspects and may include a variety of experimental models not explicitly listed in the guidelines. There is clearly no optimal approach that fits all needs since pharmacological profiling must be tailored to the needs of individual projects. The approach chosen should reflect a company's expertise and project-specific potential liabilities. Nevertheless, some general trends have emerged in the past few years.

In vitro high-throughput electrophysiological screening is a rather new element of safety pharmacology profiling for many companies, but it is here to stay. In particular, screening for hERG channel activity can and should be done rather early in the lead optimization process. Methodologies are available for reasonable throughput and the potential for interactions with hERG should be identified early enough to allow medicinal chemists the time needed to reduce this unwanted activity. Effective tools are now available and include *in silico* approaches as well as traditional manual electrophysiological studies in well-profiled test systems. The automated patch clamp technology is available for most of the major ion channels (e.g., I_{Kr}, I_{Na}, I_{CaL}, I_{Ks}) expressed in mammalian cell lines and should be applied to identify potential multi-ion channels. To complete the early safety panel, a large receptor screen is recommended to assess the pharmacological promiscuity of the new drugs (e.g., interference with autonomic nervous system via modulation of adrenergic receptors), which could influence the results of the later *in vivo* studies.[59] A second *in vitro* step that adds value to the overall electrophysiological assessment is to evaluate effects on myocardial action potential using systems mentioned previously. The initial focus on hERG is necessary from a pragmatic point of view, based on the regulatory fixation on this single-channel activity. However, there is a strong argument that ultimately only effects that result in changes on the myocardial action potential are of relevance. The models needed for assessing effects on the myocardial action potential are a bit more complex and time consuming than those used for measuring hERG activity, but they require little compound and give additional value to the overall risk assessment. Paired with results from a hERG assay, one achieves rather early on a predictive assessment for cardiovascular liability.[60] The myocardial action potential assay can also be included during early lead optimization. If one focuses on the potential for compounds to affect ventricular repolarization, one might argue that the next essential step entails an evaluation of the electrocardiogram in a nonrodent species to complement the *in vitro* evaluation. Indeed, this is what is found in the ICH S7B guideline. These studies form a valuable bridge to later studies in larger animals that are only feasible for a few drug candidates that are thought to have a chance for further development. Unexpected effects on blood pressure and heart rate can be just as devastating to a lead optimization program as are effects on the QT interval. Finally, a thorough *in vivo* assessment of both systemic hemodynamic parameters and the electrocardiogram characteristics is essential. The dog has been the most commonly used species for these assessments, and full implant technology has become the gold standard experimental approach to allow for studies in conscious animals. The minipig or the monkey species can also be successfully used for generating high-quality cardiovascular data. A guideline such as the ICH S7A must be very general in nature and cannot specify exactly what is reasonable to do for every development compound. Good pharmacological science should be the driving force behind the selection of studies performed, and the responsibility for this selection still lies with the pharmaceutical industry.

3.7 OUTLOOK

New promising methods and approaches for evaluating drug-induced cardiotoxicity assessments (i.e., beat-to-beat variation (instability) of QT, APD prolongation by triangulation, beat-to-beat instability of APD, characterization of frequency-dependence and transmural dispersion) need to be developed and validated in both already available and new *in vivo* and *in vitro* assays. If such readouts then can be correlated to similar readouts in clinical studies using ECG recordings, then the prerequisites are at hand also to convince the relevant regulatory authorities that preclinical data indeed may be used as predictors of a proarrhythmic clinical risk. With good *in vitro/in vivo* correlation of preclinical readouts, a substantial reduction in animal experiments may be achieved. Apart from this, we need to keep an eye on human stem cells, which can be differentiated into ventricular myocytes. Even though more validation work needs to be done, it is known that cardiomyocytes derived from human embryonic stem cells respond with action potential prolongation and even some kind of spontaneous triggered activities resembling EADs in the presence of hERG blockers (Figure 3.3). The ventricular cardiomyocytes derived from human embryonic stems is currently the only human designed tool that bears a tremendous potential to become a powerful *in vitro* tool to predict arrhythmia and cellular cardiotoxicity with a very high specificity.[61]

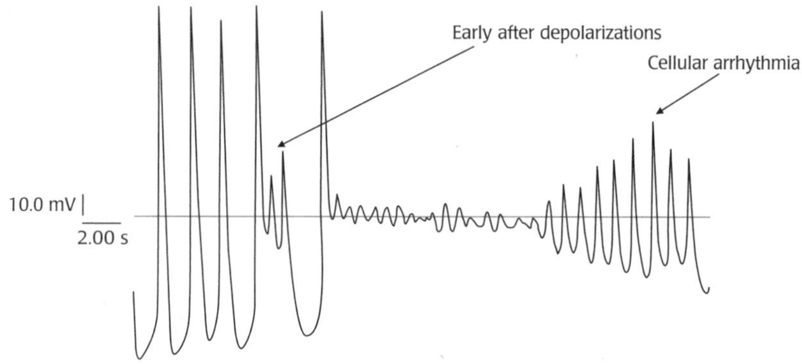

Figure 3-3: Original current-clamp recording of a spontaneous beating cardiomyocyte derived from human embryonic stem cells. The cell was superfused with 100 n*M* E-4031, a potent hERG channel blocker, which lead after an action potential prolongation to early after depolarizations and chaotic electrical behavior at the cellular level (cellular arrhythmia).

REFERENCES

1. Cahoon WD, Jr. Acquired QT prolongation. *Prog Cardiovasc Nurs*. 2009;24(1): 30–33.
2. Sager PT. Key clinical considerations for demonstrating the utility of preclinical models to predict clinical drug-induced torsades de pointes. *Br J Pharmacol*. 2008;154(7):1544–1549.
3. Bode G, Olejniczak K. ICH topic: The draft ICH S7B step 2: Note for guidance on safety pharmacology studies for human pharmaceuticals. *Fundam Clin Pharmacol*. (2002);16(2):79–81.
4. Committee for Proprietary Medicinal Product. *Points to Consider. The Assessment of QT Interval Prolongation by Non-Cardiovascular Medicinal Products*; 1997. CPMP/986/96.
5. ICH Harmonized Tripartite Guideline. *S7A Safety Pharmacology Studies for Human Pharmaceuticals*. U.S. Department of Health and Human Services, FDA; 2000. Retrieved from http://www.ich.org.
6. ICH S7B. *The Non-Clinical Evaluation of the Potential for Delayed Ventricular Repolarization (QT Interval Prolongation) by Human Pharmaceuticals*. U.S. Department of Health and Human Services, FDA; 2005. Retrieved from http://www.ich.org.
7. Lagrutta AA, Trepakova ES, Salata JJ. The hERG channel and risk of drug-acquired arrhythmia: An overview. *Current Top Med Chem*. 2008;8(13):1102–1112.
8. Sanguinetti MC, Jurkiewicz NK. Two components of cardiac delayed rectifier K+ current. Differential sensitivity to block by class III antiarrhythmic agents. *J. Gen Physiol*. 1990;96:195–215.
9. Sanguinetti MC, Jiang C, Curran, ME, et al. A mechanistic link between an inherited and an acquired cardiac arrhythmia: HERG encodes the IKr potassium channel. *Cell* 1995;81,299–307.
10. Sanchez-Chapula JA, Navarro-Polanco RA, Culberson C, et al. Molecular determinants of voltage-dependent human ether-a-go-go related gene (HERG) K+ channel block. *J Biol Chem*. 2002;277(26):23587–23595.
11. Kang J, Chen XL, Wang L, et al. Interactions of the antimalarial drug mefloquine with the human cardiac potassium channels KvLQT1/minK and HERG. *J Pharmacol Ex The*. 2001;299(1):290–296.
12. Wang Q, Curran ME, Splawski I, et al. Positional cloning of a novel potassium channel gene: KVLQT1 mutations cause cardiac arrhythmias. *Nat Genet*. 1996;12(1):17–23.
13. Crump W, Cavero I. QT interval prolongation by non-cardiovascular drugs: Issues and solutions for novel drug development. *Pharm Sci Tech Today*. 1999;2:270–280.

14. DiFrancesco D, Borer JS. The funny current: Cellular basis for the control of heart rate. *Drugs*. 2007;67(15):15–24.
15. Antzelevitch C, Shimizu W, Yan GX, et al. The M cell: Its contribution to the ECG and to normal and abnormal electrical function of the heart. *J Cardiovasc Electrophysiol*. 1999;10:1124–1152.
16. Bassani RA. Transient outward potassium current and Ca2+ homeostasis in the heart: Beyond the action potential. *Braz J Med Biol Res*. 2006;39(3):393–403.
17. Antzelevitch C. Role of spatial dispersion of repolarization in inherited and acquired sudden cardiac death syndromes. *Am J Physiol Heart Circ Physiol*. 2007;293(4):H2024–2038.
18. Zhu TG, Patel C, Martin S, et al. Ventricular transmural repolarization sequence: its relationship with ventricular relaxation and role in ventricular diastolic function. *Eur Heart J*. 2009;30(3):372–380.
19. Taggart P, Sutton PMI, Opthof T, et al. Transmural repolarisation in the left ventricle in humans during normoxia and ischaemia. *Cardiovasc Res*. 2001;50:454–462.
20. Drouin E, Charpentier F, Gauthier C, et al. Electrophysiologic characteristics of cells spanning the left ventricular wall of human heart: Evidence for presence of M cells. *JACC*. 1995;26(1):185–192.
21. Antzelevitch, C. Drug-induced spatial dispersion of repolarization. *Cardiol J*. 2008;15(2):100–121.
22. Thai KM, Ecker GF. Predictive models for HERG channel blockers: Ligand-based and structure-based approaches. *Curr Med Chem*. 2007;14(28):3003–3026.
23. Wempe MF. Quaternary ammonium ions can externally block voltage-gated K+ channels. Establishing a theortical and experimental model that predicts KDs and the selectivity of K+ over Na+ ions. *J Mol Struct*. 2001;562:63–78.
24. Ekins S, Crumb WJ, Sarazan RD, et al. Three-dimensional quantitative structure-activity relationship for inhibition of human ether-a-go-go-related gene potassium channel. *J Pharmacol Exp Ther*. 2002;301:427–434.
25. Cavalli A, Poluzzi E, De Ponti F, et al. Toward a pharmacophore for drugs inducing the long QT syndrome: Insights from a CoMFA study of HERG K(+) channel blockers. *J Med Chem*. 2002;45:3844–3853.
26. Roche O, Trube G, Zuegge J, et al. A virtual screening method for prediction of the HERG potassium channel liability of compound libraries. *Chembiochem*. 2002;3:455–459.
27. Pearlstein R, Vaz RJ, Kanga J, et al. Characterization of HERG potassium channel inhibition using CoMSiA 3D QSAR and homology modeling approaches. *Bioorg Med Chem Lett*. 2003;3:1829–1835.
28. Ermondi G, Visentin S, Caron G. GRIND-based 3D-QSAR and CoMFA to investigate topics dominated by hydrophobic interactions: The case of hERG K+ channel blockers. *Eur J Med Chem*. 2009;44:1926–1932.
29. Sanguinetti MC, Tristani-Firouzi M. hERG potassium channels and cardiac arrhythmia. *Nature*. 2002;23(440):463–469.
30. Roden, DM . Drug-induced prolongation of the QT interval. *N Engl J Med*. 2004;350(10),1013–1022.
31. Kirsch GE, Trepakova ES, Brimecombe JC, et al. Variability in the measurement of hERG potassium channel inhibition: Effects of temperature and stimulus pattern. *J Pharmacol Toxicol Methods*. 2004;50(2):93–101.
32. Stork D, Timin EN, Berjukow S, et al. State dependent dissociation of HERG channel inhibitors. *Br J Pharmacol*. 2007;151(8):1368–1376.
33. Redfern WS, Carlsson L, Davis AS, et al. Relationships between preclinical cardiac electrophysiology, clinical QT interval prolongation and torsade de pointes for a broad range of drugs: Evidence for a provisional safety margin in drug development. *Cardiovasc Res*. 2003;58,32–45.
34. Dennis A, Wang L, Wan X, et al. hERG channel trafficking: Novel targets in drug-induced long QT syndrome. *Biochem Soc Trans*. 2007;35(5):1060–1063.

35. Ficker E, Kuryshev YA, Dennis AT et al. Mechanisms of arsenic-induced prolongation of cardiac repolarization. *Mol Pharmacol.* 2004;66(1):33–44.
36. Kuryshew YA, Ficker E, Wang L, et al. Pentamidine-induced long QT syndrome and block of hERG trafficking. *J Pharmacol Exp Ther.* 2005;312(1):316–323.
37. Yuill KH, Borg JJ, Ridley JM, et al. Potent inhibition of human cardiac potassium (HERG) channels by the anti-estrogen agent clomiphene-without QT interval prolongation. *Biochem Biophys Res Commun.* 2004;318(2):556–561.
38. Dumotier B, Bastide M, Adamantidis M. Use-dependent effects of cisapride on postrest action potentials in rabbit ventricular myocardium. *Eur J Pharmacol.* 2001;422(1–3):137–148.
39. Puisieux F, Adamantidis M, Dumotier B, et al . Cisapride-induced prolongation of cardiac action potential and early after depolarizations in rabbit Purkinje fibres. *Br J Pharmacol.* 1996;117,1377–1379.
40. Franz MR. Method and theory of monophasic action potential recording. *Prog Cardiovasc Dis.* 1991;6:347–368.
41. Gintant GA, Limberis JT, McDermott JS, et al. The canine Purkinje fiber: An in vitro model system for acquired long QT syndrome and drug-induced arrhythmogenesis. *J Cardiovasc Pharmacol.* 2001;37:607–618.
42. Cavero I, Mestre M, Guillon JM, et al. Preclinical in vitro cardiac electrophysiology: A method of predicting arrhythmogenic potential of antihistamines in humans? *Drug Saf.* 1991;21(Suppl 1):19–31.
43. Li H, Zhang Y, Tian Z, et al. Genistein stimulates myocardial contractility in guinea pigs by different subcellular mechanisms. *Eur J Pharmacol.* 2008;597(1–3): 70–74.
44. Johna R, Mertens H, Haverkamp W, et al. Clofilium in the isolated perfused rabbit heart: A new model to study proarrhythmia induced by class III antiarrhythmic drugs. *Basic Res Cardiol.* 1998;93(2):127–135.
45. Hondeghem LM, Hoffman P. Blinded test in isolated female rabbit heart reliably identifies action potential duration prolongation and proarrhythmic drugs: Importance of triangulation reverse-use dependence and instability. *J Cardiovasc Pharmacol.* 2003;41:14–24.
46. Brimecombe JC, Kirsch GE, Brown AM. Test article concentrations in the hERG assay: Losses through the perfusion, solubility and stability. *J Pharmacol Toxicol Methods.* 2009;59(1):29–34.
47. Fossa AA. Assessing QT prolongation in conscious dogs: validation of a beat-to-beat method. *Pharmacol Ther.* 2008;119(2):133–140.
48. Gauvin DV, Tilley LP, Smith FW, Jr, et al. Electrocardiogram, hemodynamics, and core body temperatures of the normal freely moving cynomolgus monkey by remote radiotelemetry. *J Pharmacol Toxicol Methods.* 2006;53(2):140–151.
49. Gralinski MR. The dog's role in the preclinical assessment of QT interval prolongation. *Toxicol Pathol.* 2003;31:11–16.
50. Gauvin DV, Tilley LP, Smith FW, Jr, et al. Electrocardiogram, hemodynamics, and core body temperatures of the normal freely moving laboratory beagle dog by remote radiotelemetry. *J Pharmacol Toxicol Methods.* 2006;53(2):128–139.
51. Soloviev MV, Hamlin RL, Barrett RM, et al. Different species require different correction factors for the QT interval. *Cardiovasc Toxicol.* 2006;6(2):145–157.
52. Takahara A, Sugiyama A, Satoh Y, et al. Comparison of four rate-correction algorithms for the ventricular repolarization period in assessing net effects of IKr blockers in dogs. *J Pharmacol Sci.* 2006;102(4):396–404.
53. King A, Bailie M, Olivier NB. Magnitude of error introduced by application of heart rate correction formulas to the canine QT interval. *Ann Noninvasive Electrocardiol.* 2006;11(4):289–298.
54. Holzgrefe HH, Cavero I, Gleason CR, et al. Novel probabilistic method for precisely correcting the QT interval for heart rate in telemetered dogs and cynomolgus monkeys. *J Pharmacol Toxicol Methods.* 2007;55(2):159–175.

55. Webster R, Leishmann D, Walker D. Towards a drug concentration effect relationship for QT prolongation and torsades des pointes. *Curr Opin Drug Discov Devel.* 2002;5:116–126.
56. Hondeghem LM. QT prolongation is an unreliable predictor of ventricular arrhythmia. *Heart Rhythm.* 2008;5(8):1210–1212.
57. Gintant GA. Preclinical Torsades-de-Pointes screens: advantages and limitations of surrogate and direct approaches in evaluating proarrhythmic risk. *Pharmacol Ther.* 2008; 119(2):199–209.
58. Bass AS, Darpo B, Valentin JP, et al. Moving towards better predictors of drug-induced torsades de pointes. *Br J Pharmacol.* 2008;154(7):1550–1553.
59. Whitebread S, Hamon J, Bojanic D, et al. Keynote review: In vitro safety pharmacology profiling: an essential tool for successful drug development. *Drug Discov Today.* 2005;10(21):1421–1433.
60. Guth BD, Germeyer S, Kolb W, et al. Developing a strategy for the nonclinical assessment of proarrhythmic risk of pharmaceuticals due to prolonged ventricular repolarization. *J Pharmacol Toxicol Methods.* 2004;49(3):159–169.
61. Stummann TC, Bremer S. The possible impact of human embryonic stem cells on safety pharmacological and toxicological assessments in drug discovery and drug development. *Curr Stem Cell Res Ther.* 2008;3(2):118–311.

4 **Predicting drug-induced liver injury**

Safer patients or safer drugs?

Jinghai J. Xu

4.1 INTRODUCTION: THE PROBLEM OF DRUG-INDUCED LIVER INJURY

Liver injury or hepatotoxicity caused by medications has been a major challenge for health care professionals and drug developers alike. In the United States alone, drug-induced liver injury (DILI) is responsible for 5 percent of all hospital admissions and 50 percent of all acute liver failures.[1] DILI is the most common reason for black-box warnings among drugs previously approved for marketing, as well as drug withdrawals after regulatory approval for marketing.[2] DILI is also a leading reason for nonapproval decisions by the Food and Drug Administration (FDA) in the United States, and a major reason why drugs fail in clinical and preclinical development.[2,3]

Drugs for which development, approval, or clinical usage were significantly impacted due to hepatotoxicity include troglitazone, bromfenac, tienilic acid, temafloxacin, nomifensin, perhexiline, ibufenac, benoxaprofen, zileutin, trovafloxacin, tolcapone, felbamate, iproniazid, ticrynafen, labetalol, alpidem, ebrotidine, dilevalol, tasosartan, telithromycin, and ximelagatran.[4] Several textbooks have been published on the topic of DILI (e.g., References 5, 6). There is also an annual summary of drugs associated with hepatotoxicity, which provides excellent updates on this topic.[7]

Regulators of the pharmaceutical industry have made it a priority to provide clinical and preclinical guidance to improve detection of DILI.[8,9] Databases of potentially hepatotoxic drugs have been established,[10] interagency collaborations aimed at better prediction of DILI are underway.[11] Among the many collaborative efforts are standardization of the nomenclature and clinical diagnosis of hepatotoxicity,[12] creating a registry of carefully documented DILI cases and corresponding controls, and banking of biological specimens (DNA, plasma, and immortalized lymphocytes) to facilitate detailed genetic analyses.[13]

What are the key strategies in predicting DILI? Most of the DILI are idiosyncratic, meaning that not all patients taking the drug will experience liver toxicity. In fact, only a small percentage of patients (typically fewer than 1 in 100) will experience elevated liver enzymes in their sera (a biomarker for liver injury), and even a smaller percentage (typically fewer than 1 in 1,000 patients) will go on to develop fulminant liver injury.[14] In the broadest sense, there are two categorical strategies used to predict DILI: (a) identify safer patients and (b) identify safer drugs. This chapter will examine predictive approaches and provide critical reviews in both.

4.2 IDENTIFY SAFER PATIENTS: PATIENTS' RISK FACTORS FOR DILI

To identify safer patients for a particular medication, one needs to understand both toxicokinetic and toxicodynamic variables and their safety implications in a given patient situation. The goal is to proactively identify a subpopulation of patients whose combination of variables resulted in "unacceptable" risks for receiving such medication. As with any medical intervention, the right balance of benefit and risk should be properly addressed at the individual level by a patient's physician and pharmacist. Keeping up-to-date regarding the factors that contributes to "at risk" patients, coupled with keen awareness of a particular patient's situation, is a prerequisite of avoiding drug toxicity. Major patient risk factors for DILI, which fall into either toxicokinetic or toxicodynamic category, are discussed in the following sections.

4.2.1 Risk factors from a toxicokinetic perspective

Toxicokinetic risk factors are those that can lead to increased C_{max} (maximum concentration) and/or AUC (area under the curve of the concentration vs. time plot) of a given drug in a patient's liver. The drug in question can be the parent drug, its toxic metabolite, or a combination. The liver's increased exposure to drugs can be caused by increased drug absorption (e.g., for an orally administered medication) and/or decreased drug clearance. Some of the major causes of toxicokinetic risk factors are summarized next.

Age: Blood flow to key clearance organs such as liver and kidney decline with age.[15,16] Combined with decline in metabolic activities in these organs among aging patients, it is not surprising that drug clearance rates typically decrease with age.[17] For example, in a comprehensive compilation of therapeutic drug monitoring data for 15 antidepressant drugs in a naturalistic clinical setting, drug concentrations in the elderly patients (i.e., age 65 years of age or older) is about 40–90 percent higher than the concentrations in patients younger than 65 years of age.[18]

Gender: Men are typically larger than women in size and weight. This can result in larger distribution volumes and faster total clearance of many drugs in men compared to women. In addition, gender-specific differences in drug metabolizing enzymes and transporters and influence of sex hormones and fertility medications may further affect pharmacokinetic and toxicokinetic differences between men and women.[19] In the same published therapeutic drug monitoring of antidepressant drugs mentioned previously, drug concentrations in women is about 10–40 percent higher than those in men across many antidepressant drugs.[18]

Expression/function/regulation of metabolic enzymes and drug transporters affecting drug's local liver concentration and transit time: The expression, function, and regulation of detoxification (and sometimes toxification) enzymes, such as cytochrome P450s (CYP450s) and glutathione-S-transferases (GSTs) are influenced by both genetic (e.g., DNA polymorphism) and epigenetic (e.g., expression regulation) reasons. Likewise, the expression, function, and regulation of drug transporters are influenced by both genetic (e.g., polymorphisms of DNA sequences) and epigenetic (e.g., the available amount of transporting co-factors) causes. As a result, the affinity (e.g., K_m) and reaction rate (e.g., V_{max}) of drug metabolic enzymes, uptake, and efflux transporters can affect the local drug concentration that liver parenchymal cells "see" at a given dose at a given time.[20,21]

Drug–drug interactions: The coadministration of two or more drugs is increasingly common in today's health care. This is especially true in the elderly, whose disease management often requires concomitant usage of more than one medication. Since most drugs are metabolized by phase I and/or phase II enzymes, and the clearance of such drugs and metabolites can be mediated by various drug transporters, inhibition of these enzymes and transporters by one drug could lead to increased exposure of another drug that is a substrate for such enzyme or transporter. Drug–drug interactions and their implications in drug toxicity are discussed in greater detail in Chapter 5 of this book.

It is therefore not surprising that when therapeutic drug monitoring was carefully conducted and analyzed in large patient populations, pronounced interindividual variability was observed. The interindividual variability was typically higher than intraindividual variability. For example, in a two-year analysis of non-nucleoside reverse transcriptase inhibitors (NNRTIs) and protease inhibitors (PIs) in routine clinical practice, NNRTIs showed 55 percent interindividual coefficient of variation (CV) and 20 percent intraindividual CV, whereas PIs showed 84 percent interindividual CV and 38 percent intraindividual CV.[22] In another study, the interindividual CV for dose-normalized citalopram concentrations was about 70 percent for S-citalopram, whereas the intraindividual variations over time for the same parameter was approximately 30 percent.[23] Even when paroxetine pharmacokinetics were measured in children and adolescents (i.e., not in the elderly), the mean area under the plasma drug concentration curve was 0.09 ± 0.10 mg/mL·h (notice that the standard deviation was higher than the mean value).[24] For reasons discussed previously, such a large variability in drug levels should be expected in a real-world setting. For drugs that have narrow therapeutic indices, supra-therapeutic drug exposure levels in critical organs including liver can potentially lead to serious consequences.[25]

4.2.2 Risk factors from a toxicodynamic perspective

Toxicodynamic risk factors are those that can lead to altered host response to drugs that are independent of drug exposure. Some of the known mechanisms mediating toxicodynamic responses include (a) distribution and density of relevant receptor or enzyme for receptor- or enzyme-mediated toxicity, (b) basal and inducible levels of endogenous defense mechanisms such as endogenous antioxidants and antioxidative enzyme systems, (c) preexisting conditions such as subclinical defects that lower the threshold for further exogenous injury (e.g., subclinical mitochondrial defects), (d) a host's ability to repair an injury in time prior to the next onset of drug insult (e.g., for chronic drug treatment), and (e) a host's ability to adapt to injury sufficiently to minimize further drug-induced injury (e.g., up-regulation of repair pathways and/or down-regulation of inflammation and/or death pathways). Some of the known leading toxicodynamic risk factors that may cause decreased tolerance to toxicants may also apply to DILI. These factors include idiosyncratic immune responses (e.g., the downstream consequences of drug-induced hapten formation), intrinsic or acquired diseases having an impact on the hepatic toxic response (e.g., fatty liver diseases), nutritional or lifestyle factors (e.g., excessive alcohol, tobacco smoking), other environmental factors, and combined use of other drugs that modulate toxicodynamic responses. Some of the known toxicodynamic risk factors that are particularly relevant to DILI are summarized here.

Disease states: Non-alcoholic fatty liver disease (NAFLD) is a major hepatic manifestation of type 2 diabetes mellitus. Diabetes developed as a complication of cirrhosis is known as hepatogenous diabetes (HD). HD in early cirrhosis stages may be subclinical in manifestation. Only insulin resistance and glucose intolerance may be observed.[26] However, if these patients were further treated with a diabetic drug that happened to possess a low grade of liver injury potential, more severe liver injury may manifest. Indeed, increased incidences of hepatotoxicity have been observed in diabetic patients receiving drug therapies,[27] although the exact mechanisms have not been fully elucidated to date.

In addition to NAFLD and diabetes, other pathophysiological states that have implications in hepatotoxicity include chronic intermittent hypoxia (CIH), which occurs during a number of disease states.[28] Intermittent hypoxia activates a number of signaling pathways involved in oxygen sensing, oxidative stress, metabolism, catecholamine biosynthesis, and immune responsiveness. Specifically, in a controlled human study, CIH increases oxidative stress by increasing production of reactive oxygen species (ROS) without a compensatory increase in antioxidant activity.[29] In mice, CIH induced oxidative stress particularly in the liver. In addition, CIH greatly exacerbated acetaminophen (APAP)-induced liver toxicity, causing fulminant hepatocellular injury in an otherwise acetaminophen-resistant mice model.[30] Indeed, acetaminophen or CIH alone did not affect serum levels of liver enzymes or hepatic glutathione or nitrotyrosine levels. However, mice exposed to both CIH and APAP at the same time exhibited decreased hepatic glutathione in conjunction with a fivefold increase in nitrotyrosine levels, suggesting formation of toxic peroxynitrite in hepatocytes. Such combination also caused marked increases in proinflammatory chemokines, monocyte chemoattractant protein-1 and macrophage inflammatory protein-2, which were not observed in mice exposed to CIH or APAP alone. These preclinical findings may have important clinical implications in idiosyncratic DILI.[31]

The recommendation that, where appropriate, new animal models of human disease(s) be introduced into drug safety assessment should be an area of active research in translational medicine.[32]

Lifestyle and fat mass influences: Long-term alcohol usage and smoking is known to compromise liver functions. Alcoholic liver diseases (ALD) may be subclinical in its early stages, but it is known to induce oxidative stress and compromise mitochondrial functions.[33] In addition, excessive fat intake and storage resulting in steatosis, as in NAFLD, can sensitize the liver to lipid peroxidation and fulminant liver injury by yet another insult of toxicant.[34,35] Adipokines secreted by adipocytes can further serve as signaling molecules and modulate liver function.[36,37] Fat mass also increases the reservoir in which lipophilic drug molecules can store, further prolonging the terminal half-lives of these drugs. The combination of these host risk factors may explain the clinical observation that fatty liver diseases could predispose patients to drug-induced hepatotoxicity.[35]

Nutritional status: Many antioxidants are present in the diet (e.g., vitamin E, vitamin C, peptides for the synthesis of glutathione, trace metals, and minerals like zinc). However, poor nutrition or malabsorption leads to deficiency of these key vitamins and antioxidants. This may impair the antioxidative defense capacity, leading to drug-induced oxidative stress and lower threshold for DILI. In a preclinical study, a mere 1.6- and 2.1-fold increase in liver zinc content was associated with an increase in liver metallothionein between 50- and 200-fold.[38] Metallothionein is a key antioxidant protein *in vivo* capable of scavenging most common kinds of oxidative species.[39] It is therefore conceivable that a lack of sufficient dietary available zinc could compromise a patient's hepatic metallothionein levels and his or her antioxidant reserve capabilities in liver.

Host immune system and responses: Drug-induced hepatotoxicity is usually associated with the recruitment of immune cells to the liver accelerating an inflammatory response often initiated by activation of the Kupffer cells. As such, the host's immune system can either serve as an amplifier or attenuator of the initiating (but often silent and subclinical) liver insult. At present, the complex interplays between the drug insult and the host immune systems are still poorly understood. But some recent findings are worthy of highlighting here. In an *in vitro* co-culture study, a human hepatoma (Huh-7) and monocytic (THP-1) cell line were used to perform comparative studies on two peroxisome proliferator-activated receptor gamma (PPARgamma) agonists, troglitazone and rosiglitazone. In the cocultures, troglitazone caused an enhanced cytotoxicity as compared to single cultures of either cell line, whereas little cytotoxicity was seen after treatment with rosiglitazone.[40] In another *in vitro* study, drugs are administered to three liver cell types (primary human and rat hepatocytes, and the human hepatoma HepG2 cell line) across a landscape of inflammatory contexts containing lipopolysaccharide (LPS) and cytokines such as tumour necrosis factor (TNF), interferon (IFN) gamma, interleukin (IL) 1 alpha, and IL-6. Cytokines- enhanced toxicities for multiple idiosyncratic human hepatotoxicants (ranitidine, trovafloxacin, nefazodone, nimesulide, clarithromycin, and telithromycin), but not for their corresponding nonhepatotoxic comparator drugs (famotidine, levofloxacin, buspirone, and aspirin).[41] A larger compendium of drug–cytokine hepatotoxicity data demonstrated that drug hepatotoxicity signals were largely potentiated by TNF, IL-1 alpha, and LPS within the context of multicytokine mixes. Hence, it may be argued that the host immune responses including the inflammatory cytokine milieu may act as potentiator or at least modifier of the initial drug-induced (and often silent) hepatotoxic effects.

Interaction with other drugs: In addition to toxicokinetic drug–drug interactions as discussed earlier, drug interactions may alter the toxicodynamic response on tissues and organs. Amoxicillin–clavulanic acid is one of the most frequently implicated causes of drug-induced liver injury worldwide.[42] Recent preclinical studies suggested that additive or synergistic oxidative damage by both drugs in combination is a probable cause of such drug interaction, as the level of damage was directly correlated with the level of glutathione and lipid peroxidation, and further alleviated by pretreatment with an antioxidant.[43] Other mechanisms of toxicodynamic drug–drug interactions include additive or cooperative damage to the mammalian mitochondria,[44] synergistic potentiation of inflammatory pathways such as tumor necrosis factor-alpha (TNFa).[45]

Interaction with nutritional supplements and herbal extracts: Nutritional supplements and herbal extracts are widely used. However, their acute and long-term impact on liver homeostasis were not well characterized. In Asia, herbal compounds are the most common cause of drug-induced liver injury.[7] A worrisome trend that is now happening in the Western world is the continued use of herbal extracts with known potential to cause hepatotoxicity, due to a lack of regulatory supervision compared to medicinal products. For example, even though green tea has been safely consumed by humans over centuries, the addition of highly biological active extracts in much higher amount than naturally consumed from green tea have essentially violated the first principle of toxicology – "there is nothing that is not a poison, what differentiates poison from a medicine is its exposure." Recently, the use of oral green tea extracts (*Camellia sinensis*) has been implicated in acute hepatitis.[46] Poor quality control and contamination issues could also lead to DILI. For example, severe hepatotoxicity occurred following ingestion of Herbalife nutritional supplements contaminated with *Bacillus subtilis*.[47] Since nutritional supplement, often ingested in large quantities daily, has the potential to alter both liver's toxicokinetic and toxicodynamic responses (e.g., Reference 48), the use of these nutritional supplement should be more carefully documented in clinical DILI cases.

Genetics of receptors, transcription factors, enzymes, and transporters: The enterohepatic nuclear receptors such as farnesoid X receptor (FXR), pregnane X receptor (PXR), constitutive active/androstane receptor (CAR), liver X receptor (LXR), and estrogen receptors (ER) are important in maintaining signal transduction by endogenous chemicals including bile acids, bilirubin, cholesterol, carbohydrates, lipids, and estrogens. The regulation of these nuclear receptors is part of liver's adaptive response protecting it from toxicity caused by excessive accumulation of these endogenous signaling molecules. These receptors, once activated, in turn modulate the expression and activities of a variety of hepatic enzymes and transporters, to orchestrate what is known as "endobiotic homeostasis." For example, the activation of some of these receptors can protect the liver from cholestatic liver damage.[49] On the other hand, hepatotoxicity of estrogenic compounds are mediated by estrogen receptor.[50] In addition, transcription factors such as Stat-3, NFkB, PPARs, and Nrf2, are important modulators of toxicant responses. For example, nuclear factor erythroid 2-related factor (Nrf2) transactivates gene expression by way of the antioxidant response element (ARE), which controls the hepatic expression of glutamate–cysteine ligase subunits and glutathione (GSH) synthase, two rate-limiting enzymes in maintaining hepatic glutathione (GSH) levels. Intrahepatic GSH levels, in turn, protect the liver from oxidative damage. Polymorphisms in Nrf2 may increase hosts' susceptibility to toxicity.[51] Indeed, polymorphisms among nuclear hormone receptors, transcription factors, enzymes, and transporters are currently active areas of academic research. It is anticipated that some of these polymorphisms may lower a host's threshold for hepatotoxicity. For example, studies have found that glutathione-S-transferase m1 and t1 null genotypes increased susceptibility to idiosyncratic DILI.[52] In another example, a deletion allele of a nuclear factor kappa B1 (NFkB1) polymorphism could be associated with a higher risk of developing liver cirrhosis through an increase in inflammation.[53]

Given the complex interplay of both genetic and epigenetic factors that can affect toxicokinetic and toxicodynamic responses of human patients to drugs, is predicting a "safer" patient possible? To answer this complex question, let us examine the relative simple case of perhexiline, where the mechanism behind initially observed hepatotoxicity is well characterized, and genetic factors influencing the toxicokinetic responses are well understood.[54] Perhexiline was first introduced as an antiangina agent in the early 1970s. The hepatotoxicity of perhexiline is understood to be a direct side effect of its intended pharmacological action of inhibition of mitochondrial transport function. The rate-limiting enzyme in the clearance pathway of perhexiline is cytochrome P450 family member 2D6 (CYP2D6), one of the first and best characterized polymorphic CYP enzymes from a pharmacogenetic perspective. Individuals who are poor metabolizers of CYP2D6 are at risk for perhexiline-induced liver injury.[55] Perhexiline toxicity follows classic concentration–effect relationship, with both therapeutic (i.e., nontoxic) and toxic levels well characterized. Hence, this drug would be a perfect case to apply pharmacogenetics to predict who is a "safer" patient for perhexiline, correct? In reality, the answer is not that simple.[56] While CYP2D6 –/– homozygous subjects can be reliably predicted to be poor metabolizers of CYP2D6 (thus at higher risk for perhexiline toxicity),[57] heterozygous carriers show a large variability in CYP2D6 phenotype, and other alleles causing decreased or increased CYP2D6 activity made it even more difficult to correctly predict an individual's CYP2D6 phenotype. In addition, more than seventy different CYP2D6 alleles have been reported, which encode at least thirty-seven different proteins.[58] Furthermore, a wild type subject could be on another drug that is a potent inhibitor or inducer of CYP2D6; hence, a pharmacogenetics test based on DNA sequence alone could lead to both false positive and false negative predictions. As a result, even in the case of this single enzyme controlling the clearance of a well-understood drug, therapeutic drug monitoring (i.e., measuring the circulating level of perhexiline and its major metabolite) is still the best way (and indeed the only clinically mandated way) to minimize hepatotoxicity. In fact, when asked the question "how many drugs that were withdrawn from the market due to safety reasons in the past decade can be rescued by pharmacogenetic predictions," the answer is: none now, and probably none in the near future.[54] The reason are several: (a) Evidences supporting accurate genetic predictions per se are lacking; (b) multiple nongenetic factors play significant roles in drug toxicity; (c) if there already exists another drug in the same class with a wider therapeutic index, or such a drug is coming to market soon, the justification to resurrect an inferior drug with a narrow therapeutic index faces insurmountable challenges.

The predictive role of biomarkers should be discussed in light of predicting "safer" patients (i.e., is there a better human biomarker than the Hy's law applied currently?). The Hy's law, which basically states that elevated liver enzymes coupled with elevated bilirubin levels in a patient's blood is an ominous sign for liver injury, is a reasonably specific but imperfect biomarker for drugs capable of causing severe DILI. For example, Hy's law is too insensitive or too late for some drugs (as in the example of troglitazone),[59] while overly sensitive for other drugs (as in the case of statins used to treat hypercholesterolemia, or tacrine to treat the symptoms of Alzheimer's disease).[60] Much effort has been devoted to the identification of both more specific and sensitive biomarkers than Hy's law, and some promising research is underway.[61] However, none of these emerging biomarkers has been validated in large enough preclinical and clinical studies across enough hepatotoxic and nonhepatotoxic drugs to be able to replace or supplement Hy's law at the current time.

Given that there is a plethora of causal factors that can modulate a patient's pharmacokinetic and pharmacodynamic responses, and limitations in currently available biomarkers to predict DILI in advance of fulminant injury, identifying "safer" patients with sufficient clinical confidence may not be possible in the foreseeable future. Hence, an alternative approach must be sought to lessen the DILI burden on patient health and productivity of drug development. Identifying a safer drug with a sufficiently wide therapeutic index is a key strategy of this alternative approach. The remainder of this chapter will be devoted to the identification of safer drugs.

4.3 IDENTIFY SAFER DRUGS: RISK FACTORS OF A PROBLEMATIC DRUG

Identifying safer drugs, especially the ability to predict which drug is more likely to be safe in a realistic clinical setting with divergent pharmacokinetic and pharmacodynamic variables, is a key strategy toward minimizing DILI. As with identifying safer patients, this requires sound reasoning of both pharmacokinetic and pharmacodynamic factors for a given drug, combined with rational understanding of major mechanisms of DILI. Indeed, understanding toxicity mechanism(s) of early generation drugs can often lead to the identification of safer drugs in the next iteration of drug design and selection. This strategy, often termed "backup seeking" or "best-in-class mining," has been employed by many research-based pharmaceutical companies. In-depth understanding of the mechanisms of the original DILI, proper design of mechanism-based test systems, and improved prediction of human pharmacokinetic parameters are critical to the success of such strategy. Some of the leading DILI mechanisms frequently encountered in drug research and development include reactive metabolites, reactive oxygen species, mitochondrial damage, inhibition of biliary efflux transporters, and immunological mechanisms.

4.3.1 Multi-hit and multistep mechanisms of DILI: A contemporary understanding

The leading mechanisms of DILI have been reviewed previously and will not be repeated here (e.g., References 14, 62). Instead, a relatively recently rediscovered concept of the multi-hit hypothesis of DILI is worth highlighting. As its name implies, the multi-hit hypothesis of DILI states that a drug-induced liver injury is caused by more than one mechanism either operating in concert or in a sequential manner. The modern concept of multi-hit can be traced to the field of carcinogenesis[63–65]; however, Pessayre et al. is probably among the first to use it explicitly to describe the mechanism of steatohepatitis.[66] In this scenario, various combinations of obesity, diabetes, and hypertriglyceridemia, with insulin resistance as the common feature, cause hepatic steatosis (i.e., host factor as "first hit"). Next, drugs interfere with the normal role of mitochondria resulting in increased production of reactive oxygen species (i.e., ROS and mitochondrial damage as "second hit"). The combination of steatosis and ROS lead to lipid peroxidation, which can further trigger cytokine induction, Fas ligand induction, and fibrogenesis leading up to steatohepatitis.[66] This "2-hit" hypothesis has been used to explain steatohepatitis induced by drugs such as perhexline, amiodarone, and tamoxifen.[67]

The multi-hit hypothesis has also been used to explain the immunological potentiation of some idiosyncratic DILI. In this scenario, a preexisting inflammation in the host serves as "first hit." The drug treatment serves as "second hit." A good animal model for this scenario is rodents pretreated with bacterial membrane preparations such as lipopolysaccharide (LPS), followed by drug treatment. This model has been applied to explain idiosyncratic DILI caused by antibiotics, where the intended patients typically experience preexisting inflammation caused by bacterial infection.[68–71]

In a similar logic, the multi-hit hypothesis can be applied to rodent or other animal models with precompromised host liver functions, either by genetic knockout, knock-in, RNAi knockdown, high-fat diet, alcohol pretreatment, or other drug or chemical pretreatment. Indeed, this encompasses a large array of academic research and cannot be captured in detail by this chapter. The recent interest in the heterozygous superoxide dismutase 2 (SOD2) gene heterozygous knockout (Sod2+/-) mice serves as a good example. The Sod2+/- mice exhibit mild oxidant stress in mitochondria but remain clinically inconspicuous. Comparison of the hepatic mitochondrial proteome from Sod2+/- mice and wild type mice revealed that while both SOD 1 and 2 were down-regulated, other antioxidant enzymes and related proteins were up-regulated by less than twofold, indicative of some compensation by the antioxidant defense system.[72] Therefore, the Sod2+/- mice are suitable animal models for studying clinically silent mitochondrial abnormalities as the "first-hit" host factor. When drugs were administered to these mice as a "second-hit", uncompensated oxidative damage was observed for troglitazone[73] and nimesulide.[74] Collectively, these and other studies provide scientific merit that appropriate animal models for the intended human disease of a drug therapy should be considered and utilized in drug safety assessment.[75]

Acetaminophen provides another example of an analogous *in vitro* multi-hit process. Previously, most of the acetaminophen-induced hepatotoxicity research focused on the reactive metabolite of acetaminophen, which led to covalent protein modification (reviewed in Reference 76). Recently, it was realized that mitochondrial damage and oxidative stress may be the second-hit leading to acetaminophen-induced liver injury.[77,78] This is substantiated by animal studies where partial knockdown of SOD2 in rats, as well as mice heterozygous to SOD2 were more susceptible to acetaminophen-induced liver injury than wild type animals.[79,80]

The PPARgamma agonist, troglitazone, is probably another good example of the multi-hit hypothesis. Troglitazone was found to undergo bioactivation to form reactive metabolite and covalent glutathione adduct.[81] Troglitazone has also been shown to target mitochondria and induce mitochondria-mediated hepatocellular injury both *in vitro* and *in vivo*.[73] In addition, troglitazone and more potently, its sulfated metabolite, are inhibitors of bile salt efflux protein (BSEP), the rate-limiting protein in the transporting of bile salts from hepatocytes to bile.[82] Altered hepatobiliary transport may lead to intrahepatocyte accumulation of troglitazone.[83] The combination of these properties may contribute to a "perfect storm" in susceptible diabetic hosts, leading to ultimate liver injury.

In theory at least, the multi-hit hypothesis can explain the low incidence rate and idiosyncratic nature of DILI. Consider a simple scenario where a particular DILI requires three distinct steps or mechanisms, and the probability of each step occurring in a patient population is <10 percent (or less than 1 in 10 patients). Assuming that the probabilities of these three steps are completely independent of each other, then the overall probability of DILI becomes less than 1 in 1,000 patients. Since a combination of toxicity mechanisms may account for the final DILI, it is imperative that an integrated approach be developed and evaluated to better predict safer drugs. The remainder of this chapter will provide illustrations of such approaches.

4.3.2 Integrated approaches to predict DILI

When used blindly, any drug can generate an "adverse" signal in a single mechanism-based test at some exceedingly high concentration in an artificial system, be it *in vitro* or *in vivo*. Therefore, it is pivotal that an integrated system-based approach be applied to predict the likelihood of DILI. Such system-based approaches should, at a minimum, take into consideration the expected therapeutic drug exposure levels, the duration of the intended drug therapy, the existing standard of care, and their expected efficacy and side effects in patient populations. From a tactical perspective, any novel approaches (e.g., genomics, proteomics, metabolomics, cytomics, reactive intermediates, covalent binding assays, or any other assay model and technology) need to be validated by unbiased testing of a sufficient number of drugs that include both hepatotoxic and nonhepatotoxic ones in clinical usage.

The mixed experience with reactive metabolite formation and covalent binding is a good case in point. There is indeed a large body of academic research suggesting that the formation of reactive metabolite and covalent protein adducts may play a causal role in DILI (e.g., reviewed in References 82, 84). As a result, a panel of *in vitro* tests has been developed to interrogate this one type of mechanism only, and databases have been developed to capture the vast literature in this field.[85,86] These tests emphasized the formation of covalent protein adducts but omitted other mechanisms of DILI, namely, oxidative stress, mitochondrial damage, mechanisms relating to cholestasis and steatosis, and immune system functions.[87] It also often omitted exposure considerations, namely, the drug exposure levels at which "adverse signals" considered relevant *in vivo* were observed. Finally, and perhaps the most important of all, the false positive rate of such assay prediction is poorly characterized. Since not enough safe drugs were tested and characterized by this *in vitro* testing paradigm, the false positive rate was essentially unknown. However, we do know that drugs can be perfectly safe when used as prescribed but do form reactive metabolites *in vitro*. Such examples include meloxicam,[88] paroxetine,[89] pioglitazone,[90] and aripiprazole.[91]

In a more thorough and balanced evaluation of the *in vitro* reactive metabolite tests in both human liver microsomes and S9 fractions, Obach et al. found that a panel of safe drugs in the clinic can form as much reactive metabolites as those hepatotoxic drugs, even after corrections for drug clearance parameters.[92,93] Obviously, a more balanced and system-based approach to reactive metabolite formation and its clinical implications is needed hence forward.

Based on our current understanding, the major initiating events and/or mechanisms of DILI include (a) perturbation of mitochondrial functions leading up to mitochondrial damage; (b) oxidative stress caused either by reactive metabolite formation, glutathione depletion, and/or reactive oxygen species formation; (c) fatty liver (steatosis) especially in the presence of oxidative stress; (d) perturbation of bile salt efflux into bile, leading up to intrahepatic cholestasis. Since a single drug may perturb the liver in multiple ways, an ideal test system should be able to interrogate all of these mechanisms in an integrated fashion.

We therefore turned to whole cell–based systems, especially cellular models with a more *in vivo*-like balance of drug metabolizing enzymes and transporters, with bile canaliculi formation and bile/drug uptake and efflux functions. Amongst hepatocyte culture systems that are commonly employed for preclinical studies, primary human hepatocytes are considered the "gold standard" for evaluating drug metabolism, transport, and toxicity.[94,95] In comparison, primary rat hepatocytes, while more readily available and similarly capable of maintaining differentiated hepatic function in time scales of a few days *in vitro*, do not reproduce some aspects of human drug metabolism.[96,97] Immortalized and transformed human cell lines (e.g., HepG2 cells) are also frequently employed but have poor maintenance of liver-specific functions and are relatively insensitive to human hepatotoxicants in simple cytotoxicity assays.[98] Among the various ways of primary human hepatocyte cultures, the collagen substratum with either collagen or Matrigel overlay (i.e., the collage/collage- or collagen/Matrigel-sandwiched model) can maintain a balanced expression profile and function of hepatic metabolic enzymes and transporter functions.[99,100] In addition, adjacent hepatocytes cultured in this sandwiched model can form bile canaliculi and maintain both expression and function of hepatobiliary transporters, among which is the human BSEP, an important player in intrahepatic cholestasis.[101] Finally, sandwiched-cultured hepatocytes have been successfully used to predict *in vivo* biliary clearance of drugs, which is an important consideration for *in vitro* toxicological studies.[102]

To investigate a multitude of hepatic injury mechanisms simultaneously in this *in vitro* model, we employed live-cell imaging with a combination of biochemical probes: (a) Draq5, a lipophilic dye with strong affinity to DNA and lipids, was used to probe both nuclear morphology and lipid accumulation in the cytoplasm[103]; (b) TMRM, a mitochondrial membrane potential dye, was used to probe mitochondrial transition pore and membrane potential[104]; (c) CM-H2DCFDA, a redox-sensitive dye, was used to probe intracellular levels of reactive oxygen species[104]; (d) mBCl was used to probe intracellular concentrations of reduced glutathione[105]. Upon drug treatment, the media compartment of the treated cultures can be saved for drug-level analysis, metabonomic analysis, and protein biomarker and other soluble biomarker analysis (e.g., References 106, 107). The remaining hepatocytes can be stained briefly with these live-cell stains, and cells imaged under an automated epifluorescent microscope equipped with an environmental chamber (e.g., KineticScan from Cellomics). Normal human hepatocytes exhibited healthy mitochondria, ample glutathione, and lacking oxidative stress or lipid accumulation (Figure 4.1). Any discernable deviations from such healthy imaging patterns, either in singleton but often in combinations, provide putative "signals" of potential liver injury at the level of drugs tested in this *in vitro* system (Figure 4.1).

In order to correlate the observed "signals" or combination of "signals" observed in vitro to clinical outcome of DILI, esp. idiosyncratic DILI, two types of rationale are proposed as follows:

1. Toxicokinetic considerations

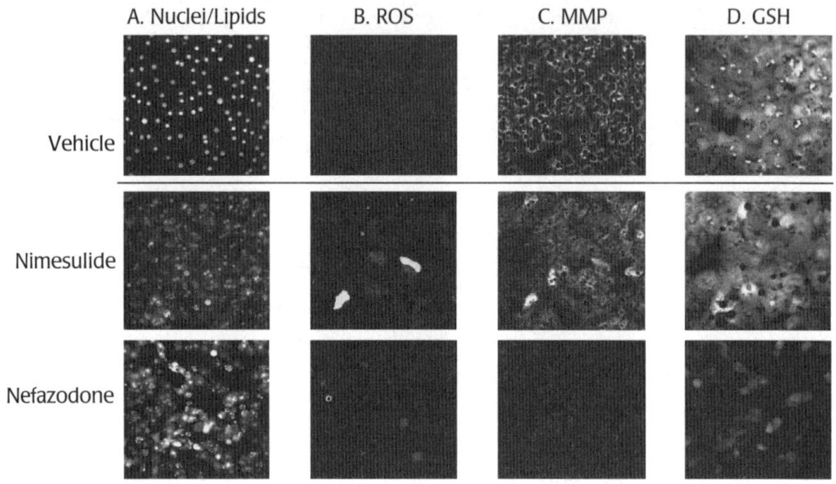

Figure 4-1: Example images from the human HIAT. Primary human hepatocytes were cultured in collagen/Matrigel-sandwiched configuration in 96-well plates to maintain hepatic uptake and efflux transporter function and inducible metabolic enzymes. Vehicle or drugs of interest were added for a period of 24 h at 100× C_{max} (oral single-dose therapeutic C_{max}). Nuclei and lipid accumulation, reactive oxygen species (ROS), mitochondrial membrane potential (MMP), and glutathione (GSH) were stained by live-cell probes, and their fluorescent images were captured and displayed in columns A, B, C, and D, respectively. Both nimesulide and nefazodone induced idiosyncratic DILI in susceptible patients after initial approval for marketing. HIAT identified ROS as a possible mechanism of nimesulide-induced hepatocyte injury. It also suggested that nefazodone could be another potential multi-hit example of DILI, as all four image patterns were significantly different from vehicle control. Reprinted with permission from Xu et al.[108]

One leading issue that needs to be addressed up front, is what concentration tested *in vitro* is relevant to the prediction of idiosyncratic DILI in a large patient population. According to the FDA, to detect a rare event occurring at 1 in 1,000 patients with 95 percent certainly requires at least 3,000 patients (i.e., known as the "rule of three"). Obviously, it is impractical to obtain primary human hepatocytes from 3,000 patients for an *in vitro* toxicological study, whether there is sufficient scientific merit or not. To increase the probability of detecting potential adverse signals in a relatively simple *in vitro* system, dose escalation is proposed. Since prediction of idiosyncratic DILI is essentially prediction of outlier response rather than an average response, a C_{max} scaling factor of 100× for potential liver effect of an oral drug is proposed based on these outlier considerations:

- 6× scaling factor to account for higher liver exposure for an oral drug (due to drug's first-pass metabolic or transporter processing by the liver)
- 6× scaling factor to account for pharmacokinetic variability in a large patient population (due to age, disease, drug interactions, genetic polymorphisms, etc.)
- 3× scaling factor to account for host sensitivity and toleration differences (i.e., a toxicodynamic safety margin)
- 6×6×3× ~ 100× (i.e., a cumulative 100× for predicting potential outlier response, as the three types of scaling factors above are independent)

Proof-of-concept studies have demonstrated that 100× C_{max} is a reasonable scaling factor to differentiate hepatotoxic (or positive) versus nontoxic (or negative) drugs.[108] For example, in a family of antidepressant drugs, nefazodone was consistently positive, whereas buspirone and fluoxetine remained negative, but all tested at 100× of their respective single-dose therapeutic C_{max}.[108]

2. Multi-hit considerations

Since the live-cell imaging approach allowed monitoring of multiple hepatotoxic mechanisms as described previously, it is possible to test the hypothesis that perhaps a combination of cellular imaging measurements can provide us with a more robust differentiators between positive versus negative drugs than a single mechanism alone. When a larger number of drugs ($N > 300$) were tested by the live-cell imaging technology, the imaging profiles were generated automatically by image analysis algorithms. These profiles were further subjected to standard machine learning algorithms. In one preferred approach, decision trees using the random forest model were generated using an iterative two-thirds of experimentally generated data for training, and the remaining one-third was used for testing. Each compound was scored by fraction of positive predictions it received from the trees on which it was not trained, to form an out-of-bag prediction score. The purpose of this is to mimic the real-world scenario of making novel predictions. The score obtained for each compound was then used to produce the receiver operator characteristic (ROC) curve. The ROC curve was generated by computing the true positive and false positive rate for all possible thresholds for any measured or derived value. The best predictions occur toward the top-left corner indicative of high true positive and low false positive rates (Figure 4.2). When more than 300 drugs including more than 100 generally considered safe drugs were tested, our hepatocyte imaging assay technology (HIAT) was able to predict clinical DILI with a 50–60 percent sensitivity and 95–100 percent specificity[108]. When combined with traditional animal testing, the integrated testing paradigm (Figure 4.3) can identify over 75 percent of hepatotoxic drugs in humans including the idiosyncratic ones with high specificity.

The imaging predictions from HIAT recapitulated previously recognized and reported mechanisms of DILI for some drugs, such as steatohepatitis mechanism of perhexiline and oxidative stress by nimesulide. In addition, HIAT substantiated the hypothesis that many positive drugs can initiate hepatotoxic signals in more than one mechanism (i.e., multi-hit hypothesis). For example, steatosis, oxidative stress, and mitochondrial damage may underlie DILI by nefazodone (Figure 4.1). The logic flow of such an integrated approach of investigating and predicting DILI, anchored on multiparametric cellular imaging, is depicted in Figure 4.3.

4.3.3 The need for more predictive human hepatotoxicity models

Obviously, even with a combinatorial assessment of hepatotoxic mechanisms, a relatively simple *in vitro* system cannot recapitulate all of the mechanisms

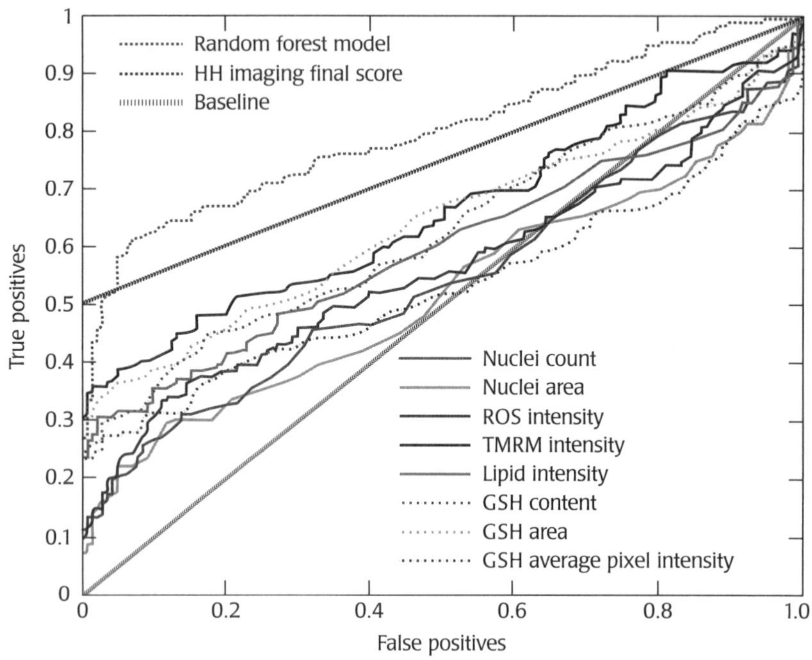

Figure 4-2: Receiver operator characteristic (ROC) curve showing the fractions of both true positives and false positives at any given threshold of HIAT imaging parameters. Automated image analysis and standard machine learning algorithms were applied to generate the ROC curves, for both individual imaging readout and various combined readouts. The best threshold yielded data point toward the top left of the curve (i.e., high true positive rate and low false positive rate). The combined human hepatocytes imaging score and random forest model produced the best balance of true positive (50–60 percent) and false positive rates (0–5 percent). Reprinted with permission from Xu et al.[108] *See color plates.*

behind every DILI. How to further improve assay sensitivity, while maintaining its high specificity, will be the focus of future research. There are several ways one may extend the research direction of HIAT.

1. Challenge the hepatocyte culture model with more complexity.

Traditionally, researchers have been using hepatocytes cultures in relatively simple culture media. Adding more complexity to the culture system, while mimicking important *in vivo* considerations relevant to hepatotoxicity, may be a fruitful research direction. Recently, we introduced immune complexity by adding proinflammatory cytokines. Indeed, In the presence of a mixture of proinflammatory cytokines, an additional seven out of forty-three idiosyncratic hepatotoxic drugs elicited more hepatotoxicity synergy, whereas zero out of thirty-six in nonhepatotoxic drugs did so.[41] Specifically, in primary human hepatocytes cultures, telithromycin and trovafloxacin both induced only one type of sublethal injury, mitochondrial membrane potential depletion. But they elicited markedly patterns of cytokine synergy as assayed by caspase 3/7 activity in the presence of cytokine mixture. Adding other cell types (e.g., Kupffer cells) to be cocultured with hepatocytes is another potentially promising area of research.[109]

Models, Measurements	**Approximate Fraction of Human DILI Identified**
Cell lines, simple readouts (e.g., ATP)	~10%
↓	
Primary hepatocytes, simple readouts (e.g., ATP)	~20%
↓	
Primary hepatocytes, imaging readouts (i.e., HIAT)	~50–60%
↓	
Combined animal testing, serum biomarkers and histopath	~50–60%
↓	
Combined clinical trials in phases 1–4, serum biomarkers	~90%

Figure 4-3: An integrated testing paradigm of applying various *in vitro* and *in vivo* models and measurements to predict human DILI. The approximate fractions of human DILI identified, including idiosyncratic DILI, were also listed. Since live-cell imaging based on primary human hepatocyte cultures (i.e., HIAT) identified 50–60 percent of human DILI in a short-term *in vitro* setting using 96-well plates, it forms the most cost-effective core of this testing paradigm. When *in vitro* HIAT based on human hepatocytes and *in vivo* preclinical predictions based on animal testing in rodents and nonrodents were combined, more than 75 percent of human DILI were identified. This was due to the fact that each model identified an overlapping subset of 50–60 percent of human DILI, and each had a low false positive rate.

2. Extend the drug-treatment time while maintaining the metabolic and transport functions of hepatocytes.

In our relatively simple *in vitro* system, we applied short-term treatment (24 h) and an aggressive dose-escalation schema to increase the probability of predicting idiosyncratic DILI in the clinic. If we can prolong the drug treatment while maintaining the metabolic and transport functions of hepatocytes, we can conceivably lower drug exposure levels and study hepatocytes' adaptive (or lack thereof) responses to subtoxic levels of drug treatment. Recently, several laboratories have independently published promising data to extend the lifetime of primary hepatocyte cultures while maintaining their differentiated functions. These culturing methodologies include micropatterned cocultures,[110] three-dimensional cultures with controlled flow,[111] and higher oxygen content.[112] The rational combination of these culturing approaches (medium composition, oxygen, co-culture with other cell types, and fluid flow) and their applications in subchronic hepatotoxicity testing should be a fruitful area of future research.

4.4 CONCLUDING REMARKS AND OUTLOOK

Hepatotoxicity is a major cause of drug development failures in both clinical trial and postapproval phases, thus posing a major challenge for the pharmaceutical industry. Furthermore, DILI poses a serious public health challenge as the leading cause of acute liver failure in the United States. Idiosyncratic drug hepatotoxicity – a hepatotoxicity subset that occurs in a very small fraction of human patients (<1 in 1,000), is poorly predicted by standard preclinical animal models or even clinical trials. The development and validation of novel preclinical tools that demonstrate successful identification of idiosyncratic drug hepatotoxicity is a paramount need for the industry and public at large.

As illustrated in this chapter, predicting DILI requires an integrated approach in pharmaceutical research and development. Even though predicting a safer patient remains a lofty goal, predicting safer drugs will provide a higher probability of success in the foreseeable future. The identification of DILI based on human hepatocyte models coupled with human pharmacokinetic data should form the core of an iterative preclinical–clinical toxicity assessment paradigm. Recent publications have demonstrated the utility of a physiologically relevant drug dosing limit of 100× C_{max} to obtain a low false positive rate, while maintaining a sufficient true positive rate. Future work will build on this *in vitro–in vivo* correlation and employ more sophisticated cell-culture methodologies from the bioengineering field. The ultimate goal of predicting safer drugs will require even more focused collaborations among toxicologists and pharmacologists, metabolism and pharmacokinetic scientists, and bioengineers and medicinal chemists.

REFERENCES

1. Ostapowicz G, Fontana RJ, Schiodt FV, et al. Results of a prospective study of acute liver failure at 17 tertiary care centers in the United States. *Ann Intern Med.* 2002;137(12):947–954.
2. Temple RJ. Hepatotoxicity through the years impact on the FDA. Paper presented at Drug-Induced Liver Toxicity, Silver Spring, Maryland; 2001.
3. Schuster D, Laggner C, Langer T. Why drugs fail – A study on side effects in new chemical entities. *Curr Pharm Des.* 2005;11(27):3545–3559.
4. Peters TS. Do preclinical testing strategies help predict human hepatotoxic potentials? *Toxicol Pathol.* 2005;33(1):146–154.
5. Zimmerman H. *Hepatotoxicity: The Adverse Effects of Drugs and Other Chemicals on the Liver.* 2nd ed. Philadelphia: Lippincott Williams & Wilkins; 1999.
6. Stricker BHC, ed. *Drug-Induced Hepatic Injury.* 2nd ed. Amsterdam: Elsevier; 1992.
7. Norris W, Paredes AH, Lewis JH. *Drug-induced liver injury in 2007. Curr Opin Gastroenterol.* 2008;24(3):287–297.
8. FDA. Drug-Induced Liver Injury: Premarketing Clinical Evaluation. http://www.fda.gov/downloads/Drugs/GuidanceComplianceRegulatoryInformation/Guidances/UCM174090.pdf. Accessed 2010.
9. EMEA. Non-clinical Guideline on Drug-Induced Hepatotoxicity. http://www.ema.europa.eu/pdfs/human/swp/15011506en.pdf. Accessed 2010.
10. Guo JJ, Wigle PR, Lammers K, Vu O. Comparison of potentially hepatotoxic drugs among major US drug compendia. *Res Social Adm Pharm.* 2005;1(3):460–479.
11. Fontana RJ, Watkins PB, Bonkovsky HL, et al. Drug-induced liver injury network (DILIN) prospective study: Rationale, design and conduct. *Drug Saf.* 2009;32(1):55–68.

12. Rochon J, Protiva P, Seeff LB, et al. Reliability of the Roussel Uclaf Causality Assessment Method for assessing causality in drug-induced liver injury. *Hepatology.* 2008;48(4):1175–1183.
13. DILIN. DILIN Overview. https://dilin.dcri.duke.edu/for-researchers/. Accessed 2010.
14. Kaplowitz N. Idiosyncratic drug hepatotoxicity. *Nat Rev Drug Discov.* 2005; 4(6):489–499.
15. Wynne H. Drug metabolism and ageing. *J Br Menopause Soc.* 2005;11(2):51–56.
16. Muhlberg W, Platt D. Age-dependent changes of the kidneys: Pharmacological implications. *Gerontology.* 1999;45(5):243–253.
17. Cusack BJ. Pharmacokinetics in older persons. *Am J Geriatr Pharmacother.* 2004;2(4):274–302.
18. Reis M, Aamo T, Spigset O, Ahlner J. Serum concentrations of antidepressant drugs in a naturalistic setting: Compilation based on a large therapeutic drug monitoring database. *Ther Drug Monit.* 2009;31(1):42–56.
19. Schwartz JB. The influence of sex on pharmacokinetics. *Clin Pharmacokinet.* 2003;42(2):107–121.
20. Feng B, Xu JJ, Bi YA, et al. Role of hepatic transporters in the disposition and hepatotoxicity of a HER2 tyrosine kinase inhibitor CP-724,714. *Toxicol Sci.* 2009;108(2):492–500.
21. Fukudo M, Yano I, Yoshimura A, et al. Impact of MDR1 and CYP3A5 on the oral clearance of tacrolimus and tacrolimus-related renal dysfunction in adult living-donor liver transplant patients. *Pharmacogenet Genomics.* 2008;18(5):413–423.
22. Fabbiani M, Di Giambenedetto S, Bracciale L, et al. Pharmacokinetic variability of antiretroviral drugs and correlation with virological outcome: 2 years of experience in routine clinical practice. *J Antimicrob Chemother.* 2009;64(1):109–117.
23. Reis M, Cherma MD, Carlsson B, Bengtsson F. Therapeutic drug monitoring of escitalopram in an outpatient setting. *Ther Drug Monit.* 2007;29(6):758–766.
24. Findling RL, Reed MD, Myers C, et al. Paroxetine pharmacokinetics in depressed children and adolescents. *J Am Acad Child Adolesc Psychiatry.* 1999;38(8): 952–959.
25. Ebbesen J, Buajordet I, Erikssen J, et al. Drug-related deaths in a department of internal medicine. *Arch Intern Med.* 2001;161(19):2317–2323.
26. Garcia-Compean D, Jaquez-Quintana JO, Maldonado-Garza H. Hepatogenous diabetes. Current views of an ancient problem. *Ann Hepatol.* 2009;8(1):13–20.
27. Wang T, Shankar K, Ronis MJ, Mehendale HM. Mechanisms and outcomes of drug- and toxicant-induced liver toxicity in diabetes. *Crit Rev Toxicol.* 2007;37(5):413–459.
28. Douglas RM, Haddad GG. Can O2 dysregulation induce premature aging? *Physiology (Bethesda).* 2008;23:333–349.
29. Pialoux V, Hanly PJ, Foster GE, et al. Effects of exposure to intermittent hypoxia on oxidative stress and acute hypoxic ventilatory response in humans. *Am J Respir Crit Care Med.* 2009;180(10):1002–1009.
30. Savransky V, Nanayakkara A, Vivero A, et al. Chronic intermittent hypoxia predisposes to liver injury. *Hepatology.* 2007;45(4):1007–1013.
31. Savransky V, Reinke C, Jun J, et al. Chronic intermittent hypoxia and acetaminophen induce synergistic liver injury in mice. *Exp Physiol.* 2009;94(2):228–239.
32. Dixit R, Boelsterli UA. Healthy animals and animal models of human disease(s) in safety assessment of human pharmaceuticals, including therapeutic antibodies. *Drug Discov Today.* 2007;12(7–8):336–342.
33. Wu D, Cederbaum AI. Oxidative stress and alcoholic liver disease. *Semin Liver Dis.* 2009;29(2):141–154.
34. Donthamsetty S, Bhave VS, Mitra MS, Latendresse JR, Mehendale HM. Nonalcoholic fatty liver sensitizes rats to carbon tetrachloride hepatotoxicity. *Hepatology.* 2007;45(2):391–403.

35. Tarantino G, Conca P, Basile V, et al. A prospective study of acute drug-induced liver injury in patients suffering from non-alcoholic fatty liver disease. *Hepatol Res.* 2007;37(6):410–415.
36. Musso G, Gambino R, Durazzo M, et al. Adipokines in NASH: Postprandial lipid metabolism as a link between adiponectin and liver disease. *Hepatology.* 2005;42(5):1175–1183.
37. Musso G, Gambino R, Pacini G, De Michieli F, Cassader M. Prolonged saturated fat-induced, glucose-dependent insulinotropic polypeptide elevation is associated with adipokine imbalance and liver injury in nonalcoholic steatohepatitis: Dysregulated enteroadipocyte axis as a novel feature of fatty liver. *Am J Clin Nutr.* 2009;89(2):558–567.
38. Liu J, Zhou ZX, Zhang W, Bell MW, Waalkes MP. Changes in hepatic gene expression in response to hepatoprotective levels of zinc. *Liver Int.* 2009;29(8):1222–1229.
39. Li X, Chen H, Epstein PN. Metallothionein protects islets from hypoxia and extends islet graft survival by scavenging most kinds of reactive oxygen species. *J Biol Chem.* 2004;279(1):765–771.
40. Edling Y, Sivertsson LK, Butura A, Ingelman-Sundberg M, Ek M. Increased sensitivity for troglitazone-induced cytotoxicity using a human in vitro co-culture model. *Toxicol In Vitro.* 2009;23(7):1387–1395.
41. Cosgrove BD, King BM, Hasan MA, et al. Synergistic drug-cytokine induction of hepatocellular death as an in vitro approach for the study of inflammation-associated idiosyncratic drug hepatotoxicity. *Toxicol Appl Pharmacol.* 2009;237(3):317–330.
42. Chang CY, Schiano TD. Review article: Drug hepatotoxicity. *Aliment Pharmacol Ther.* 2007;25(10):1135–1151.
43. El-Sherbiny GA, Taye A, Abdel-Raheem IT. Role of ursodeoxycholic acid in prevention of hepatotoxicity caused by amoxicillin-clavulanic acid in rats. *Ann Hepatol.* 2009;8(2):134–140.
44. Upreti VV, Eddington ND, Moon KH, Song BJ, Lee IJ. Drug interaction between ethanol and 3,4-methylenedioxymethamphetamine ("ecstasy"). *Toxicol Lett.* 2009;188(2):167–172.
45. Shaw PJ, Hopfensperger MJ, Ganey PE, Roth RA. Lipopolysaccharide and trovafloxacin coexposure in mice causes idiosyncrasy-like liver injury dependent on tumor necrosis factor-alpha. *Toxicol Sci.* Nov 2007;100(1):259–266.
46. Verhelst X, Burvenich P, Van Sassenbroeck D, Gabriel C, Lootens M, Baert D. Acute hepatitis after treatment for hair loss with oral green tea extracts (*Camellia sinensis*). *Acta Gastroenterol Belg.* 2009;72(2):262–264.
47. Stickel F, Droz S, Patsenker E, Bogli-Stuber K, Aebi B, Leib SL. Severe hepatotoxicity following ingestion of Herbalife nutritional supplements contaminated with *Bacillus subtilis*. *J Hepatol.* 2009;50(1):111–117.
48. Foti RS, Dickmann LJ, Davis JA, et al. Metabolism and related human risk factors for hepatic damage by usnic acid containing nutritional supplements. *Xenobiotica.* 2008;38(3):264–280.
49. Uppal H, Saini SP, Moschetta A, et al. Activation of LXRs prevents bile acid toxicity and cholestasis in female mice. *Hepatology.* 2007;45(2):422–432.
50. Yamamoto Y, Moore R, Hess HA, et al. Estrogen receptor alpha mediates 17alpha-ethynylestradiol causing hepatotoxicity. *J Biol Chem.* 2006;281(24):16625–16631.
51. Osburn WO, Kensler TW. Nrf2 signaling: An adaptive response pathway for protection against environmental toxic insults. *Mutat Res.* 2008;659(1–2):31–39.
52. Lucena MI, Andrade RJ, Martinez C, et al. Glutathione S-transferase m1 and t1 null genotypes increase susceptibility to idiosyncratic drug-induced liver injury. *Hepatology.* 2008;48(2):588–596.
53. Marcos M, Pastor I, Gonzalez-Sarmiento R, Laso FJ. A functional polymorphism of the NFKB1 gene increases the risk for alcoholic liver cirrhosis in patients with alcohol dependence. *Alcohol Clin Exp Res.* 2009;33(11):1857–1862.

54. Shah RR. Can pharmacogenetics help rescue drugs withdrawn from the market? *Pharmacogenomics*. 2006;7(6):889–908.
55. Gardiner SJ, Begg EJ. Pharmacogenetics, drug-metabolizing enzymes, and clinical practice. *Pharmacol Rev*. Sep 2006;58(3):521–590.
56. Gardiner SJ, Begg EJ. Pharmacogenetic testing for drug metabolizing enzymes: Is it happening in practice? *Pharmacogenet Genomics*. 2005;15(5):365–369.
57. Barclay ML, Sawyers SM, Begg EJ, et al. Correlation of CYP2D6 genotype with perhexiline phenotypic metabolizer status. *Pharmacogenetics*. 2003;13(10): 627–632.
58. Gaedigk A, Simon SD, Pearce RE, Bradford LD, Kennedy MJ, Leeder JS. The CYP2D6 activity score: Translating genotype information into a qualitative measure of phenotype. *Clin Pharmacol Ther*. 2008;83(2):234–242.
59. Lewis JH. 'Hy's law,' the 'Rezulin rule,' and other predictors of severe drug-induced hepatotoxicity: Putting risk-benefit into perspective. *Pharmacoepidemiol Drug Saf*. 2006;15(4):221–229.
60. Kaplowitz N. Rules and laws of drug hepatotoxicity. *Pharmacoepidemiol Drug Saf*. 2006;15(4):231–233.
61. Ozer J, Ratner M, Shaw M, Bailey W, Schomaker S. The current state of serum biomarkers of hepatotoxicity. *Toxicology*. 2008;245(3):194–205.
62. Lee WM. Drug-induced hepatotoxicity. *N Engl J Med*. 2003;349(5):474–485.
63. Armitage P, Doll R. A two-stage theory of carcinogenesis in relation to the age distribution of human cancer. *Br J Cancer*. 1957;11(2):161–169.
64. Emmelot P, Scherer E. Multi-hit kinetics of tumor formation, with special reference to experimental liver and human lung carcinogenesis and some general conclusions. *Cancer Res*. 1977;37(6):1702–1708.
65. Ashley DJ. The two "hit" and multiple "hit" theories of carcinogenesis. *Br J Cancer*. 1969;23(2):313–328.
66. Pessayre D, Berson A, Fromenty B, Mansouri A. Mitochondria in steatohepatitis. *Semin Liver Dis*. 2001;21(1):57–69.
67. Begriche K, Igoudjil A, Pessayre D, Fromenty B. Mitochondrial dysfunction in NASH: Causes, consequences and possible means to prevent it. *Mitochondrion*. 2006;6(1):1–28.
68. Zou W, Beggs KM, Sparkenbaugh EM, et al. Sulindac metabolism and synergy with tumor necrosis factor-alpha in a drug-inflammation interaction model of idiosyncratic liver injury. *J Pharmacol Exp Ther*. 2009;331(1):114–121.
69. Shaw PJ, Ganey PE, Roth RA. Trovafloxacin enhances the inflammatory response to a Gram-negative or a Gram-positive bacterial stimulus, resulting in neutrophil-dependent liver injury in mice. *J Pharmacol Exp Ther*. 2009;330(1):72–78.
70. Shaw PJ, Ditewig AC, Waring JF, et al. Coexposure of mice to trovafloxacin and lipopolysaccharide, a model of idiosyncratic hepatotoxicity, results in a unique gene expression profile and interferon gamma-dependent liver injury. *Toxicol Sci*. 2009;107(1):270–280.
71. Deng X, Liguori MJ, Sparkenbaugh EM, et al. Gene expression profiles in livers from diclofenac-treated rats reveal intestinal bacteria-dependent and -independent pathways associated with liver injury. *J Pharmacol Exp Ther*. 2008;327(3): 634–644.
72. Lee YH, Boelsterli UA, Lin Q, Chung MC. Proteomics profiling of hepatic mitochondria in heterozygous Sod2+/- mice, an animal model of discreet mitochondrial oxidative stress. *Proteomics*. 2008;8(3):555–568.
73. Lee YH, Chung MC, Lin Q, Boelsterli UA. Troglitazone-induced hepatic mitochondrial proteome expression dynamics in heterozygous Sod2(+/-) mice: Two-stage oxidative injury. *Toxicol Appl Pharmacol*. 2008;231(1):43–51.
74. Ong MM, Wang AS, Leow KY, Khoo YM, Boelsterli UA. Nimesulide-induced hepatic mitochondrial injury in heterozygous Sod2(+/-) mice. *Free Radic Biol Med*. 2006;40(3):420–429.

75. Boelsterli UA. Animal models of human disease in drug safety assessment. *J Toxicol Sci.* 2003;28(3):109–121.
76. James LP, Mayeux PR, Hinson JA. Acetaminophen-induced hepatotoxicity. *Drug Metab Dispos.* 2003;31(12):1499–1506.
77. Reid AB, Kurten RC, McCullough SS, Brock RW, Hinson JA. Mechanisms of acetaminophen-induced hepatotoxicity: Role of oxidative stress and mitochondrial permeability transition in freshly isolated mouse hepatocytes. *J Pharmacol Exp Ther.* 2005;312(2):509–516.
78. Hanawa N, Shinohara M, Saberi B, Gaarde WA, Han D, Kaplowitz N. Role of JNK translocation to mitochondria leading to inhibition of mitochondria bioenergetics in acetaminophen-induced liver injury. *J Biol Chem.* 2008;283(20):13565–13577.
79. Yoshikawa Y, Morita M, Hosomi H, et al. Knockdown of superoxide dismutase 2 enhances acetaminophen-induced hepatotoxicity in rat. *Toxicology.* 2009;264(1–2):89–95.
80. Fujimoto K, Kumagai K, Ito K, et al. Sensitivity of liver injury in heterozygous Sod2 knockout mice treated with troglitazone or acetaminophen. *Toxicol Pathol.* 2009;37(2):193–200.
81. Alvarez-Sanchez R, Montavon F, Hartung T, Pahler A. Thiazolidinedione bioactivation: A comparison of the bioactivation potentials of troglitazone, rosiglitazone, and pioglitazone using stable isotope-labeled analogues and liquid chromatography tandem mass spectrometry. *Chem Res Toxicol.* 2006;19(8):1106–1116.
82. Funk C, Pantze M, Jehle L, et al. Troglitazone-induced intrahepatic cholestasis by an interference with the hepatobiliary export of bile acids in male and female rats. Correlation with the gender difference in troglitazone sulfate formation and the inhibition of the canalicular bile salt export pump (Bsep) by troglitazone and troglitazone sulfate. *Toxicology.* 2001;167(1):83–98.
83. Lee JK, Marion T, Abe K, Lim C, Pollack GM, Brouwer KL. Hepatobiliary disposition of troglitazone and metabolites in rat and human sandwich-cultured hepatocytes: Use of Monte Carlo simulations to assess the impact of changes in biliary excretion on troglitazone sulfate accumulation. *J Pharmacol Exp Ther.* 2010:332(1):26–34.
84. Uetrecht J. Idiosyncratic drug reactions: Past, present, and future. *Chem Res Toxicol.* 2008;21(1):84–92.
85. Evans DC, Baillie TA. Minimizing the potential for metabolic activation as an integral part of drug design. *Curr Opin Drug Discov Devel.* 2005;8(1):44–50.
86. Hanzlik RP, Koen YM, Theertham B, Dong Y, Fang J. The reactive metabolite target protein database (TPDB) – A web-accessible resource. *BMC Bioinformatics.* 2007;8:95.
87. Antoine DJ, Williams DP, Park BK . Understanding the role of reactive metabolites in drug-induced hepatotoxicity: State of the science. *Expert Opin Drug Metab Toxicol.* 2008;4(11):1415–1427.
88. Obach RS, Kalgutkar AS, Ryder TF, Walker GS. In vitro metabolism and covalent binding of enol-carboxamide derivatives and anti-inflammatory agents sudoxicam and meloxicam: Insights into the hepatotoxicity of sudoxicam. *Chem Res Toxicol.* 2008;21(9):1890–1899.
89. Zhao SX, Dalvie DK, Kelly JM, et al. NADPH-dependent covalent binding of [3H] paroxetine to human liver microsomes and S-9 fractions: Identification of an electrophilic quinone metabolite of paroxetine. *Chem Res Toxicol.* 2007;20(11): 1649–1657.
90. Masubuchi Y. Metabolic and non-metabolic factors determining troglitazone hepatotoxicity: A review. *Drug Metab Pharmacokinet.* 2006;21(5):347–356.
91. Bauman JN, Frederick KS, Sawant A, et al. Comparison of the bioactivation potential of the antidepressant and hepatotoxin nefazodone with aripiprazole, a structural analog and marketed drug. *Drug Metab Dispos.* 2008;36(6):1016–1029.
92. Obach RS, Kalgutkar AS, Soglia JR, Zhao SX. Can in vitro metabolism-dependent covalent binding data in liver microsomes distinguish hepatotoxic from nonhepatotoxic drugs? An analysis of 18 drugs with consideration of intrinsic clearance and daily dose. *Chem Res Toxicol.* 2008;21(9):1814–1822.

93. Bauman JN, Kelly JM, Tripathy S, et al. Can in vitro metabolism-dependent covalent binding data distinguish hepatotoxic from nonhepatotoxic drugs? An analysis using human hepatocytes and liver S-9 fraction. *Chem Res Toxicol.* 2009;22(2):332–340.
94. LeCluyse EL, Alexandre E, Hamilton GA, et al. Isolation and culture of primary human hepatocytes. *Method Mol Biol.* 2005;290:207–229.
95. Hewitt NJ, Lechon MJ, Houston JB, et al. Primary hepatocytes: Current understanding of the regulation of metabolic enzymes and transporter proteins, and pharmaceutical practice for the use of hepatocytes in metabolism, enzyme induction, transporter, clearance, and hepatotoxicity studies. *Drug Metab Rev.* 2007;39(1):159–234.
96. Li AP. Human hepatocytes as an effective alternative experimental system for the evaluation of human drug properties: General concepts and assay procedures. *ALTEX.* 2008;25(1):33–42.
97. Li N, Bi YA, Duignan DB, Lai Y. Quantitative expression profile of hepatobiliary transporters in sandwich cultured rat and human hepatocytes. *Mol Pharm.* 2009;6(4):1180–1189.
98. Xu JJ, Diaz D, O'Brien PJ. Applications of cytotoxicity assays and pre-lethal mechanistic assays for assessment of human hepatotoxicity potential. *Chem Biol Interact.* 2004;150(1):115–128.
99. Schmelzer E, Acikgoez A, Fruhauf NR, et al. Biotransformation of cyclosporin in primary rat, porcine and human liver cell co-cultures. *Xenobiotica.* 2006;36(8):693–708.
100. Dong JQ, Smith PC. Glucuronidation and covalent protein binding of benoxaprofen and flunoxaprofen in sandwich-cultured rat and human hepatocytes. *Drug Metab Dispos.* 2009;37(12):2314–2322.
101. Kostrubsky SE, Strom SC, Kalgutkar AS, et al. Inhibition of hepatobiliary transport as a predictive method for clinical hepatotoxicity of nefazodone. *Toxicol Sci.* 2006;90(2):451–459.
102. Abe K, Bridges AS, Brouwer KL. Use of sandwich-cultured human hepatocytes to predict biliary clearance of angiotensin II receptor blockers and HMG-CoA reductase inhibitors. *Drug Metab Dispos.* 2009;37(3):447–452.
103. Smith PJ, Blunt N, Wiltshire M, et al. Characteristics of a novel deep red/infrared fluorescent cell-permeant DNA probe, DRAQ5, in intact human cells analyzed by flow cytometry, confocal and multiphoton microscopy. *Cytometry.* 2000;40(4):280–291.
104. Donato MT, Martinez-Romero A, Jimenez N, et al. Cytometric analysis for drug-induced steatosis in HepG2 cells. *Chem Biol Interact.* 2009;181(3):417–423.
105. Stevenson D, Wokosin D, Girkin J, Grant MH. Measurement of the intracellular distribution of reduced glutathione in cultured rat hepatocytes using monochlorobimane and confocal laser scanning microscopy. *Toxicol In Vitro.* 2002;16(5):609–619.
106. Dambach DM, Andrews BA, Moulin F. New technologies and screening strategies for hepatotoxicity: Use of in vitro models. *Toxicol Pathol.* 2005;33(1):17–26.
107. Gao J, Ann Garulacan L, Storm SM, et al. Identification of in vitro protein biomarkers of idiosyncratic liver toxicity. *Toxicol In Vitro.* 2004;18(4):533–541.
108. Xu JJ, Henstock PV, Dunn MC, Smith AR, Chabot JR, de Graaf D. Cellular imaging predictions of clinical drug-induced liver injury. *Toxicol Sci.* 2008;105(1):97–105.
109. Tukov FF, Maddox JF, Amacher DE, Bobrowski WF, Roth RA, Ganey PE. Modeling inflammation-drug interactions in vitro: A rat Kupffer cell-hepatocyte coculture system. *Toxicol In Vitro.* 2006;20(8):1488–1499.
110. Khetani SR, Bhatia SN. Microscale culture of human liver cells for drug development. *Nat Biotechnol.* 2008;26(1):120–126.
111. Sivaraman A, Leach JK, Townsend S, et al. A microscale in vitro physiological model of the liver: Predictive screens for drug metabolism and enzyme induction. *Curr Drug Metab.* 2005;6(6):569–591.
112. Kidambi S, Yarmush RS, Novik E, Chao P, Yarmush ML, Nahmias Y. Oxygen-mediated enhancement of primary hepatocyte metabolism, functional polarization, gene expression, and drug clearance. *Proc Natl Acad Sci USA.* 2009;106(37):15714–15719.

5 *In vitro* evaluation of metabolic drug–drug interactions

Albert P. Li

5.1 INTRODUCTION

Simultaneous coadministration of multiple drugs to a patient is a highly probable event. A patient may be coadministered multiple drugs for the treatment of a single disease (e.g., cancer, HIV infection) or for the treatment of multiple diseases or disease symptoms (e.g., type 2 diabetes, cholesterol elevation, high blood pressure). It is now known that drug–drug interactions may have serious, sometimes fatal consequences. Serious drug–drug interactions have led to the necessity of a drug manufacturer to withdraw or limit the use of marketed drugs. Examples of fatal drug–drug interactions are shown in Table 5.1. As illustrated by the examples in Table 5.1, a major mechanism of adverse drug–drug interactions is the inhibition of the metabolism of a drug by a coadministered drug, thereby elevating the systemic burden of the affected drug to a toxic level.

Besides toxicity, loss of efficacy can also result from drug–drug interactions. In this case, the metabolic clearance of a drug is accelerated due to the inducing effects of a coadministered drug on drug metabolism. A well-known example is the occurrence of breakthrough bleeding and contraceptive failures of women taking oral contraceptives who were coadministered with the enzyme inducer rifampin[1]. Examples of drug–drug interactions leading to the loss of efficacy are shown in Table 5.2.

Estimation of drug–drug interaction potential is therefore an essential element of drug development. Screening for drug–drug interaction in early phases of drug development allows the avoidance of the development of drug candidates with high potential for adverse drug interactions. Estimation of drug–drug interaction potential is a regulatory requirement – it is required for New Drug Applications (NDA) to the U.S. Food and Drug Administration (FDA).[2] In this chapter, the scientific principles, technologies, and experimental approaches for the preclinical evaluation of drug–drug interactions are reviewed.

Table 5-1. Drugs that have been withdrawn from the market due to fatal interactions with coadministered drugs

Drug–drug interaction	Mechanism of interactions	Reference
Terfenadine and ketoconazole interaction, leading to fatal arrhythmia (torsade de pointes). Terfenadine was withdrawn from the market in January 1997 and replaced by a safer alternative drug (fexofenadine), which is the active metabolite of terfenadine.	Terfenadine is metabolized mainly by CYP3A4 and has been found to interact with CYP3A4 inhibitors (e.g., ketoconazole) leading to elevation of plasma terfenadine level to cardiotoxic levels.	44–46; www.fda.gov/bbs/topics/answers/ans00853.html
Mibefradil interaction with multiple drugs, leading to serious adverse effects. Mibefradil interactions with statins has led to rhabdomyolysis. Mibefradil was withdrawn from the market in June 1998, less than a year after it was introduced to the market in August 1997.	Mibefradil is a potent CYP3A4 inhibitor known to elevate the plasma levels of over 25 coadministered drugs to toxic levels. Statins, especially simvastatin and cerivastatin, are known to cause rhabdomyolysis.	47; www.fda.gov/bbs/topics/answers/ans00876.html
Sorivudine and 5-fluorouracil (5-FU) interaction, leading to severe or fatal gastrointestinal and bone marrow toxicities. Soruvidine was withdrawn from the market in 1993.	Sorivudine inhibits dihydropyrimidine dehydrogenase, an enzyme pathway responsible for fluoropyrimidine metabolism.	48
Gemfibrozil and cerivastatin interaction leads to rhabdimyolysis. Cerivastatin was withdrawn from the market in August 2001.	Inhibition of cerivastatin metabolism by gemfibrozil, apparently due to CYP2C8 inhibitory effects of gemfibrozil.	49; www.fda.gov/medwatch/safety/2001/Baycol2.html

5.1.1 Mechanisms of adverse drug–drug interactions

Adverse effects in a patient due to coadministration of multiple drugs can be caused by pharmacological or pharmacokinetic drug–drug interactions defined as follows:

Pharmacological interactions are adverse effects that occur due to combined pharmacological activities, leading to exaggerated pharmacological effects. An example of pharmacological interactions is serious, sometimes fatal drop in blood pressure due to coadministration of nitroglycerin and sildenafil.[3]

Pharmacokinetic interactions are adverse effects that occur due to altered body burden of a drug as a result of a coadministered drug that can occur because of the ability of one drug to alter the absorption, distribution, metabolism, and excretion (ADME properties) of the coadministered drug. Of the ADME properties, drug metabolism represents the most important and prevalent mechanism for pharmacokinetic interactions.

Table 5-2. Drug–drug interactions leading to loss of efficacy

Drug–drug interaction	Mechanism	Reference
Oral contraceptive–rifampin interactions, leading to the breakthrough bleeding and contraceptive failure	Rifampin accelerates the metabolism of the estrogenic component (e.g., 17 alpha-ethinylestradiol) of oral contraceptives via induction of the metabolizing enzymes (CYP3A4 and estrogen sulphotransferases).	1, 50
Cyclosporin and rifampin interaction, leading to rejection of transplanted organs	Rifampin induces CYP3A, leading to accelerated metabolic clearance of cyclosporine to nonimmunosuppressive level.	51
St. John's wort (SJW) interactions with prescribed drugs, leading to loss of efficacy	SJW (*Hypericum perforatum*) is an herbal medicine found to contain ingredients that can induce CYP3A4, CYP2C9, CYP1A2, and various transporters, leading to clinically observed accelerated metabolic clearance and/or loss of efficacy of a large number of drugs including warfarin, phenprocoumon, cyclosporine, HIV protease inhibitors, theophylline, digoxin, and oral contraceptives. The incidents with SJW illustrate the importance of the evaluation of potential drug–drug interaction potential of herbal medicines.	52

5.1.2 Drug metabolism

All drugs administered to a patient are subject to biotransformation. Orally administered drugs are first subjected to metabolism by the intestinal epithelium and, upon absorption into the portal circulation, metabolized by the liver before entering the systemic circulation. While multiple tissues have certain degree of biotransformation capacity, it is generally accepted that hepatic metabolism represent the most important aspect of drug metabolism.

Drug metabolism can be classified into two major categories.

Phase I oxidation

Phase I oxidation generally is described as the addition of an oxygen atom (e.g., as an hydroxyl moiety) to the parent molecule. Phase I oxidation is carried out by multiple enzyme pathways, including the various isoforms of the cytochrome P450 (CYP) family and the non-P450 biotransformation enzymes such as flavin-containing monooxygenase (FMO) and monamine oxidase (MAO).

Phase II conjugation

Phase II conjugation represents enzyme reactions that lead to the addition of a highly water soluble molecule to the chemical that is being metabolized, leading to highly water soluble "conjugates" to allow efficient excretion. Examples of Phase II enzymes are UDP-glucuronyl transferase (UGT), sulfotransferase (ST),

Table 5-3. Major pathways for drug metabolism, enzymes, subcellular locations, and *in vitro* experimental system containing the enzymes

Major classification	Enzyme	Subcellular location	Representative *in vitro* experimental system
Phase I oxidation	Cytochrome P450 mixed function monooxygenases	Endoplasmic reticulum	Microsomes; S9; hepatocytes
	Monoamine oxidase	Mitochondria	Hepatocytes
	Flavin-containing monooxygenase	Endoplasmic reticulum	Microsomes; S9; hepatocytes
	Alcohol/aldehyde dehydrogenase	Cytosol	S9; hepatocytes
	Esterases	Cytosol and endoplasmic reticulum	Microsomes; S9; hepatocytes
Phase II conjugation	UDP-dependent glucuronyl transferase	Endoplasmic reticulum	Microsomes; S9; hepatocytes
	Phenol sulfotransferases; estrogen sulfotransferase	Cytosol	S9; hepatocytes
	N-acetyl transferase	Endoplasmic reticulum	Microsomes; S9; hepatocytes
	Soluble glutathione-S-transferases (GST)	Cytosol	S9; hepatocytes
	Membrane-bound GST	Endoplasmic retuculum	Microsomes; S9; hepatocytes

Note: These enzymes are grouped into Phase I oxidation and Phase II conjugation enzymes, although it is now believed that such classification may not be possible for all drug-metabolizing enzymes. Representative *in vitro* experimental systems containing these enzymes are shown to guide the selection of the most relevant approach for specific enzyme pathways. It is apparent that intact hepatocytes represent the most complete *in vitro* system for drug metabolism studies as they contain all the key hepatic drug-metabolizing enzyme pathways.

and glutathione-S-transferase (GST). Conjugation reactions often occur with the hydroxyl moiety of the parent structure or with the oxidative metabolites.

The major drug-metabolizing enzymes and subcellular locations are summarized in Table 5.3.

5.1.3 CYP isoforms

Cytochrome P450-dependent monooxygenases are the drug-metabolizing enzymes often involved in metabolic drug–drug interactions. The CYP family is represented by a large number of isoforms, with each having selectivity for certain chemical structures. The major hepatic human CYP isoforms are CYP1A2, CYP2A6, CYP2B6, CYP2C8, CYP2C9, CYP2C19, CYP2D6, CYP2E1, and CYP3A4. Of these isoforms, the CYP3A isoforms are the most important in drug metabolism. CYP3A isoforms (CYP3A4 and CYP3A5) collectively represent the most abundant hepatic CYP isoforms (approximately 26 percent), followed by CYP2C

Table 5-4. Major human P450 isoforms involved in drug metabolism

CYP isoform	Substrate	Inhibitor	Inducer
CYP1A2	Phenytoin	Furafylline	Omeprazole
CYP2A6	Coumarin	Tranylcypromine	Rifampin
CYP2B6	Bupropion	Ticlopidine	Rifampin
CYP2C8	Taxol	Quercetin	Rifampin
CYP2C9	Tolbutamide	Sulfaphenazole	Rifampin
CYP2C19	*s*-Mephenytoin	Omeprazole	Rifampin
CYP2D6	Dextromethorphan	Quinidine	none
CYP2E1	Chlorzoxazone	Diethyldithiocarbamate	Ethanol
CYP3A4	Testosterone	Ketoconazole	Rifampin

Note: The individual isoforms and examples of isoform-specific substrates, inhibitors, and inducers are shown.

isoforms (approximately 17 percent). In terms of the isoforms involved in drug metabolism, CYP3 isoforms are known to be involved in the metabolism of the most number of drugs (approximately 33 percent), followed by CYP2C isoforms (approximately 25 percent).[4]

P450 isoforms are known to have specific substrates, inhibitors, and inducers (Table 5.4).

5.1.4 Human *in vitro* experimental systems for drug metabolism

Substantial species–species differences occur in drug metabolism pathways, especially for CYP isoforms. Because of the species–species differences, human *in vitro* hepatic experimental systems rather than nonhuman animals are viewed as the most relevant to the evaluation of xenobiotic properties, including human drug metabolism and metabolism-based drug–drug interactions.[5–8] The following are the commonly used *in vitro* experimental systems for the evaluation of metabolism-based drug–drug interactions.

Hepatocytes

Hepatocytes are the parenchymal cells of the liver responsible for hepatic biotransformation of xenobiotics. Isolated hepatocytes contain virtually all the major hepatic drug-metabolizing enzyme pathways and cofactors. Further, unlike cell fractions such as liver postmitochondrial supernatant or microsomes, the drug-metabolizing enzymes and cofactors in the hepatocytes are undisrupted and present at physiological concentrations. Freshly isolated hepatocytes and cryopreserved hepatocytes are generally believed to represent the most complete *in vitro* system for the evaluation of hepatic drug metabolism.[9,10]

In the past, the use of human hepatocytes was severely limited by their availability, as studies would be performed only if human livers were available for hepatocyte isolation. Further, hepatocyte isolation from human livers is not a technology available to most drug metabolism laboratories. This limitation has

Table 5-5. Viability and plateability (ability of hepatocytes to be cultured as monolayer cultures) of the various lots of cryopreserved human hepatocytes[a]

Lot #	Yield (cells/vial)	Viability (trypan blue)	Plating	Confluency (%)
HU4003	**4.5×10^6**	**86%**	**YES**	**100**
HU4001	6.0×10^6	80%	NO	20
HU4004	6.0×10^6	80%	NO	30
HU4000	**7.2×10^6**	**93%**	**YES**	**100**
HU4013	**7.3×10^6**	**92%**	**YES**	**75**
HU4016	**6.2×10^6**	**81%**	**YES**	**100**
HU4021	**5.4×10^6**	**89%**	**YES**	**70**
HU4022	**5.5×10^6**	**91%**	**YES**	**80**
HU4026	5.85×10^6	91%	NO	10
HU4027	5.9×10^6	92%	NO	30
HU4028	**3.2×10^6**	**83%**	**YES**	**50**
HU4023	2.1×10^6	89%	NO	20
HU4029	**6.0×10^6**	**90%**	**YES**	**80**

[a] Hepatocytes manufactured by APSciences, Inc. in partnership with CellzDirect-Life Technologies.

been overcome in the past decade due to the advancements in the procurement of human livers for research and the commercial availability of isolated human hepatocytes. The application of human hepatocytes in drug metabolism studies is also greatly aided by the successful cryopreservation of human hepatocytes to retain drug metabolism activities.[10,11] Recently, the usefulness of cryopreserved human hepatocytes is further extended through the development of technologies to cryopreserve human hepatocytes to retain their ability to be cultured as attached cultures ("plateable" cryopreserved hepatocytes), which can be used for longer-term studies such as enzyme induction studies.[10] Examples of the viability and plateability of cryopreserved human hepatocytes prepared in our laboratory are shown in Table 5.5.

Liver postmitochondrial supernatant

Liver postmitrochondrial supernatant (PMS) is prepared by first homogenizing the liver followed by centrifuging the homogenate at a speed of either 9,000 × g or 10,000 × g to generate the supernatants S9 or S10, respectively. Liver PMS contains both cytosolic and microsomal drug-metabolizing enzymes but lacks mitochondrial enzymes. Via the use of appropriate cofactors, PMS can be used to evaluate drug metabolism by both microsomal and cytosolic drug metabolizing enzymes.

Liver microsomes

Liver microsomes are the 100,000 × g pellet from the PMS. Microsome preparation procedures in general involve the homogenization of the liver, dilution of the homogenate with approximately four volumes of sample weight with a buffer[12] (e.g., 0.1 *M* Tris-HCl, pH 7.4, 0.1 *M* KCl, 1.0 m*M* EDTA, 1.0 m*M* PMSF)

Table 5-6. A comparison of the key *in vitro* drug-metabolizing experimental systems in their contents of the major drug-metabolizing enzymes)

In vitro system	P450	MAO	UGT	ST	GST
Liver microsomes	+	–	+[a]	–	+[b]
S9	+	–	+[a]	+[a]	+
Liver cytosol	–	–	–[a]	+[a]	+[c]
Hepatocytes	+	+	+	+	+

Notes: S9, liver postmitochondrial supernatant; P450, cytochrome P450 isoforms; MAO, monoamine oxidase; UGT, UDP-glucuronsyl transferase; ST, sulfotransferase; GST, glutathione-S-transerase.

[a] Activity of this drug-metabolizing enzyme requires the addition of specific cofactors, for instance, UDP-glucuronic acid (UDPGA) for UGT activity, and 3′-phosphoadenosine 5′-phosphosulfate (PAPS) for ST activity.

[b] Membrane-bound GST but not the soluble GST are found in the microsomes.

[c] Soluble GST but not membrane-bound GST are found in the cytosol.

followed by centrifugation at 9,000–14,000 × g to remove nonmicrosomal membranes, and then at 100,000–138,000 × g to pellet the microsomes.[13] Microsomes contain the smooth endoplasmic reticulum, which is the site of the major phase I oxidation pathway, the P450 isoforms, esterases, as well as a major conjugating pathway, UGT. Liver microsomes are routinely used for the evaluation of P450 and UGT related drug metabolism.

Recombinant P450 isoforms

Recombinant P450 isoforms (rCYP) are microsomes derived from organisms transfected with genes for individual human P450 isoforms (e.g., bacteria, yeast, mammalian cells[14–16]); therefore, they contain only one specific human isoform. The major human P450 isoforms involved in drug metabolism are available commercially as rCYP. This experimental system is widely used to evaluate the drug-metabolizing activities of individual P450 isoforms.[15]

Cytosol

The supernatant after the 100,000 × g centrifugation for microsome preparation is the cytosol that is practically devoid of all membrane-associated enzymes. N-acetyl transferases, sulfotransferases, and dehydrogenases are examples of cytosolic enzymes. Although drug–drug interaction studies are mainly studied using liver microsomes, there are cases of drug–drug interactions involving phase II pathways that can be studied using liver cytosol.[17]

The different *in vitro* experimental systems in their drug-metabolizing enzymes are compared in Table 5.6.

5.2 MECHANISMS OF METABOLIC DRUG–DRUG INTERACTIONS

Metabolic drug–drug interaction results from the alteration of the metabolic clearance of one drug by a coadministered drug. There are two major pathways of metabolic drug–drug interactions.

Inhibitory drug–drug interaction

When one drug inhibits the drug metabolism enzyme responsible for the metabolism of a coadministered drug, the result is a decreased metabolic clearance of the affected drug, resulting in a higher than desired systemic burden. For drugs with a narrow therapeutic index, this may lead to serious toxicological concerns. Most fatal drug–drug interactions are due to inhibitory drug–drug interactions.

Inductive drug–drug interactions

Drug–drug interactions can also be a result of the acceleration of the metabolism of a drug by a coadministered drug. Acceleration of metabolism is usually due to the induction of the gene expression, leading to higher rates of protein synthesis and therefore higher cellular content of the induced drug-metabolizing enzyme and a higher rate of metabolism of the substrates of the induced enzyme. Inductive drug–drug interactions can lead to a higher metabolic clearance of the affected drug, leading to a decrease in plasma concentration and loss of efficacy. Inductive drug–drug interactions can also lead to a higher systemic burden of metabolites, which, if toxic, may lead to safety concerns.

5.2.1 Mechanism-based approach for the evaluation of drug–drug interaction potential

Due to the realization that it is physically impossible to evaluate empirically the possible interaction between one drug and all marketed drugs, and that most drug-metabolizing enzyme pathways are well defined, a mechanism-based approach is used for the evaluation of drug–drug interaction potential of a new drug or drug candidate.[6,7,18] This mechanistic-based approach is now also recommended by the U.S. FDA (www.fda.gov/cber/gdlns/interactstud.htm). The approach consists of the following major studies.

Metabolic phenotyping

Metabolic phenotyping is defined as the identification of the major pathways involved in the metabolism of the drug in question. The reasoning is that if the pathways are known, then one can estimate potential interaction of the drug in question with known inhibitors or inducers of the pathway.

Evaluation of inhibitory potential for drug-metabolizing enzymes

The ability of the drug in question to inhibit the activities of known pathways for drug metabolism is evaluated. If a drug is an inhibitor of a drug-metabolizing enzyme pathway, it will have the potential to cause inhibitory drug interactions with coadministered drugs that are substrates of the inhibited pathway.

Induction potential for drug-metabolizing enzymes

The ability of the drug in question to induce drug-metabolizing enzyme activities is evaluated. If the drug in question is an inducer of a specific pathway, it will have the potential to cause inductive drug interactions with coadministered drugs that are substrates of the induced pathway.

5.2.2 Experimental approaches for the *in vitro* evaluation of drug–drug interaction potential

Because of the known species–species differences in drug metabolism, it is now believed that *in vitro*, human-based, experimental systems are more appropriate than nonhuman animal models for the evaluation of drug–drug interactions. *In vitro* positive findings are usually confirmed with *in vivo* clinical studies. The typical preclinical studies for drug–drug interactions follow.

Study 1: Metabolic phenotyping 1 – metabolite identification

The objective of this study is to identify the major metabolites of the drug in question. For this study, the drug in question is incubated with an appropriate *in vitro* metabolic system to allow the formation of metabolites. Metabolites are then identified using analytical chemical approaches. The *in vitro* experimental system of choice is human hepatocytes, with high-performance liquid chromatography/mass spectrometry (HPLC/MS) or tandem mass spectrometry (HPLC/MS/MS) as the most convenient analytical tool to identify the metabolites.

The metabolites are generally identified as metabolites of Phase I oxidation or Phase II conjugation. If Phase I oxidation is concluded as the major pathway for the oxidative metabolism of the drug, a second study will be performed to evaluate which of the several oxidative pathways are involved. Phase II conjugation pathways can be generally recognized by the identity of the metabolite, and subsequent experiments to further identify the pathways may not be necessary. For instance, if the metabolite is a glucuronide, UGT can be identified as the enzyme involved.

A typical experimental design is as follows:

- *In vitro* system: Cryopreserved human hepatocytes pooled from two donors (male, female)
- Three drug concentrations: 1, 10, and 100 μ*M*
- Hepatocyte concentration: 0.5 to 1.0 million hepatocytes per mL
- Three incubation times: 1, 2, and 4 h (suspension culture); up to 24 h (attached culture)
- Incubation in 24-well plates at 37°C
- Organic solvent (e.g., acetonitrile) to terminate reaction and to extract medium and intracellular metabolites
- Stored frozen until analysis
- Analytical chemistry: HPLC/MS/MS
- Quantification of disappearance of parent chemical in all samples
- Identification of metabolites from 100 μ*M* samples
- Detection of metabolites in 1 and 10 μ*M* samples

Table 5-7. Experimental conditions to reduce the activity of the major drug-metabolizing enzyme pathways using the *in vitro* experimental systems for drug metabolism

In vitro system[a]	Condition	Inactivated pathway(s)[b]
Microsomes	NADH omission	PCYP, FMO
Microsomes or hepatocytes	1-aminobenzotriazole treatment	PCYP
Microsomes	Heat (45°C) inactivation	FMO
S9	Pargyline treatment	MAO

Source: Table adapted from http://www.fda.gov/cder/guidance/6695dft.pdf.
[a] Microsomes, liver microsomes; S9, postmitochondrial supernatant.
[b] PCYP, P450 isoforms; FMO, flavin-containing monooxygenases; MAO, monoamine oxidase.

Study 2: Metabolic phenotyping 2 – identification of major metabolic pathways

If oxidative metabolites are found to be the major metabolites, it is necessary to evaluate which major oxidative pathways are involved in the metabolism. This is performed via the use of liver microsomes and experimental conditions that would inhibit a specific pathway. The major pathways and experimental conditions are shown in Table 5.7.

As P450 pathways are considered the most important for metabolic drug–drug interactions, the study with the general P450 inhibitor, 1-aminobenzotriazole (ABT), is one that should be performed. ABT is known to inhibit all eight human P450 isoforms involved in drug metabolism.[19] Inhibition of metabolism of a test article by ABT would indicate that the test article is metabolized by the P450 pathway. A typical study with ABT is as follows:

- Human liver microsomes (0.5 mg protein/mL)
- Experiment 1: Evaluation of experimental conditions for the accurate quantification of metabolic clearance
- Incubation with three concentrations of test article (e.g. 0.1, 1, and 10 μ*M*) and three incubation times (e.g., 15, 30, and 60 min)
- Quantification of test article disappearance
- Experiment 2: Reaction phenotyping
- Incubation with 1 concentration of the test article at 1 incubation time (chosen from Experiment 1) in the presence and absence of three concentrations of ABT (100, 200, and 500 μ*M*)
- Quantification of test article disappearance and evaluate the effects of ABT treatment

Study 3: Metabolic phenotyping 3 – identification of P450 isoform pathways (P450 phenotyping)

Observation of ABT inhibition of the metabolism of the drug or drug candidate in Study 2 would imply the involvement of P450. The next step is to identify which P450 isoforms are involved in the metabolism, a process termed P450 phenotyping.[20] There are three major approaches for this study.

Table 5-8. Preferred and acceptable P450 isoform-specific inhibitors suggested by FDA in the September 2006 draft guidance document for drug–drug interaction evaluation and preferred inhibitors used at *In Vitro* ADMET Laboratories (IVAL)

CYP	FDA preferred inhibitor	FDA acceptable inhibitor	IVAL preferred inhibitor
1A2	Furafylline	alpha-Napthoflavone	Furafylline
2A6	Tranylcypromine, methoxsalen	Pilocarpine, tryptamine	Tranylcypromine
2B6		Ticlopidine, sertraline	Ticlopidine
2C8	Quercetin	Trimethorprim, gemfibrozil, rosiglitazone	Quercetin
2C9	Sulfaphenazole	Fluconazole	Sulfaphenazole
2C19		Ticlopidine	Omeprazole
2D6	Quinidine		Quinidine
2E1		Diethyldithiocarbamate	Diethyldithiocarbamate
3A4/5	Ketoconazole, itraconazole	Troleandomycin, verapamil	Ketoconazole

Liver microsomes and isoform-selective inhibitors. In this experiment, the test article is incubated with human liver microsomes in the presence and absence of individual selective inhibitors for the eight major CYP isoforms. The ability of an inhibitor to impede metabolism of the test article would indicate that the pathway obstructed by the inhibitor is involved in metabolism. For instance, if ketoconazole, a potent CYP3A4 inhibitor, is found to interfere with the metabolism of the test article, then CYP3A4 is concluded to be involved in the metabolism of the test article. It is also a common practice to assign the degree of involvement by the maximum percent inhibition. For instance, if the maximum inhibition, expressed as percentages of the total metabolism in the absence of inhibitor, by sulfaphenazole (CYP2C9 inhibitor) and ketoconazole (CYP3A4 inhibitor) are 20 percent and 80 percent, respectively, it can be concluded that the CYP2C9 is involved in 20 percent and CYP3A4 in 80 percent of the metabolism of the test article. It is important to realize that the inhibitors are isoform-selective rather than isoform-specific, so data interpretation must be performed carefully to avoid an inaccurate assignment of enzyme pathways.[21] It is always prudent to confirm the results of this study with results using a different approach (e.g., using rCYP).

The preferred and acceptable P450 isoform-specific inhibitors per U.S. FDA are shown in Table 5.8.

Incubation with individual rCYPs. In this experiment, individual rCYPs are used to evaluate which P450 isoforms are involved in test article metabolism.[20] The test article is incubated with each rCYP, and its disappearance is quantified. A rCYP that would lead to the disappearance of the test article would indicate that the isoform is involved in the metabolism of the test article. For instance, if rCYP2C19 incubation leads to the disappearance of the test article, then CYP2C19 is concluded to be involved in the metabolic clearance of the test article. It is important to realize that these studies are performed with a single P450 isoform and therefore lack competing enzyme pathways. Metabolism by a rCYP isoform may not be relevant *in vivo* because of higher-affinity pathways.

Correlation study with human liver microsomes. In this experiment, the test article is incubated with multiple lots of human liver microsomes, which have been previously characterized for the activities of the individual CYPs.[22] The rate of metabolic clearance of the test article is then plotted against the CYP activities of the different lots of microsomes. A linear correlation between activity and rate of disappearance for a specific CYP would indicate that this pathway is involved in the metabolism of the test article. This study requires the evaluation of at least ten liver microsome lots with a well-distributed gradations of activities.

Liver microsome/inhibitor study design

In general, studies with liver microsomes are believed to be more relevant than that with rCYP, as studies with individual rCYP does not allow competition in metabolism for isoforms with different affinities for the substrate, and therefore may over-emphasize the participation of low-affinity pathways. It is important to use substrate concentrations similar to expected plasma concentrations. An artefactually high concentration would cause the substrate to be metabolized similarly by high- and low-affinity enzyme pathways.[23] Using liver microsomes with physiologically relevant substrate concentrations should provide the best results. A typical liver microsome experiment with inhibitors is as follows:

- Human liver microsomes (0.5 mg/mL)
- Experiment 1: Metabolic Stability Study
- Incubation with three concentrations of test article (e.g., 0.1, 1, 10 μ*M*) and three incubation times (e.g. 15, 30, and 60 minutes)
- Quantification of test article disappearance
- Experiment 2: Reaction Phenotyping
- Incubation with one concentration of the test article at one incubation time (chosen from Experiment 1) in the presence and absence of isoform-specific inhibitors
- Quantification of test article disappearance

The isoform-specific inhibitors suggested by the FDA are shown in Table 5.6.

Evaluation of CYP isoform contributions using both liver microsomes and rCYPs. It is also possible to calculate the relative contribution of individual isoforms using data from both liver microsomes and rCYPs using the following approach.[24,25]

First, the relative activity factor for individual isoforms (using isoform-specific substrates) is calculated. This is necessary as each lot of liver microsome would have different relative amounts of each P450 isoform. V_{max} and K_m values are determined for each isoform using isoform-specific substrates for both liver microsomes and rCYP. The Relative Activity Factor (RAF) is calculated using the following equation:

$$\text{RAF} = (V_{max}/K_m \text{ of CYP in microsomes})/V_{max}/K_m \text{ of rCYP}$$

Contribution of a specific CYP isoform to metabolism of a test article is then calculated using the following equation:

$$\text{Contribution of CYP (\%)} = \text{RAF} \times (V_{rCYP})/(V_{microsomes})$$

Study 4: CYP inhibitory potential

The objective of this study is to evaluate if the drug or drug candidate in question is an inhibitor of a specific P450 isoform. This study can be performed with rCYP, human liver microsomes, and human hepatocytes.

rCYP studies. rCYP studies represent the most convenient and rapid study for the evaluation of CYP inhibitory potential. As the study involves substrates that form metabolites that can be quantified by fluorescence, the laborious and time-consuming HPLC or LC/MS sample analysis is not required. For this reason, most drug development laboratories would perform rCYP inhibition assays as a screen for P450 inhibitory potential of their drug candidates. The study involves the incubation of individual rCYP isoforms with the test article at various concentrations (e.g., seven concentrations plus solvent control) in triplicate, and a substrate that can be metabolized by the specific isoform. As the reaction only contains one single isoform, isoform-specific substrates are not required to be used. The requirement is that the substrate would generate metabolites that can be measured by a plate reader with the capability to quantify florescence.

Liver microsome studies. Liver microsomes represent the most appropriate experimental system for the evaluation of the interaction of a drug with P450 isoforms. For the evaluation of CYP inhibitory potential, the test article is incubated with liver microsomes in the presence of individual isoform-specific substrates. The isoform-specific substrates and the metabolites quantified are shown in Table 5.7.

Human hepatocyte studies. rCYP and human liver microsomes are cell-free systems, allowing direct interaction of the test article with the P450 isoforms. *In vivo*, the inhibitor is initially absorbed into the systemic circulation and then interacts with the enzymes after penetration through the hepatocyte plasma membrane. Once inside the cytoplasm, the inhibitor may be metabolized by Phase I and/or Phase II metabolism and/or actively transported out of the hepatocytes, for instance, via bile excretion. Furthermore, there may be transporters present to actively uptake the inhibitor. The result is that the intracellular concentration of the inhibitor may be substantially different from the plasma concentration. Results with rCYP and human liver microsomes may not be useful to estimate *in vivo* inhibitory effects based on plasma concentrations if the intracellular concentration of the inhibitor is not known.

The use of intact human hepatocytes may allow a more accurate extrapolation of *in vitro* results to *in vivo*. The study is performed using intact human hepatocytes incubated with isoform-specific substrate and the test article. The intact plasma membrane and the presence of all hepatic metabolic pathways and cofactors allow distribution and metabolism of the test article. The resulting inhibitory effect therefore should be physiologically more relevant to the *in vivo* situation than results with cell-free systems.

It is recommended that inhibition studies with intact hepatocytes be performed if inhibitory effects of a drug or drug candidate have been observed with rCYP or liver microsomes to allow a more accurate prediction of the extent of *in vivo* inhibitory effects. Time-dependent inhibition of P450 can also be studied using intact human hepatocytes.[26] One precaution with the use of intact hepatocytes is to concurrently measure also cytotoxicity. As dead hepatocytes are not active in drug metabolism, without cytotoxicity information, cytotoxic drug concentrations could be interpreted as inhibitory concentrations.

A recent advancement is to use intact hepatocytes suspended in whole human plasma for inhibition studies to allow correction for plasma protein binding.[27] As drugs *in vivo* are always in contact with 100 percent human blood, this is conceptually sound and therefore deserves further investigation on its general applicability. One disturbing finding in our laboratory is that testosterone, a compound that is readily metabolized *in vivo*, is not metabolized by intact human hepatocytes in whole plasma (A. P. Li, unpublished).

The P450 isoform-specific substrates and their respective metabolites to be quantified are presented in Table 5.9. These substrates can be used for both liver microsomes and hepatocytes.

IC_{50}, K_i, K_{inact}, and $[I]/K_i$ determinations

Enzyme inhibition data are often presented as IC_{50}, the concentration of the inhibitor to cause 50 percent inhibition at one chosen substrate concentration; K_i, the inhibition constant (dissociation constant from the inhibitor–enzyme complex) determined by enzyme kinetic analysis (e.g., Dixon plot); and K_{inact}, the time-dependent inhibition constant for mechanism-based inhibitors. IC_{50} values can be estimated from the study described earlier. A positive inhibition, defined as dose-dependent inhibition, with the inhibited activity lower than 50 percent of that of the negative control, will require further experimentation to define K_i for a better evaluation of *in vivo* inhibitory potential. Further, a study to determine K_{inact} may be performed to evaluate if the inhibitor acts via covalent binding to the active site of the enzyme, leading to time-dependent irreversible inhibition.

Table 5-9. P450 isoform-specific substrates and their respective metabolites

CYP	Substrate	Metabolite
1A2	Phenacetin Ethoxyresorufin	Acetaminophen Resorufin
2A6	Coumarin	7-OH-Coumarin
2B6	Bupropion	Hydroxypropion
2C8	Taxol	6-alpha-hydroxypaclitaxel
2C9	Tolbutamide	4′-Hydroxytolbutamide
2C19	*s*-Mephenytoin	4-OH-Mephenytoin
2D6	Dextromethorphan	Dextrophan
2E1	Chlorzoxazone	6-Hydroxychlorzoxazone
3A4/5	Testosterone	6-beta-Hydroxytestosterone

Note: These substrates are used for the evaluation using *in vitro* experimental systems such as liver microsomes, liver S9, or hepatocytes in which multiple isoforms are expressed.

IC_{50} is generally determined by plotting the log of the relative activity (activity in the presence of the inhibitor as a percent of the activity of the negative control (solvent control), and then estimate the concentration yielding 50 percent relative activity using linear regression analysis. IC_{50} can also be calculated from the relationship between inhibitor concentrations and percent of control activity with the aid of a nonlinear regression program such as SCIENTIST (Micromath, Salt Lake City, UT).[28]

K_i can be determined using Dixon plot with the reciprocal of the activity as the y-axis, and inhibitor concentration as the x-axis. Results with at least two substrate concentrations below $V_{\max}$ are plotted, with K_i calculated as the negative of the x-intercept.[29] K_i can also be estimated with the aid of nonlinear regression analysis software such as SYSTAT (SPPS, Inc., Chicago, IL).[30]

Most P450 inhibitors act via reversible (competitive or noncompetitive mechanisms) with which their inhibitory potential can be estimated from their IC_{50} or K_i values. Some inhibitors are "mechanism-based" or "time-dependent" inhibitors, which can cause irreversible inhibition due to the formation of reactive metabolites by the CYP isoform, leading to covalent binding to the active site and thereby causing irreversible inhibition of the affected enzyme molecule.[31] Irreversible inhibitors therefore will have prolonged inhibition of the enzyme even after clearance of the drug in question. K_{inact} is a measurement of the potency of such "mechanism-based" inhibitors.

K_{inact} can be determined using the following approach[32]:

1. Plot the natural logarithm of the relative activity (activity in the presence of the inhibitor as a percent of the activity of the solvent or negative control) versus time and determine the slope at each inhibitor concentration. The slope, $k_{observed}$, is a measurement of the rate of enzyme inactivation at each concentration of the inhibitor.

2. Plot 1/ $k_{observed}$ versus 1/inhibitor concentration (Lineweaver-Burk plot). K_{inact} is calculated as the reciprocal of the y-intercept, and K_i as the negative of the reciprocal of the x-intercept. Alternatively, Plot the Kitz-Wilson plot of $t_{1/2}$ (calculated as 0.692/ $k_{observed}$) versus the reciprocal of the inhibitor concentration and estimate K_{inact} as the y-intercept, and K_i as the reciprocal of the x-intercept.

$[I]/K_i$, the ratio of the anticipated or known steady state plasma drug concentration to K_i, is generally used to determine the likelihood of clinical drug–drug interactions.[33,34] A general rule of thumb suggested by the FDA (http://www.fda.gov/cder/guidance/6695dft.pdf) is as follows:

- **$[I]/K_i < 0.1$: Unlikely to cause *in vivo* drug–drug interactions**
- **$[I]/K_i = 1$: Possible to cause *in vivo* drug–drug interactions**
- **$[I]/K_i > 1$: Likely to cause *in vivo* drug–drug interactions**

K_i is estimated by an experiment with varying inhibitor and substrate concentrations. A typical K_i study is as follows:

- *In vitro* experimental system: rCYP; human liver microsomes, or hepatocytes.
- Inhibitor concentration: Five (ideally yielding 10–90 percent inhibition of activity)
- Substrate concentration: Minimum of two for the Dixon plot; three is recommended.
- Timepoint: One (within the linear time course) if time course is known; multiple (e.g., 5, 10, and 15 minutes) if time course under the experimental conditions has not been established.
- K_i is determined by Dixon plot, plotting the reciprocal of activity versus inhibitor concentration. The negative of the x-coordinate value corresponding to the intercept of the plots for the low and high substrate concentrations is the K_i.

For mechanism-based inhibitors, K_{inact} is estimated by an experiment with varying inhibitor concentration and preincubation time. A typical K_{inact} study is as follows:

- *In vitro* experimental system: rCYP; human liver microsomes, or hepatocytes
- Preincubation time (preincubation of enzyme with inhibitor): Five (e.g., 5, 10, 15, 20, 30 minutes)
- Inhibitor concentration: Five (ideally yielding 10–90 percent inhibition of activity)
- Substrate concentration: One
- Substrate incubation time: One (within the linear time course) if time course is known; multiple (e.g., 5, 10, and 15 minutes) if time course under the experimental conditions has not been established
- K_{inact} is determined as described previously.

Study 5: Enzyme Induction potential

Enzyme induction is a major mechanism for drug–drug interactions. Induction of a drug-metabolizing enzyme by one drug would lead to the enhanced metabolism of coadministered drugs that are substrates of the induced enzyme.

Experimental evaluation of enzyme induction involves the treatment of human hepatocytes for several days with the test article followed by evaluation of enzyme activities using P450 isoform-specific substrates.[35,36] As freshly isolated hepatocytes possess endogenous activities, which may be the result of inducers present in the donor's systemic circulation, the isolated hepatocytes are cultured for 2–3 days to allow the P450 enzyme activities to return to a basal level. Testing for induction potential is that initiated by treatment of the cultured hepatocytes for 2–3 days to allow full expression of the induced enzyme. Induction is generally evaluated by measuring enzyme activity as activity represents the most relevant endpoint for drug–drug interaction. Both freshly isolated and plateable cryopreserved human hepatocytes can be used for the induction study.[10,37,38]

As of this writing, all known inducers of P450 isoforms *in vivo* are inducers *in vitro*.[10] The known human P450 inducers are shown in Table 5.8.

The typical experimental procedures for an enzyme induction study are as follows:

- Day 0: Plate human hepatocytes (freshly isolated or plateable cryopreserved human hepatocytes)
- Day 1: Refresh medium
- Day 2: Refresh medium
- Day 3: Change medium to that containing test article, solvent control, or positive controls
- Minimum of three test article concentrations, with the high concentration at least one order of magnitude greater than expected plasma concentration
- If plasma concentration not known, evaluate concentrations ranging over at least two orders of magnitude (e.g., 1, 10, 100 μM)
- Day 4: Refresh treatment medium
- Day 5: Refresh treatment medium
- Day 6: Measure activity (*in situ* incubation with isoform-specific substrates)

The isoform-specific substrates described earlier for CYP inhibition studies are generally used for enzyme induction studies.

The known CYP inducers have been determined to induce either CYP1A and/or CYP3A, with inducers of other inducible isoforms such as CYP2A6, CYP2C9, CYP2C19 found also to be CYP3A inducers. For general enzyme induction evaluation for drug–drug interactions, it may be adequate to simply screen for CYP1A and CYP3A induction. If CYP3A induction is observed, then investigations into CYP2A6, CYP2C9, and CYP2C19 induction are warranted.

The two most common confounding factors for P450 induction studies are as follows:

1. Inducers that are also inhibitors: The co-occurrence of P450 inhibition and induction (i.e., the compound is both an inhibitor and inducer) can confound induction results. Ritonavir is an example of a CYP3A4 inducer[39] which is also a potent CYP3A4 inhibitor.[40] The inhibitory effects can overcome any induction effects using activity as an endpoint. For the evaluation of enzyme induction potential of inhibitors, western blotting for the amount of enzyme proteins would be most appropriate. Studies with mRNA expression would provide data to distinguish between induction of gene expression or protein stabilization as mechanisms. As in the case of ritonavir, induction effects persist after the clearance of the drug from the systemic circulation, leading to enhanced clearance of drugs that are substrates of the induced pathways. It is important to define the induction potential of a drug even if it is found to be an enzyme inhibitor.
2. Cytotoxic compounds: Induction effects can be masked by the decrease of cell viability, as most induction assays quantify substrate metabolism *in situ* (in the same cell culture plate that the cells are cultured) and assume that there is no change in cell number. Cytotoxicity evaluation therefore should always be performed concurrently with induction studies. In the presence of cytotoxicity, activity should be corrected by the viability for comparison with negative control activity to assess induction potential.

A compound is concluded to be an inducer if reproducible, statistically significant, and dose-dependent induction effects are observed. The FDA recommends the use of the criterion of "40% of higher of the activity of positive controls" as a positive response (www.fda.gov/cber/gdlns/interactstud.htm).

Drugs with P450 induction potential in humans are shown in Table 5.10. It is interesting to note that most of these inducers are also found to have clinically significant hepatotoxicity.

Study 6: In vitro empirical drug–drug interactions

The physiological significance of the findings based on the mechanistic approach may be substantiated by *in vitro* drug–drug interactions between frequently coadministered drugs that are likely to have interaction with the drug in question.[18] This is particularly important if the drug in question is either a CYP3A4 substrate or is a CYP3A4 inhibitor. As CYP3A4 is now known to have different affinities for different substrates and inhibitors,[41] the interaction potential for a drug and a particular coadministered drug may be substantially different from that estimated by using a surrogate substrate of CYP3A4.

This study can be performed with liver microsomes or hepatocytes. The use of hepatocytes probably would allow the development of data more relevant to humans *in vivo*.

Table 5-10. Clinically demonstrated human enzyme inducers and their respective *in vitro* induction results as well as their association with severe hepatotoxicity

In vivo enzyme inducer	*In vitro* human hepatocyte induction finding	Severe clinical hepatotoxicity
Carbamazepine	+	+
Dexamethasone	+	−
Isoniazid	+	+
Omeprazole	+	+
Phenobarbital	+	+
Phenytoin	+	+
Rifampin	+	+
Rifapentine	+	−
Rifabutin	+	−
Troglitazone	+	+
St. John's wort	+	+

5.3 DATA INTERPRETATION

The studies described in this chapter allow one to develop data for the estimation of drug–drug interaction potential of the drug or drug candidate in question. Accurate prediction of *in vivo* effects is possible only through thorough and scientifically sound interpretation of the data. Although every novel chemical structure will provide a unique set of data and therefore requires individualized data interpretation and/or further experimentation, the following guidelines can be use to aid the evaluation of the data generated.

Pathway evaluation

The following are the possible outcome of the study:

1. The test article is not metabolized by liver microsomes, or hepatocytes: This is indicated by the lack of either metabolite formation or parent disappearance in Studies 1 and 2. Hepatic metabolism is not involved in the metabolic clearance of the compound. There should be no concern with coadministered drugs that can alter drug-metabolizing enzyme activities.
2. The test article is metabolized but not metabolized by P450 isoforms: As P450-related drug–drug interactions are the most prevalent, non-P450 drug–drug interactions should be considered on a case-by-case basis. For instance, MAO interaction may be important if the drug in question may be coadministered with known MAO substrates or inhibitors. UGT substrates, for instance, may have drug interactions with UGT inhibitory drugs such as probenacid.
3. The test article is metabolized by a single P450 isoform: This represents the easiest data to interpret, albeit not a good scenario for a drug candidate.

A drug that is metabolized predominantly by a single P450 isoform will be very likely to have drug–drug interactions with inhibitors of the isoform. The known cases of serious drug–drug interactions often involve a single P450 pathway, with CYP3A4 being the most prominent. Drugs that have been withdrawn due to fatal drug–drug interactions are often CYP3A4 substrates or potent CYP3A4 inhibitors. Because of the role of CYP2C8 in the metabolism of statins that are widely prescribed to combat hypercholesterolemia, CYP2C8 has become a second most important isoform for drug–drug interactions. Cerivastatin, a CYP2C8 substrate, was withdrawn from the market in August 2001 after reports of fatal interactions with the CYP2C8 inhibitor gemfibrozil.[42]

4. The test article is metabolized by multiple P450 isoforms: This is generally interpreted that the test article may not have serious interactions with a specific inhibitor of one of the P450 isoforms, as the metabolic clearance can be carried out by the unaffected pathways. However, there are examples of drugs that have been found to be metabolized by multiple pathways but would later be found in clinical or postmarketing studies to have interactions with potent inhibitors of a specific pathway. An example is the antifungal terbinafine, which has been characterized using human liver microsomes and rCYPs to be metabolized by multiple P450 isoforms: CYP1A2, CYP2C8, CYP2C9, CYP2C19, CYP2D6, and CYP3A4, leading to the author's conclusion that "the potential for terbinafine interaction with other drugs is predicted to be insignificant."[43] In the same study, as terbinafine was a competitive inhibitor of CYP2D6, it was concluded that terbinafine would have interactions with CYP2D6 substrates. *In vivo* studies confirmed the CYP2D6 inhibitory effects as predicted by *in vitro* studies; however, it was also observed clinically that rifampin, a CYP3A4 inducer, caused a 100 percent increase terbinafine clearance (www.fda.gov/medwatch/safety/2004/jan_PI/Lamasil_PI.pdf). One possible explanation of this is that, upon CYP3A4 induction, the total metabolism of terbinafine is greatly enhanced due to the high capacity of CYP3A4 for this substrate. It is therefore important to realize that although a drug is metabolized by multiple isoforms, it may still have significant drug interactions with inducers of isoforms with high capacity for the metabolism of the drug.

P450 inhibition

The outcomes of P450 inhibition studies may include the following:

1. No inhibition observed: If no inhibitory effects are observed with rCYP, microsomes and hepatocytes, the substance in question is considered not to have the potential to cause inhibitory metabolic drug–drug interactions *in vivo*. As of now, there are no examples of *in vivo* enzyme inhibitors that are not inhibitors *in vitro*.

2. Significant inhibition observed: A practical definition of significant inhibition is that the test article is found to cause dose-dependent and >50 percent inhibition of one or more P450 isoforms at the concentrations evaluated. The conclusion is that the test article is a potent inhibitor. As described earlier, the physiological significance is determined by the $[I]/K_i$ value, with any $[I]/K_i$ value of 0.1 or higher as possible or likely to cause *in vivo* drug–drug interactions. It is recommended that $[I]/K_i$ values obtained from cell-free systems (microsomes and rCYP) be confirmed by that with intact hepatocytes to aid an accurate prediction of *in vivo* effects. If the results with hepatocytes are also determined to be significant, *in vivo* studies will need to be performed to estimate human *in vivo* drug–drug interaction potential.
3. No time-dependent inhibition observed: The inhibitor is not a mechanism-based inhibitor.
4. Time-dependent inhibition observed: The inhibitor is a time-dependent inhibitor. *In vivo* studies will need to be performed to further define its drug–drug interaction potential.
5. Additional safety concern: A time-dependent inhibitor may need to be further studied to define its hepatotoxic potential, as a number of time-dependent P450 inhibitors are found to cause idiosyncratic hepatotoxicity.

P450 induction

The following outcome may be observed:

1. No induction observed: The substance evaluated is not an enzyme inducer if P450 inhibitory and cytotoxic potential are eliminated as confounding factors.
2. Induction observed: The substance evaluated is observed to cause dose-dependent and physiologically significant induction (e.g., induced activity over twofold of negative control activity). If the doses found to be positive are within clinical plasma concentrations (e.g., within 10× of plasma C_{max}), *in vivo* studies may be needed to further define the test article's *in vivo* enzyme induction and the subsequent drug–drug interaction potential.
3. Additional safety concern: Enzyme inducers may need to be further evaluated for their hepatotoxic potential, as a large number of enzyme-inducing drugs are found to cause severe hepatotoxicity.

5.4 NUCLEAR RECEPTORS AND DRUG–DRUG INTERACTIONS

Nuclear receptors (NR) function as ligand-activated transcription factors that regulate expression of a host of genes, including those coding for key drug-metabolizing enzymes and transporters. It is now known that the induction of drug-metabolizing enzymes and transporters involved three major nuclear receptors, namely, the pregnane X receptor (PXR), the constitutive andorstane receptor (CAR), and the aryl hydrocarbon receptor (AhR). The properties of these receptors in drug–drug interactions are reviewed here:

1. PXR, a nuclear receptor, was discovered in virtually all mammalian species studied, including mouse, rat, rabbit, dog, pig, monkey, and man. PXR is activated by a variety of steroids, drugs, and xenobiotics and is inhibited by interleukin-6. Species differences have been discovered for PXR, which lead to the known species differences in response to inducers. Although PXR activation is generally linked to CYP3A induction, it is now known that the receptor is also associated with the induction of CYP2B, CYP2C, UGT and the transporters MDR1 and OATP2. A cell line transfected with PXR linked to a luciferase reporter gene is now used commonly as a relatively high throughput screening assay for PXR activators.
2. CAR is mainly associated with CYP2B induction. CAR is a cytoplasmic enzyme, which, upon activation, would translocate to the nucleus, leading to gene activation. One of the earliest discovered enzyme inducer, phenobarbital, is believed to activate CYP2B via CAR activation. CAR is found in mouse, rat, monkey, and man. CAR activity and cytoplasmic-nuclear translocation is enhanced by activators of gluccocorticoid receptor (GR), a process called nuclear receptors cross-talk. As for PXR, substantial differences have been observed for CAR. The chemical 1,4-bis[2-(3,5-dichloropyridyloxy)] benzene (TCPOBOP), one of the strongest CYP2B inducers and CAR activators in mouse, is substantially inactive in man. The species differences are believed to be due to the divergent ligand-binding domain of the CAR orthologs from the different animal species. One of the major differences between primary human hepatocytes and human hepatocyte cell lines such as HepG2 is that CAR resides in the cytoplasm in the primary hepatocytes similar to the hepatocytes *in vivo*, but it resides abnormally in the nucleus in hepatocyte cell lines. For this reason, data generated from induction studies with hepatocyte cell lines may not be relevant to that observed *in vivo*.
3. AhR is known to mediate mainly CYP1A induction. As its name implies, the ligands of AhR are mainly aryl hydrocarbons such as 3-methylcholanthrene and 2,3,7-tetrachlorodibenzo-p-dioxin (TCDD). Substantial species differences in AhR have been reported, leading to species differences in response to various AhR ligands. Omeprazole, a potent AhR activator and CYP1A inducer in human hepatocytes, for instance, is substantially less active in rodent hepatocytes. Conversely, TCDD and another polyhalogenated biphenyl, polybrominated biphenyl (PBB), are more potent in CYP1A induction in rodents than in man. AhR is not as important as PXR and CAR for drug–drug interactions, but it is involved in myriad toxicological phenomenon including developmental errors and carcinogenesis.

5.5 CONCLUSION

Drug–drug interactions can have serious adverse consequences and therefore should be evaluated accurately before a new drug is introduced to the human populations. Due to the scientific advances in the understanding of the key human drug-metabolizing pathways, and the availability of human *in vitro* systems for drug metabolism studies, human drug–drug interaction evaluations, especially drug metabolism related interactions, can be performed rapidly and efficiently. A scientific, mechanism-based approach to evaluate drug–drug interactions remains the most appropriate approach:

1. Via the understanding of the major drug-metabolizing pathways in the metabolism of the drug or drug candidate in question to assess its potential interactions with existing drugs that are inhibitors or inducers of the pathways involved.
2. A careful and exhaustive evaluation of the inhibitory potential of the drug or drug candidate in question toward the major human drug metabolism enzymes will allow the assessment of its potential to cause interactions with existing drugs that are substrates of the inhibited enzymes.
3. Evaluation of induction potential of the drug or drug candidate in question for the inducible human drug-metabolizing enzymes will allow the assessment of potential interactions with drugs that are substrates of the induced enzymes.

This approach is currently mainly applied towards P450 isoforms, but it can also be applied to non-P450 drug-metabolizing enzyme pathways. The next wave of major advances in drug–drug interactions is anticipated to be approaches for the evaluation of the interactions between drugs and drug transporters.

The success achieved with the scientific-based approaches in the evaluation of drug–drug interactions is a result of the extensive scientific research in the identification and characterization of drug–metabolizing enzymes, the definition of the mechanisms of metabolic-based drug–drug interactions, and the development, characterization, and intelligent application of the human-based *in vitro* experimental models for drug metabolism. Similar approaches should be adopted for the evaluation of other major adverse drug effects (e.g., idiosyncratic drug toxicity), which so far have eluded the routine drug safety evaluation approaches. It is through an open mind – a willingness to venture toward the development of hypothesis, the testing of the hypothesis, and the development and adoption of approaches to investigate a problem based on the best science – that the field of drug safety evaluation can move forward.

REFERENCES

1. Zang H, Cui D, Wang B, et al. Pharmacokinetic drug interactions involving 17alpha-ethinylestradiol: A new look at an old drug. *Clin Pharmacokinet*. 2007; 46:133–157.

2. Huang SM, Lesko LJ, Williams RL. Assessment of the quality and quantity of drug–drug interaction studies in recent NDA submissions: Study design and data analysis issues. *J Clin Pharmacol.* 1999;39:1006–1014.
3. Schalcher C, Schad K, Brunner-La Rocca HP, et al. Interaction of sildenafil with cAMP-mediated vasodilation in vivo. *Hypertension.* 2003;40:763–767.
4. Guengerich FP. Cytochrome P450s and other enzymes in drug metabolism and toxicity. *AAPS J.* 2006; 8:E101–E111.
5. Li, AP . Primary hepatocyte cultures as an in vitro experimental model for the evaluation of pharmacokinetic drug–drug interactions. *Adv Pharmacol.* 1997;43:103–130.
6. Li AP. Screening for human ADME/Tox drug properties in drug discovery. *Drug Discov Today.* 2001;6:357–366.
7. Li AP. In vitro approaches to evaluate ADMET drug properties. *Curr Top Med Chem.* 2004;4:701–706.
8. MacGregor JT, Collins JM, Sugiyama Y, et al. In vitro human tissue models in risk assessment: Report of a consensus-building workshop. *Toxicol Sci.* 2001;59:17–36.
9. Hewitt NJ, Lechon MJ, Houston JB, et al. Primary hepatocytes: Current understanding of the regulation of metabolic enzymes and transporter proteins, and pharmaceutical practice for the use of hepatocytes in metabolism, enzyme induction, transporter, clearance, and hepatoxicity studies. *Drug Metab Rev.* 2007;39:159–234.
10. Li AP. Human hepatocytes: Isolation, cryopreservation and applications in drug development. *Chem Biol Interact.* 2007;168:16–29.
11. Li AP, Lu C, Brent JA, et al. Cryopreserved human hepatocytes: Characterization of drug-metabolizing enzyme activities and applications in higher throughput screening assays for hepatotoxicity, metabolic stability, and drug–drug interaction potential. *Chem Biol Interact.* 1999;121:17–35.
12. Raucy J, Lasker JM . Isolation of P450 enzymes from human livers. *Method Enzymol.* 1991;206:577–594.
13. Nelson AC, Huang W, Moody DE. Human liver microsome preparation: impact on the kinetics of L-α-acetylmethadol (LAAM) *N*-demethylation and dextromethorphan *O*-demethylation. *Drug Metab Disp.* 2001;29:319–325.
14. Barnes HJ, Arlotto MP, Waterman MR. Expression and enzymatic activity of recombinant cytochrome P450 17-alpha-hydroxylase in Escherichia coli. *Proc Natl Acad Sci.* 1991;88:5597–5601.
15. Friedberg T, Pritchard MP, Bandera M, et al. Merits and limitations of recombinant models for the study of human P450-mediated drug metabolism and toxicity – An intralaboratory comparison. *Drug Metab Rev.* 1999;31:523–544.
16. Donato MT, Jimenez N, Castell JV, et al. Fluorescence-based assays for screening nine cytochrome P450 (P450) activities in intact cells expressing individual human P450 enzymes. *Drug Metab Disp.* 2004;32:699–706.
17. Vtric F, Haefeli WE, Drewe, J, et al. Interaction of ibuprofen and probenecid with metabolizing enzyme phenotyping procedures using caffeine as the probe drug. *Br J Clin Pharmacol.* 2003;55:191–198.
18. Li AP. Scientific basis of drug–drug interactions: Mechanism and preclinical evaluation. *Drug Inf J.* 1998;32:657–664.
19. Emoto C, Murase S, Sawada Y, et al. In vitro inhibitory effects of 1-aminobenzotriazole on drug oxidations catalyzed by human cytochrome P450 enzymes: A comparison with SKF-525A and ketoconazole. *Drug Metab Pharmacokinet.* 2003;18:287–295.
20. Rodriques AD. Integrated cytochrome P450 reaction phenotyping: Attempting to bridge the gap between cDNA-expressed cytochromes P450 and native human liver microsomes. *Biochem Pharmacol.* 1999;57:465–480.
21. Lu, AYH, Wang RW, Lin JH. Commentary: Cytochrome P450 in vitro reaction phenotyping: A re-evaluation of approaches for P450 isoform identification. *Drug Metab Disp.* 2003; 31:345–350.
22. Ring BJ, Gillespie JS, Eckstein JA, et al. Identification of human cytochromes P450 responsible for atomozetine metabolism. *Drug Metab Disp.* 2002;30:319–323.

23. Renwick AB, Surry D, Price RJ, et al. Metabolism of 7-benzyloxy-4-trifluoromethylcoumarin by human hepatic cytochrome P450 isoforms. *Xenobiotica*. 2004;30:955–969.
24. Crespi CL. Xenobiotic-metabolizing human cells as tools for pharmacological and toxicological research. *Adv Drug Res*. 1995;26:179–235.
25. Uttamsingh V, Lu C, Miwa G, et al. Relative contributions of the five major human cytochromes P450, 1A2, 2C9, 2C19, 2D6, and 3A4, to the hepatic metabolism of the proteasome inhibitor bortezomib. *Drug Metab Disp*. 2005;33:1723–1728.
26. McGinnity DF, Berry AJ, Kenny JR, et al. Evaluation of time-dependent cytochrome P450 inhibition using cultured human hepatocytes. *Drug Metab Disp*. 2006;34:1291–1300.
27. Lu C, Miwa GT, Prakash SR, et al. A novel model for the prediction of drug–drug interactions in humans based on in vitro cytochrome p450 phenotypic data. *Drug Metab Disp*. 2007; 35:79–85.
28. Chiba M, Jin L, Neway W, et al. P450 interaction with HIV protease inhibitors: Relationship between metabolic stability, inhibitory potency, and P450 binding spectra. *Drug Metab Disp*. 2001; 29:1–3.
29. Kim JY, Baek M, Lee S, et al. Characterization of the selectivity and mechanism of cytochrome P450 inhibition by dimethyl-4,4′-dimethoxy-5,6,5′,6′-dimethylenedioxybiphenyl-2,2′-dicarboxylate. *Drug Metab Disp*. 2001;29:1555–1560.
30. Wen X, Wang JS, Backman JT, et al. Gemfibrozil as an inhibitor of human cytochrome P450 2C9. *Drug Metab Disp*. 2001;29:1359–1361.
31. Walsh CT. Suicide substrates, mechanism-based enzyme inactivators: Recent developments. *Ann Rev Biochem*. 1984;53:493–535.
32. Madeira M, Levine M, Chang TKH, et al. The effect of cimetidine on dexromethorphan *O*-demethylase activity of human liver microsomes and recombinant CYP2D6. *Drug Metab Disp*. 2004;32:460–467.
33. Brown HS, Galetin A, Hallifax D, et al. Prediction of in vivo drug–drug interactions from in vivo data: Factors affecting prototypic drug–drug interactions involving CYP2C9, CYP2D6 and CYP3A4. *Clin Pharmacokinet*. 2006;45:1035–1050.
34. Kato M, Tachibana T, Ito K, et al. Evaluation of methods for predicting drug–drug interactions by Monte Carlo simulation. *Drug Metab Pharmacokinet*. 2003;18:121–127.
35. Li AP, Rasmussen A, Xu L, et al. Rifampicin induction of lidocain metabolism in cultured human hepatocytes. *J Pharmacol Exp Ther*. 1995;274:673–677.
36. Li AP, Maurel P, Gomez-Lechon MJ, et al. Applications of primary human hepatocytes in the evaluation of P450 induction. *Chem. Biol Interact*. 1997;107:5–16.
37. Roymans D, Van Looveren C, Leone A, et al. Determination of cytochrome P450 1A2 and P450 3A4 induction in cryopreserved human hepatocytes. *Biochem Pharmacol*. 2004;67:427–437.
38. Roymans D, Annaert P, Van Houdt J, et al. Expression and induction potential of cytochromes P450 in human cryopreserved hepatocytes. *Drug Metab Disp*. 2005;33:1004–1016.
39. Hariparsad N, Nallani S, Sane RS, et al. Induction of CYP3A4 by efavirenz in primary human hepatocytes: Comparison with rifampin and phenobarbital. *J Clin Pharmacol*. 2004;44:1273–1281.
40. Lillibridge JH, Liang BH, Kerr BM, et al. Characterization of the selectivity and mechanism of human cytochrome P450 inhibition by the human immunodeficiency virus-protease inhibitor nelfinavir mesylate. *Drug Metab Disp*. 1998;26:609–616.
41. Wang RW, Newton DJ, Liu N, et al. Human cytochrome P-450 3A4: In vitro drug–drug interaction patterns are substrate-dependent. *Drug Metab Disp*. 2000;28:360–366.
42. Backman JT, Kyrklund C, Neuvonen M, et al. Gemfibrozil greatly increases plasma concentrations of cerivastatin. *Clin Pharmacol Ther*. 2002;72:685–691.
43. Vickers AE, Sinclair JR, Zollinger M, et al. Multiple cytochrome P450s involved in the metabolism of terbinafine suggest a limited potential for drug–drug interactions. *Drug Metab Disp*. 1999;27:1029–1038.
44. Vazquez E, Whitfield L. Seldane warnings. *Posit Aware*. 1997;8:12.

45. Carlson AM, Morris LS. Coprescription of terfenadine and erythromycin or ketoconazole: an assessment of potential harm. *J Am Pharm Assoc (Wash).* 1996;NS36:263–269.
46. Von Moltke LL, Greenblatt DJ, Duan SX, et al. Inhibition of terfenadine metabolism in vitro by azole antifungal agents and by selective serotonin reuptake inhibitor antidepressants: Relations to pharmacokinetic interactions in vivo. *J Clin Psychopharmacol.* 1996;16:104–112.
47. Omar MA, Wilson JP. FDA adverse event reports on statin associated rhabdomyolysis. *Ann Pharmacother.* 2002;36:288–295.
48. Diasio RB. Sorivudine and 5-fluorouracil; A clinically significant drug–drug interaction due to inhibition of dihydropyrimidine dehydrogenase. *Br J Clin Pharmacol.* 1998;46:1–4.
49. Ozdemir O, Boran M, Gokce V, et al . A case with severe rhabdomyolysis and renal failure associated with cerevastatin-gemfibrozil combination therapy – A case report. *Angiology.* 2000;51:695–697.
50. Li AP, Hartman NR, Lu C, et al. Effects of cytochrome P450 inducers on 17 alpha-ethinyloestradiol (EE2) conjugation by primary human hepatocytes. *Br J Clin Pharmacol.* 1999;48:733–742.
51. Capone D, Aiello C, Santoro GA, et al. Drug interaction between cyclosporine and two antimicrobial agents, josamycin and rifampicin, in organ-transplanted patients. *Int J Clin Pharmacol Res.* 1996;16:73–76.
52. Henderson L, Yue QY, Berqquist C, et al. St. John's wort (*Hypericum perforatum*): Drug interactions and clinical outcomes. *Br J Clin Pharmacol.* 2002;54:349–356.

6 Reliability of reactive metabolite and covalent binding assessments in prediction of idiosyncratic drug toxicity

Amit S. Kalgutkar

6.1 INTRODUCTION

Safety-related attrition continues to be a major concern in the pharmaceutical industry.[1] Of a total of 548 drugs approved in the period from 1975 to 1999, 45 drugs (8.2 percent) acquired 1 or more black box warnings and 16 (2.9 percent) were withdrawn from the market owing to idiosyncratic adverse drug reactions (IADRs) *that were not predicted from animal testing and/or clinical trials.*[2] IADRs (also known as type B ADRs) are unrelated to known drug pharmacology, and are generally dose-independent. Because the frequency of occurrence of IADRs is very low (1 in 10,000 to 1 in 100,000), these reactions are often not detected until the drug has gained broad exposure in a large patient population. *Importantly, standard regulatory animal toxicity studies have traditionally shown a poor concordance with occurrence of IADRs in humans.*[3] Life-threatening IADRs noted for drugs include hepatotoxicity, severe cutaneous reactions, aplastic anemia, and blood dyscrasias. Recognizing these issues, many pharmaceutical companies are increasing their efforts in implementing predictive *in vitro* tools to identify potential safety liabilities earlier in the drug discovery process so that they can be eliminated via chemical intervention or the compound suspended from further development. One component of such assays is aimed at understanding a drug candidate's propensity to undergo reactive metabolite formation.

6.2 LINKING METABOLISM WITH TOXICITY

Drugs are metabolized via oxidative, reductive, and hydrolytic pathways (phase I reactions), which lead to a modest increase in aqueous solubility; phase II conjugations modify the newly introduced functionality to form *O*- and *N*-glucuronides, sulfate and acetate esters, all with increased hydrophilicity relative to the unconjugated metabolite. In most cases, metabolism results in the loss of biological activity of the parent drug, and such metabolic reactions are therefore regarded as detoxication pathways. However, depending on the structural features present in some compounds, the same metabolic events on occasion can generate electrophilic, reactive metabolites, a process referred to

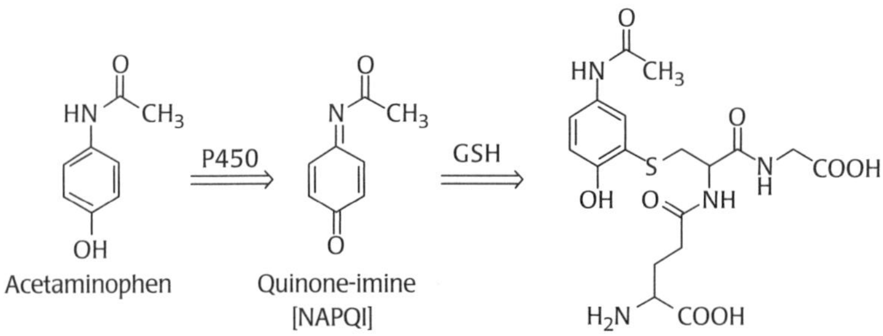

Figure 6-1: P450-catalyzed bioactivation of the anti-inflammatory agent acetaminophen.

as bioactivation. Inadequate detoxication of reactive metabolites is thought to represent a pathogenic mechanism for tissue necrosis, carcinogenicity, teratogenicity, and/or certain immune-mediated idiosyncratic toxicities.

The concept of xenobiotic bioactivation leading to toxicity can be traced back to the work of the Millers, whose studies in the 1940s demonstrated the bioactivation of aminoazo dyes into protein reactive metabolites[4]. Subsequent extension of this concept to the field of drug metabolism was demonstrated in studies with the anti-inflammatory agent acetaminophen.[5–8] The studies that revealed the cytochrome P450-mediated bioactivation of acetaminophen to a reactive quinone-imine metabolite (NAPQI),[9] capable of depleting levels of the endogenous antioxidant glutathione (GSH) and binding covalently to liver macromolecules (Figure 6.1) has served as a paradigm for drug toxicity assessment over the decades.

6.3 REACTIVE METABOLITES AND IDIOSYNCRATIC DRUG TOXICITY – KEY CHALLENGES IN DRUG DISCOVERY

Alkylation of DNA by reactive metabolites has clear implications in terms of the potential for mutagenesis, teratogenesis, and carcinogenesis; however, the consequences of covalent binding of reactive drug metabolites to proteins as it relates to IADRs remain poorly understood, even after some 40 years of research. In the case of acetaminophen, the dose-dependent hepatotoxicity observed in humans can be replicated in animals. For most other drugs this is not the case; ADRs observed in humans cannot be reproduced in animals, which implies that there are no preclinical models to predict IADR potential of drug candidates. In addition, the downstream *in vivo* consequences of reactive metabolite formation and protein covalent modification as it relates to IADRs are poorly understood. Several hypotheses, however, have been proposed to explain these phenomena. The basic hypothesis that links the formation of reactive metabolites with IADRs (especially those with a possible immune component) is the process of haptenization wherein low molecular weight (< 1000 Da) reactive metabolites are converted to immunogens via binding to high molecular weight proteins, as is the case with penicillin-induced anaphylactic reactions.[10] Immune-mediated IADRs can also result from drug-specific T-lymphocytes via presentation of the hapten to T-cells as demonstrated in the course of β-lactam- and sulfamethoxazole-induced skin rash. In the case of the antibacterial agent sulfamethoxazole, the immune activation is thought to involve a P450-catalyzed bioactivation of the aniline group to a reactive nitroso metabolite capable of covalently binding to cellular constituents.[11] Additional examples of drugs associated with haptenization include halothane, tienilic acid, and dihydralazine, all of which are bioactivated to reactive metabolites and display mechanism-based inactivation of the P450 isozymes responsible for their metabolism. Consistent with these observations, antibodies detected in sera of patients exposed to these drugs specifically recognize P450 isozymes, as being responsible for their metabolism.[12–14]

6.4 EVALUATING BIOACTIVATION POTENTIAL OF NEW COMPOUNDS IN DRUG DISCOVERY

Given lack of an in-depth understanding of the mechanisms of IADRs, the absence of animal models and relevant clinical safety biomarkers to detect these rare side effects, it is currently impossible to accurately predict which new drugs will be associated with a significant incidence of IADRs. Under the assumption that reactive metabolites, as opposed to the parent molecules from which they are derived, can be responsible for the pathogenesis of certain IADRs, most pharmaceutical companies have implemented assays to evaluate bioactivation potential of new compounds with the goal of eliminating or minimizing reactive metabolite formation by rational structural modification of the problematic chemical series.

6.4.1 Experimental methodology to evaluate reactive metabolite formation

Reactive metabolite trapping. With the possible exception of acyl glucuronides and cyclic iminium ions, most reactive metabolites are short-lived and are not detectable in circulation. Their formation can be inferred from the characterization of stable conjugates formed via reaction with GSH. The presence of the soft nucleophilic thiol group in GSH ensures efficient conjugation to soft electrophilic centers on some reactive metabolites (e.g., Michael acceptors, epoxides, arene oxides, and alkyl halides) yielding stable sulfydryl conjugates.[15,16] Qualitative *in vitro* assessment of reactive metabolite formation usually involves "trapping" studies conducted with NADPH-supplemented human liver microsomes and exogenously added GSH or its corresponding ethyl ester.[17,18] Considering that drug-metabolizing enzymes other than cytochrome P450 (e.g., monoamine oxidases, aldehyde oxidase, alcohol dehydrogenases, myeloperoxidase, uridine 5′-diphosphoglucuronosyl transferase (UGT), and sulfotransferases) are also capable of catalyzing bioactivation, due consideration has to be given to the use of alternate metabolism vectors (e.g., liver cytosol, liver S-9 fractions, hepatocytes, and neutrophils), which support the activity of these enzymes. To detect GSH conjugates, mass spectrometry is the preferred tool, and the constant neutral loss of 129 Da corresponding to loss of the pyroglutamate group can be used to provide relatively sensitive detection.[19] GSH conjugate formation can also be analyzed in the negative scan mode using the precursors of m/z 272.[20] Efforts to maximize sensitivity, while providing semiquantitative data have been executed with stable isotope-labeled, fluorescent or fixed-charge GSH derivatives with some degree of success.[21–23] It is noteworthy to point out that not all reactive metabolites can be trapped with GSH. Hard electrophiles including DNA-reactive metabolites (e.g., electrophilic carbonyl compounds) will preferentially react with hard nucleophiles such as amines (e.g., semicarbazide and methoxylamine), amino acids (e.g., lysine), and DNA bases (e.g., guanine and cytosine) affording the corresponding Schiff base.[24,25] Likewise, the cyanide anion is a "hard" nucleophile that can be used to trap electrophilic iminium species that are generated via metabolism of acyclic and cyclic tertiary amines.[26,27] Overall, characterization of the sulfydryl, amine, or cyanide conjugate structures provides an insight into the reactive metabolite structure and the bioactivation pathway(s) responsible for its formation.

With acyl glucuronides, their reactivity with biological nucleophiles has been correlated with their intrinsic chemical stability, a feature that can be assessed by comparison of pseudo first-order degradation half-live values of the 1-*O*-acyl glucuronides and rate of acyl migration in *in vitro* studies.[28,29] This approach allows a rank ordering of acyl glucuronide stability, providing a preliminary assessment of their potential for covalent adduct formation leading to toxicity.[30,31] A limitation of this exercise is that, often times, efforts need to be invested in the chemical (or biochemical) preparation of the glucuronide metabolites.

Covalent binding. Assessment of the amount of *in vitro* metabolism-dependent covalent binding to biological tissue (e.g., microsomes, S-9, hepatocytes, neutrophils, and DNA) is possible if radiolabeled drug is available.[32] The assay provides quantitative estimates of radioactivity irreversibly bound to tissue but does not provide information about the nature of covalently modified proteins. Covalent binding studies can be performed *in vivo* as well. Either tissue or blood/plasma can be examined for the degree of covalent binding. However, covalent binding may require multiple dosing to establish the true impact of the compound. Reactive metabolites formed after the first dose may be efficiently trapped by GSH and eliminated from the body. After GSH is depleted, the extent of covalent binding with cellular macromolecules may increase rapidly, resulting in toxicity as seen in the case of acetaminophen.[6]

An example of this overall approach in elucidating novel bioactivation pathways is highlighted with studies on the potassium channel opener, maxipost (BMS-204352) (Figure 6.2), which undergoes a unique P450-mediated bioactivation reaction in rats, dogs, and humans to yield an electrophilic *o*-quinone-methide intermediate, which covalently binds to albumin *in vivo* in animals and human.[33,34] Acidic hydrolysis of plasma collected after intravenous administration of [^{14}C]-BMS-204352 to rats and human led to the characterization of a

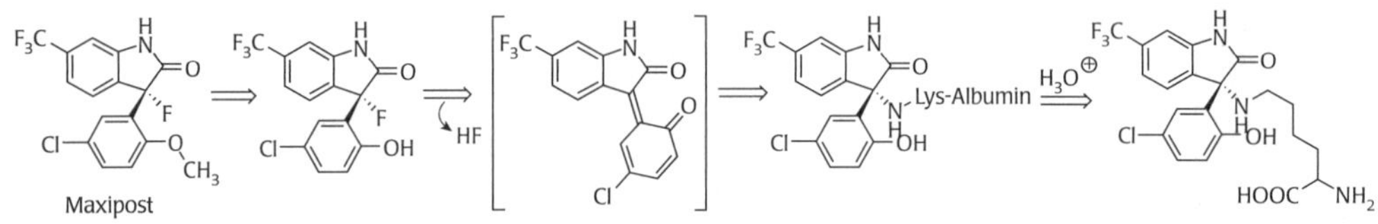

Figure 6-2: Bioactivation of the calcium channel opener maxipost in rat and human to a reactive quinone-methide, which covalently binds to albumin *in vivo*.

novel lysine conjugate of des-fluoro des-*O*-methyl BMS-204352 (see Figure 6.2). The relevance of the *in vivo* covalent binding observations with regards to maxipost toxicity remains unknown.

6.4.2 *In silico* and experimental tools for assessment of bioactivation potential of new compounds

To date, there are no examples where *in silico* tools have been utilized in a proactive fashion to predict reactive metabolite formation with small molecules. There are virtual or experimental techniques that can predict metabolic outcomes including the potential for forming reactive metabolites to some degree or the other. At best, these techniques have been used to rationalize published experimental observations on bioactivation pathways. Exploitation of these tools in drug discovery in a proactive fashion would necessitate additional experimental studies to validate the predictions.

Electrochemical oxidations. Electrochemistry has been used to mimic diverse phase I oxidative reactions such as aromatic hydroxylations, dehydrogenations, *O*- and *N*-dealkylations via the introduction of the compound into an electrochemical cell and applying a potential to the solution.[35,36] Several studies have also utilized electrochemical oxidations for mimicking reactive metabolite formation. Acetaminophen was one of the first examples wherein enzymatic two-electron oxidation to NAPQI was replicated via nonenzymatic, electrochemical means.[37] Since then, many enzymatic oxidation reactions, leading to reactive metabolites derived from, for example, electron-rich functional groups such as phenols, catechols, and aminophenols, have been mimicked by this technique.[38–42] In a prototypic process, a buffered solution of the compound (10–20 μ*M*) is infused through the electrochemical cell and a potential (0 – 600 – 1,000 mV) is applied continuously or in intervals. The experiment can be conducted in the presence of exogenous trapping agents such as GSH or *N*-acetylcysteine, which allows further structural characterization of the GSH conjugates. Specific examples of drugs where this approach has proven successful include amodiaquine, tolcapone and its downstream amine and acetanilide metabolites, diclofenac and its downstream 5-hydroxy- and 4′-hydroxy metabolites, clozapine, trimethoprim, and troglitazone (Figure 6.3).[38–42] All of these drugs are associated with some form of immune-mediated idiosyncratic toxicity[43–48] and a circumstantial link between toxicity and reactive metabolite formation has been demonstrated in

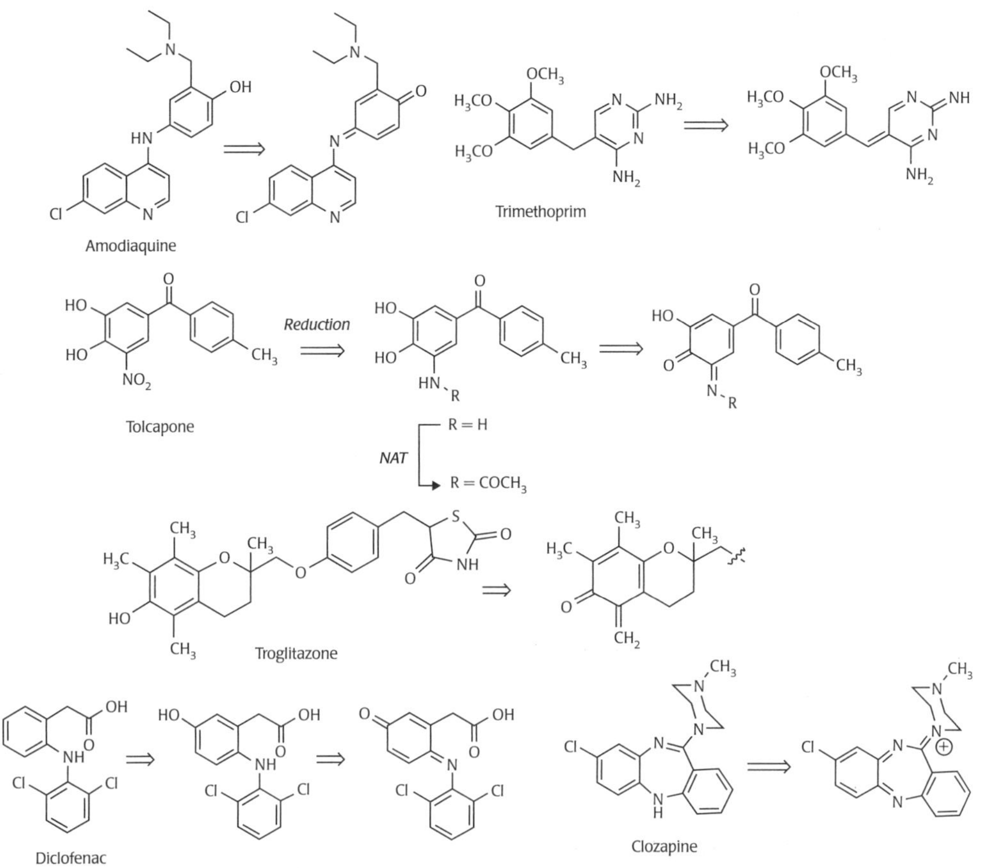

Figure 6-3: Examples of drugs evaluated for reactive metabolite formation via electrochemical and enzymatic oxidation processes.

each case.[39,49–54] In all cases, the GSH conjugates formed via electrochemical means were identical to the ones obtained by enzymatic reactions. Even though these findings suggest a commonality between enzymatic and nonenzymatic oxidative processes and a general correlation with oxidation potential, it is noteworthy to point out that most compounds typically chosen as substrates to highlight the utility of electrochemical oxidation are those that contain chemical architecture prone to a two-electron oxidation process leading to reactive quinonoid species. A limitation of this approach in terms of predicting reactive metabolite formation for new compounds becomes evident in the published studies on troglitazone and the related antidiabetic agents rosiglitazone and pioglitazone.[42] Electrochemical oxidation mimicked the P450-catalyzed oxidation of the chromane ring in troglitazone to afford the electrophilic quinone-methide, but the methodology failed to mimic the well-established P450-catalyzed bioactivation pathway involving thiazolidinedione ring scission in troglitazone, rosiglitazone, and pioglitazone,[54–56] as judged from the lack of formation of GSH conjugates of thiazolidinedione ring-opened metabolites.

Virtual predictions of metabolic (bioactivation) sites in molecules. The *in silico* tool *MetaSite* can identify the "most likely" sites of P450-mediated

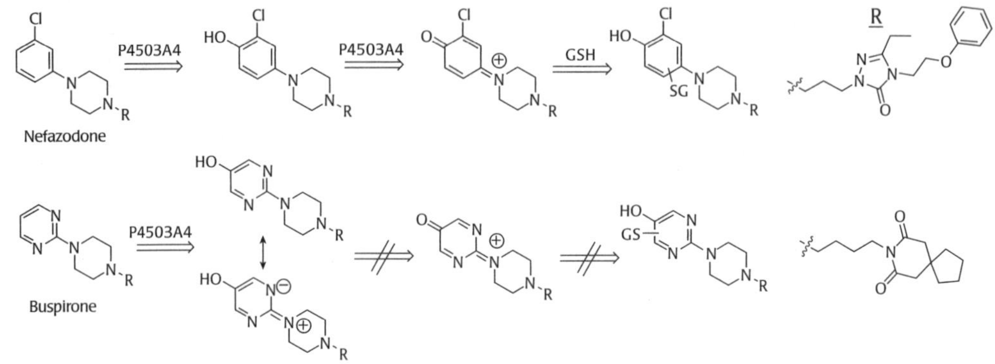

Figure 6-4: Differences in oxidative stability of the *para*-hydroxyphenyl-piperazinyl and -pyrimidinyl motifs in nefazodone and buspirone, respectively.

oxidative metabolism in structurally diverse compounds with a high degree of accuracy (> 80 percent success rate)[57] and has witnessed some success with regards to optimizing pharmacokinetic attributes (e.g., improvements in metabolic stability) of pharmacologic compounds and has potential utility to guide drug design efforts especially when prior information on metabolic fate does not exist.[58–60] There also appears to be some value in predicting reactive metabolite formation with new compounds, judging from our work using the software to optimize the metabolic stability of some neutral indomethacin amide derivatives.[60,61]

***Ab initio* calculations of oxidation potential**. Analogous to electrochemical oxidations, utility of theoretical quantum chemical calculations has focused mainly on estimating the ease with which certain electron-rich aromatic systems (e.g., catechols, hydroquinones, and *para*-hydroxyacetanilides) undergo enzyme-catalyzed two-electron oxidations to reactive metabolites. The impact of adjacent aromatic substituents on the relative rates of oxidation can also be taken into account to rationalize differences in oxidation profiles. This approach has seen some success as demonstrated in the retrospective *ab initio* analysis of acetaminophen oxidation,[62,63] and more recently, with the atypical neuroleptic drug remoxipride.[64] Although not explored in great detail, there may be some additional scope for *ab initio* calculations in early discovery toward predicting oxidative instability of electron-rich aromatic ring systems as demonstrated in our studies on the hepatotoxic and non-hepatotoxic drugs, nefazodone and buspirone, respectively.[65] While the *para*-hydroxyphenylpiperazine motif in *para*-hydroxynefazodone, a major circulating metabolite of nefazodone in man, was oxidized by P450 to the reactive quinone-imine, the corresponding *para*-hydroxypyrimidinylpiperazine metabolite of buspirone did not demonstrate this liability as judged from the lack of GSH adduct formation (Figure 6.4). The hypothesis that two-electron oxidation of *para*-hydroxybuspirone to the quinone-imine is less favorable due to differences in the protonation state at physiological pH and due to weaker resonance stabilization of the oxidation products (see Figure 6.4) was precisely predicted from *ab initio* measurements

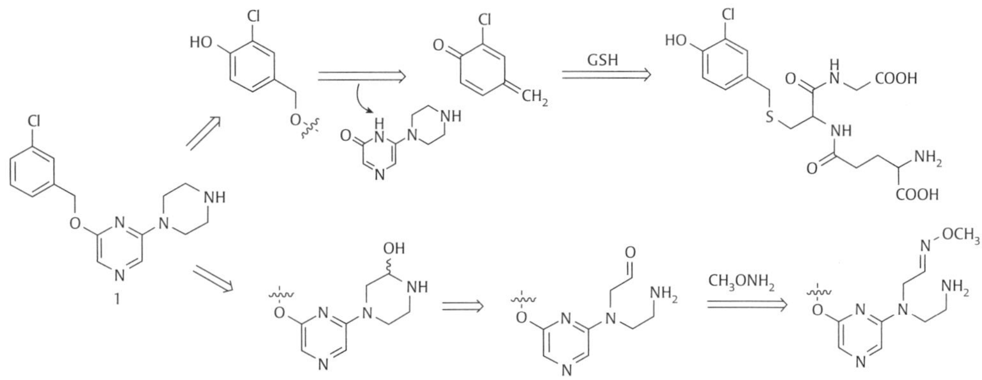

Figure 6-5: Proposed mechanism of bioactivation of the 5-HT_{2C} agonist 1, which leads to the formation of DNA-reactive metabolites.

on the relative oxidative stability of *N*-substituted *para*-hydroxynefazodone and -buspirone analogs.[65]

6.5 STRUCTURAL ALERT PREDICTIONS

A key requirement for reactive metabolite formation with any given molecule is the presence of a functionality and/or chemical architecture (referred to as structural alert/toxicophore) that is susceptible to bioactivation. The availability of methodology to assess bioactivation potential of drugs has clearly aided to replace a vague perception of a chemical class effect with a sharper picture of individual molecular peculiarity. Information to qualify certain functional groups as structural alerts also has been inferred from such studies based on numerous examples of drugs containing these motifs, which are metabolized to reactive metabolites and are associated with IADRs.[15,16] The presence or absence of a structural alert/toxicophore within a chemical structure can be inspected visually or via the use of the DEREK software. DEREK for Windows is a knowledge-based expert system that is often used to identify structural alerts in a chemical. Its predictions are based largely on common occurrences of structural features or toxicophores in literature compounds associated with reactive metabolite formation and ensuing toxicological response.[66] Consequently, if the software is not up to date with the current literature, there is a strong likelihood that chemical architecture associated with novel and complex bioactivation pathways leading to reactive metabolites will be missed. This is illustrated with two examples: first our work elucidating the bioactivation mechanism for the 5-hydroxytryptamine (5-HT)$_{2C}$ agonist and potential antiobesity agent 2-(3-chlorobenzyloxy)-6-(piperazin-1-yl)pyrazine (**1**) (Figure 6.5).[67] The S-9/NADPH-dependent genotoxic effects of **1** in the bacterial *Salmonella* Ames assay, which led to its discontinuation from clinical development, were unanticipated especially since visual inspection and/or presentation of the structure of **1** into the DEREK software did not reveal the presence of a structural alert(s). Reactive metabolite

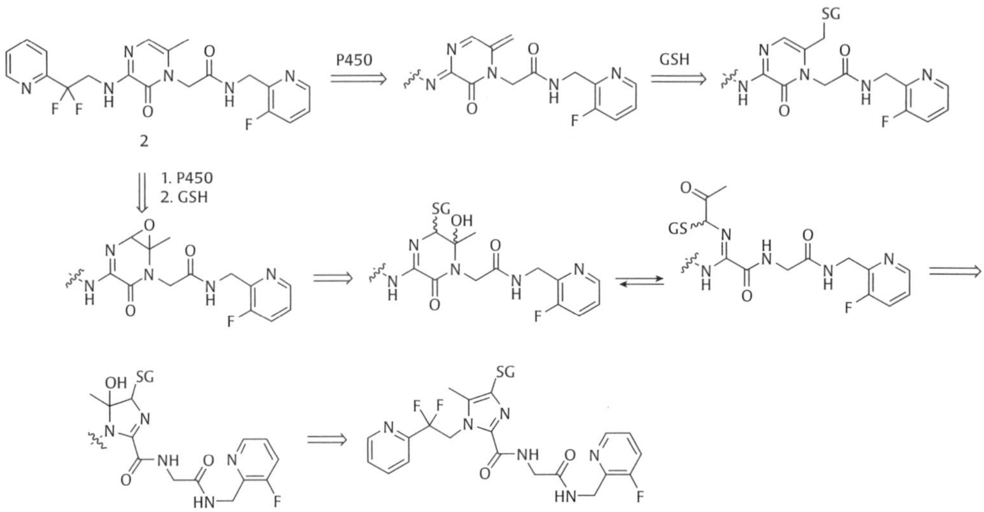

Figure 6-6: Unique pathways of bioactivation deciphered with the pyrazinone-based thrombin inhibitor *2*.

trapping studies in S-9/NADPH incubations containing exogenously added hard and soft nucleophilic trapping agents methoxylamine and GSH, respectively, led to the detection of several conjugates of **1** and its downstream metabolites; structural elucidation of these conjugates allowed an insight into fairly unique bioactivation pathways on the 3-chlorobenzyloxy and the piperazine ring system in **1**, which led to the formation of DNA-reactive metabolites (Figure 6.5). It is interesting to note that the bioactivation pathway on the 3-chlorobenzyloxy motif leading to the reactive quinone-methide is not easy to envision even for an expert mechanistic biotransformation scientist. Likewise, the role of the piperazine ring system in forming DNA-reactive metabolites is fairly unanticipated given the wide usage of this motif in medicinal chemistry and its presence in commercially successful drugs like sildenafil.

A second example is evident from the work of Singh et al.[68] on the pyrazinone-containing thrombin inhibitor **2**, which is associated with irreversible incorporation of radioactivity to human microsomal tissue and *in vivo* in the rat. Visual inspection of the structure as well as analysis in the DEREK program does not raise any concern with regards to the presence of structural alerts. However, mechanistic studies on reactive metabolite formation depict *de novo* metabolic routes of bioactivation on the latent pyrazinone-ring system, leading to the formation of reactive metabolites that adduct to GSH (Figure 6.6).

6.6 STRUCTURAL ALERTS AND DRUG DESIGN

Anecdotal evidence obtained from visual analysis of structures of several closely related toxic and nontoxic drugs suggests that drugs that lack toxicophores have a superior safety record, especially with regards to IADRs.[15] The evidence

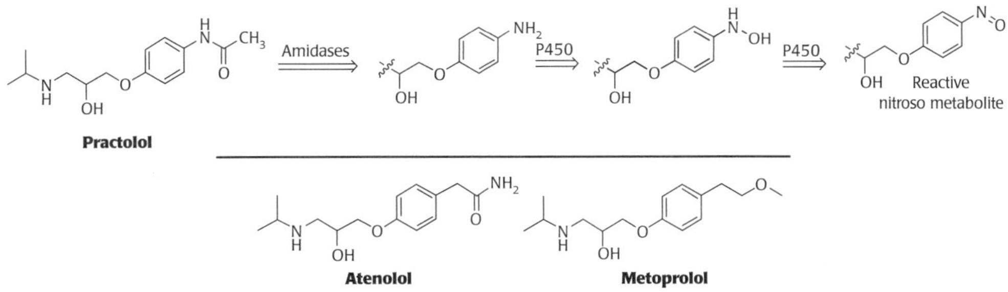

Figure 6-7: Structure-toxicity relationships with -adrenoceptor antagonists practolol, atenolol, and metoprolol.

becomes even more compelling when metabolism data supports the hypothesis as illustrated with the cardioselective β-adrenoceptor antagonists practolol, atenolol, and metoprolol. The mechanism of severe skin rashes induced by practolol is uncertain; however, a role for antinuclear antibodies, elicited by protein adducts of a reactive nitroso metabolite obtained from practolol biotransformation has been suspected (Figure 6.7),[69,70] in keeping with the observation that *cutaneous IADRs are not observed with atenolol and metoprolol, which lack the anilide toxicophore.* Consistent with this hypothesis are the findings that atenolol and metoprolol are metabolized by completely different pathways and are also subject to extensive urinary excretion as parent drugs.[71]

A second example is provided with the dibenzodiazepine derivatives and antipsychotic agents clozapine and quetiapine (Seroquel). While clozapine use is limited by a high incidence of agranulocytosis and hepatotoxicty, quetiapine does not cause these toxic events. As demonstrated earlier (see Figure 6.3), evidence that links clozapine toxicity to its propensity to form a reactive metabolite has been presented.[51,52] Proteins covalently modified with clozapine were also observed in neutrophils of patients being treated with clozapine, which reaffirms the relevance of the *in vitro* studies.[72] In the case of quetiapine, the bridging nitrogen in the benzodiazepine ring is replaced with a sulfur atom; consequently, this drug is not bioactivated to the reactive iminium species as shown with clozapine analogs.[73] Despite administration at doses comparable to clozapine, cases of agranulocytosis with quetiapine are extremely rare.

A final and perhaps an even more intriguing example of the influence that a subtle structural change can have on toxicity is highlighted with ibuprofen and ibufenac. Even though ibuprofen is considered to be one of the safest over-the-counter nonsteroidal anti-inflammatory drug (NSAID) in the market, its close-in analog ibufenac was withdrawn due to severe hepatotoxicity.[74] The daily doses of both NSAIDs were comparable, and the only structural difference between the two drugs is the presence of the additional α-methyl substituent adjacent to the carboxylic acid moiety in ibuprofen (Figure 6.8). Glucuronidation of the carboxylic acid moiety in most NSAIDs to the potentially electrophilic acyl glucuronide constitutes the principal elimination mechanism *in vivo* in humans.[29–31] As mentioned earlier, the proposed pathway of acyl glucuronide adduction with proteins involves condensation between the aldehyde group of a rearranged acyl

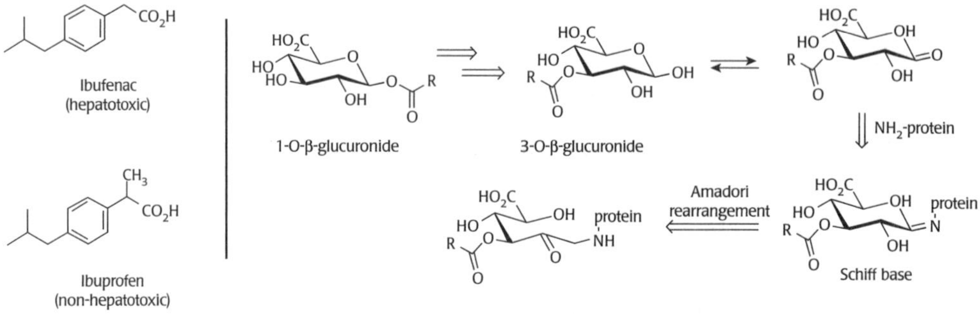

Figure 6-8: Reaction of acylglucuronides with proteins.

glucuronide and a lysine residue or an amine group of the *N* terminus, leading to the formation of a glycated protein. The formation of the iminium species is reversible but may be followed by an Amadori rearrangement of the imino sugar to the more stable 1-amino-2-keto product.[28,30,75] A structural relationship between acyl glucuronide degradation to the Schiff base and covalent binding has been established.[28,75] Acyl glucuronides of ibufenac and other acetic acid-based NSAIDs such as tolmetin and zomepirac, all of which have been withdrawn due to toxicity, exhibit the highest level of rearrangement and covalent binding, whereas mono-α-substituted acetic acids (2-substituted propionic acids) such as ibuprofen exhibit intermediate level of acyl glucuronide rearrangement and covalent binding. Overall, these observations imply that inherent electronic and steric properties must modulate the rate of acyl glucuronide rearrangement. Thus, in the case of ibuprofen, it is likely that presence of the α-methyl substituent slows the rearrangement of the acyl glucuronide to the electrophilic carbonyl intermediate.

In retrospect, the examples discussed previously imply that by avoiding toxicophores in drug design, one would lessen the odds that a drug candidate will lead to toxicity via a bioactivation mechanism. From a medicinal chemistry standpoint, this seems to be an attractive option and a path forward toward the discovery of safer drugs, especially given the lack of methodology to predict IADRs. However, it is noteworthy to point out that an exhaustive listing of structural alerts is far too comprehensive and also includes the phenyl ring that forms an electrophilic epoxide intermediate in the course of metabolism to a phenol.[16] Certainly, this is the mechanism underlying the toxicity of the organic solvents benzene and bromobenzene.[76,77] Likewise, avoiding structural alerts altogether can lead to missing out on potentially important medicines, as illustrated with atorvastatin (Lipitor), which contains the acetanilide structural alert; however, its metabolism by P450 results in the formation of acetaminophen-like metabolites (Figure 6.9).[78] Furthermore, glucuronidation of its carboxylic acid moiety results in the formation of the potentially electrophilic acyl glucuronide[79] in a manner similar to that discerned with NSAIDs (see Figure 6.9).

Finally, it is pivotal to point out that several blockbuster drugs contain toxicophores, which form reactive metabolites and covalently adduct to proteins, which in some cases is essential for pharmacological activity. For instance, the

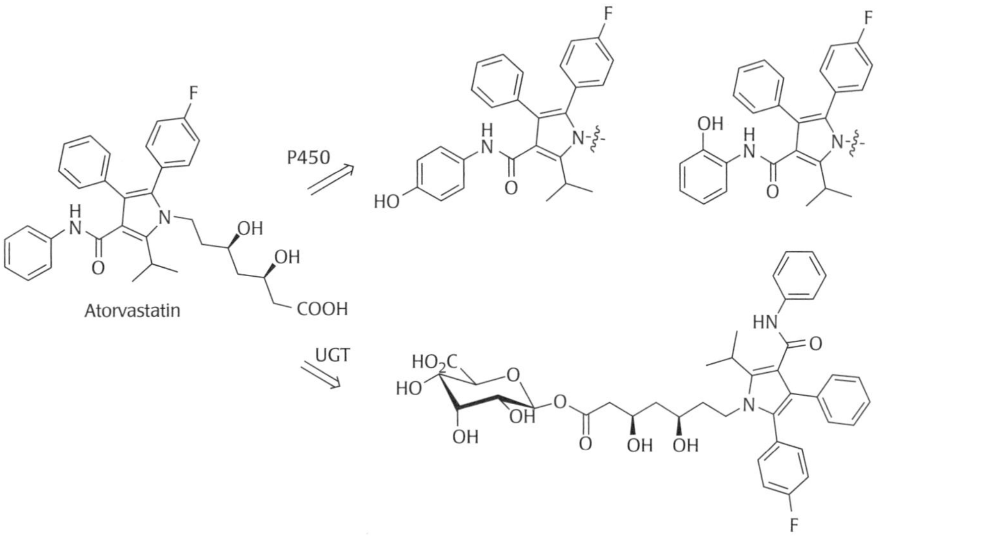

Figure 6-9: Chemical structures of atorvastatin and its metabolites derived from oxidative and conjugation pathways.

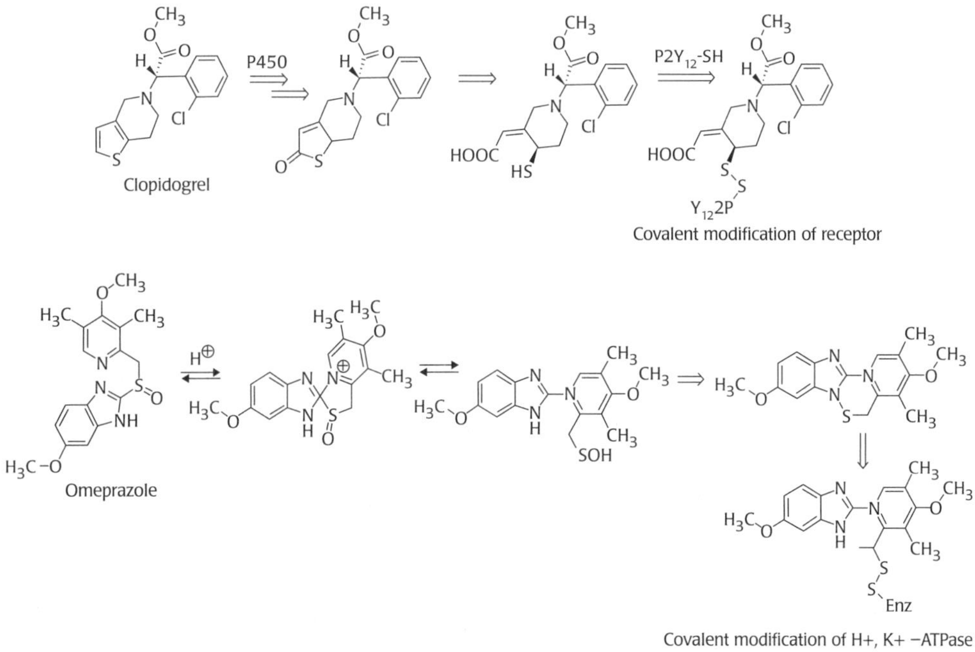

Figure 6-10: Examples of commercial blockbuster drugs, which require reactive metabolite formation for their pharmacologic action.

blockbuster cardiovascular drug and $P2Y_{12}$ antagonist clopidogrel (Plavix) by itself is inactive and requires P450-catalyzed bioactivation of its thiophene ring to form a reactive thiol metabolite, which forms a covalent disulfide bond with a cysteinyl residue on the $P2Y_{12}$ receptor in platelets (Figure 6.10), a phenomenon that gives rise to its beneficial cardiovascular effects.[80–82] Likewise, the benzimidazole class of proton-pump inhibitors used to treat gastric disorders, exemplified by omeprazole (one of the most profitable drugs during the late 1990s, with peak sales reaching $6 billion/year) by itself have no *in vitro* ability to inhibit the enzyme H^+, K^+-ATPase but are converted to a reactive sulfenamide intermediate in the acidic environment of the stomach. Covalent disulfide bond formation of this reactive species with an active site cytseine residue results in enzyme inactivation (see Figure 6.10).[83] Irreversible enzyme inhibition on account of covalent binding[84] is one pharmacokinetic benefit that contributes to making omeprazole clinically superior to H_2-receptor antagonists initially used to treat gastric acid disorders.

6.7 ARE REACTIVE METABOLITE TRAPPING AND COVALENT BINDING STUDIES RELIABLE PREDICTORS OF TOXICITY POTENTIAL OF DRUG CANDIDATES?

The examples discussed earlier in this chapter pose a significant challenge to the reliability of structural alerts, reactive metabolite trapping, and covalent binding measurements, as indicators of idiosyncratic drug toxicity. With regards to reactive metabolite formation potential, it is very important to consider factors that will influence the process for compounds containing a structural alert. These factors include (a) the presence of an alternate metabolic soft spot within the molecule that competes with structural alert bioactivation and (b) the existence of metabolic pathways that efficiently scavenge the reactive metabolite and/or its precursor. An example of the importance of the first point becomes evident upon comparison of the bioactivation potential of the benzodiazepine receptor ligands alpidem and zolpidem. Alpidem is hepatotoxic and has been withdrawn from the market; however, the commercial blockbuster zolpidem (Ambien) is devoid of the toxicity. A key structural difference in the two drugs is the replacement of the two chlorine atoms on the imidazopyridine nucleus in alpidem with two methyl groups in zolpidem. In alpidem, the imidazopyridine ring is bioactivated by P450 leading to the formation of a reactive arene oxide that reacts with GSH to yield sulfydryl conjugates (Figure 6.11), which have been detected in human excreta.[85] Even though bioactivation via epoxidation is also likely in zolpidem, the molecule does not undergo this metabolic fate; instead, the two methyl groups function as metabolic soft spots and are oxidized to the corresponding alcohol and carboxylic acid metabolites (Figure 6.11).

With respect to the importance of detoxication pathways, reactive metabolite formation may be discernible in standard *in vitro* systems, but the principal clearance mechanism of the drug *in vivo* may involve a distinctly different and perhaps more facile metabolic fate that does not yield reactive intermediates. This is illustrated with the selective estrogen receptor modulator raloxifene, which is known to undergo *in vitro* P4503A4-catalyzed bioactivation on its phenolic groups to yield reactive quinonoid species (Figure 6.12);[86] however, *in vivo*, glucuronidation of the same phenolic groups in the gut and liver constitute the

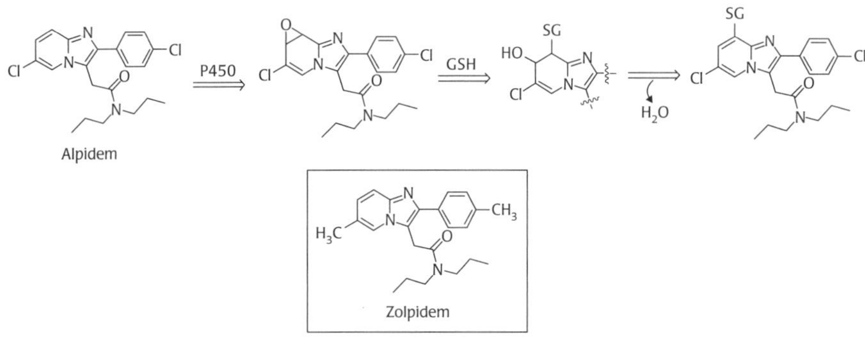

Figure 6-11: Differential metabolism of the anxiolytic agents alpidem (hepatotoxin) and zolpidem (non-hepatotoxin).

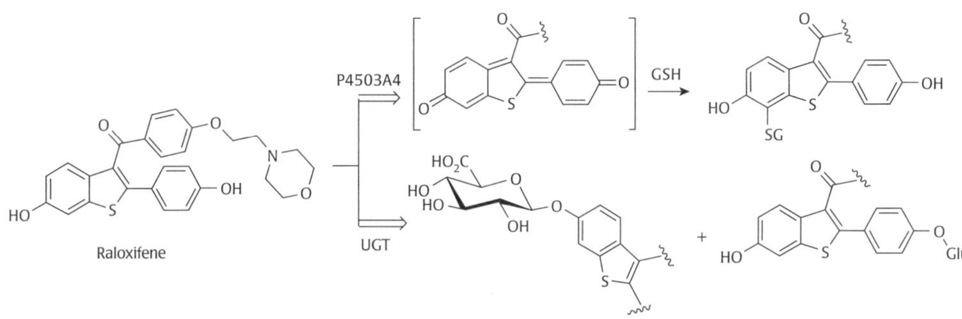

Figure 6-12: Bioactivation and competing detoxication pathways of the selective estrogen receptor modulator raloxifene.

principal elimination mechanism of raloxifene in humans (Figure 6.12).[87] Thus, the likelihood of raloxifene bioactivation *in vivo* is in question when compared with the phase II glucuronidation process, a phenomenon that may provide an explanation for the extremely rare occurrence of IADRs.

Although covalent binding data can provide a quantitative estimate of covalently bound radiolabeled drug to proteins and therefore an indirect measure of reactive metabolite formation, *no studies to date have shown a correlation between amount of reactive metabolite formed and/or extent of covalent binding and the probability that a drug will be associated with toxicity.* An example of this phenomenon is evident with the acetaminophen regioisomer, 3′-hydroxyacetanilide, which undergoes bioactivation yielding reactive metabolites that covalently adduct to GSH and proteins.[88] However, despite dose normalization to provide comparable levels of covalent binding *in vivo* in mice, 3′-hydroxyacetanilide does not exhibit the hepatotoxicity observed with acetaminophen. Furthermore, from a predictive standpoint, as a property itself, covalent binding *in vitro* has not been rigorously tested for its ability to distinguish between toxic and nontoxic drugs, primarily because nontoxic drugs have not been tested in covalent binding studies.[32,89]

We have tested the ability of covalent binding measurements in predicting idiosyncratic hepatotoxicity by examining the binding of eighteen drugs (nine hepatotoxins and nine nonhepatotoxins) to human hepatic tissue,

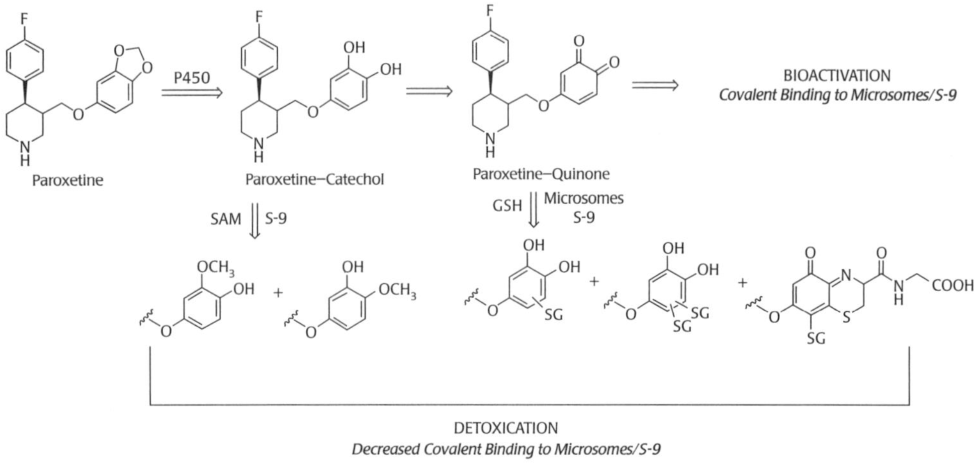

Figure 6-13: Parallel detoxication pathways that compete with the P450-catalyzed bioactivation pathway of the antidepressant paroxetine as explanation for its wide safety margin.

taking into consideration key factors such as reactive metabolite detoxication, relative importance of bioactivation leading to covalent binding versus overall metabolism, and daily dose for each drug.[90,91] Although most of the hepatotoxic drugs (e.g., acetaminophen, nefazodone, and tienilic acid) demonstrated covalent binding to some degree or the other, of great surprise were the findings that several non-hepatotoxic, commercially successful drugs such as buspirone, diphenhydramine, meloxicam, paroxetine, propranolol, raloxifene, and simvastatin demonstrated covalent binding. A quantitative comparison of covalent binding *in vitro* intrinsic clearance did not separate the two groups of compounds: in fact, paroxetine and diphenhydramine, both nonhepatotoxins, showed the greatest amount of covalent binding in microsomes. Including factors such as the fraction of total metabolism comprised by covalent binding and the total daily dose of each drug improved the discrimination between hepatotoxic and non-hepatotoxic drugs in liver microsomes, S-9, and hepatocytes; *however, the approach still would falsely identify some agents as potentially hepatotoxic.*

In the case of paroxetine, mechanistic studies further confirmed the importance of parallel metabolic and detoxication pathways in attenuating covalent binding to proteins.[92] As shown in Figure 6.13, the catechol metabolite obtained via ring scission of the 1,3-benzdioxole group in paroxetine can partition between *O*-methylation by catechol-*O*-methyl transferase or undergo oxidation to the reactive quinone intermediate, which is efficiently detoxicated by GSH; both pathways lead to a significant reduction in covalent binding. In humans, the *O*-methylated catechol derivatives constitute the principal metabolic fate of the drug. When coupled with the fact that the daily dose of paroxetine is low (20 mg), one gets some insight into the excellent safety record of this drug despite the bioactivation liability.

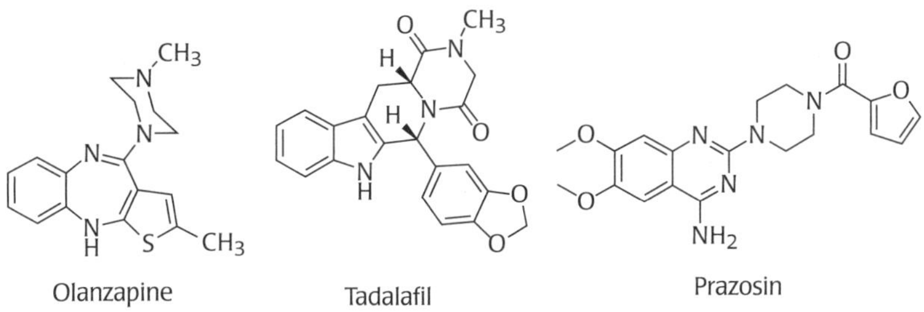

Figure 6-14: Examples of low daily dose drugs devoid of IADRs despite bioactivation liability.

6.8 DOSE AS AN IMPORTANT MITIGATING FACTOR FOR IADRS

A single most important factor in migrating IADR risks appears to be the daily dose of the drug. There are no examples of drugs that are dosed at < 20 mg/day that cause IADRs (whether or not these agents are prone to bioactivation). There are instances of two structurally related drugs that possess identical structural alerts susceptible to bioactivation, but the one administered at the lower dose is safer than the one given at a higher dose. It is likely that the improved safety of low-dose drugs arises from a marked reduction in the total body burden to reactive metabolite exposure; therefore, it is unlikely to exceed the threshold needed for toxicity. For example, the dibenzodiazepine derivative olanzapine (Zyprexa) (Figure 6.14) forms a reactive iminium metabolite very similar to the one observed with clozapine, yet olanzapine is not associated with a significant incidence of agranulocytosis. One difference between the two drugs is the daily dose; clozapine is given at a dose of > 300 mg/day, whereas the maximum recommended daily dose of olanzapine is 10 mg/day. Additional examples of this phenomenon are illustrated with tadalafil (Cialis), and the antihypertensive prazosin (Minipress) (see Figure 6.14). The methylenedioxyphenyl group in tadalafil undergoes P4503A4-catalyzed bioactivation to an electrophilic catechol, a process that also leads to the suicide inactivation of P4503A4 activity *in vitro*.[93] However, to date there are no reports of IADRs or P4503A4 drug–drug interactions associated with tadalafil use at the recommended dose of 10–20 mg/day. Likewise, there are no reports of IADRs with prazosin at the recommended daily dose of 1 mg/day, despite the bioactivation of the pendant furan ring to electrophilic intermediates, trapped with GSH and semicarbazide.[94]

6.9 CONCLUDING REMARKS

The issue of reactive metabolites continues to receive widespread interest in the pharmaceutical industry. Should evidence for reactive metabolite formation cause abandonment of an otherwise attractive drug candidate or initiate the often times challenging and time-consuming task of eliminating/minimizing their formation via rational chemical modifications? The current evidence suggests that detection of reactive metabolites for a chemical series does not warrant an instant demise of the compounds per se, but it does trigger some additional due diligence including the evaluation of competing detoxication pathways of the reactive metabolite and its precursor by phase I/phase II enzymes and an estimation of the human dose based on pharmacokinetic/pharmacodynamic studies in preclinical species. It is noteworthy to point out that the adduction of GSH with reactive metabolites is not necessarily a bad attribute; instead, it confirms the ability of the endogenous sulfydryl antioxidant to efficiently scavenge the electrophilic reactive intermediate. It is only in cases where the concentration of the reactive metabolite formed is so high that it depletes the endogenous antioxidant pool leading to toxicity as has been demonstrated with acetaminophen. It is important to emphasize that bioactivation is only one aspect of the overall risk–benefit assessment for advancing a drug candidate into development. Consequently, data from reactive metabolite trapping and covalent binding studies need to be placed in proper and broader context with previously discussed factors such as the daily dose and alternate routes of metabolism/detoxication. Likewise, appropriate consideration needs to be given for drug candidates for potential treatment options for unmet and urgent medical need.

The ability to predict the potential of a drug candidate to cause IADRs is dependent on a better understanding of the pathophysiological mechanisms of such reactions. IADRs are too complex to duplicate in a test tube, and their idiosyncratic nature precludes prospective clinical studies. Genetic factors also appear to have a crucial role in the induction of IADRs. A fruitful approach may therefore lie in focused and well-controlled phenotype/genotype studies of the rare patients who have survived this type of injury. For instance, results of a 500,000 single nucleotide polymorphism analysis in population exposed to the HIV agent abacavir-associated hypersensitivity reaction suggest that the known HLA-B gene region could be identified with as few as 15 cases and 200 population controls in a sequential analysis and as such has been instituted in practice to avoid the side effects.[95] An additional area of research includes studies on the identities of the protein targets of reactive metabolites discerned with toxic versus nontoxic drugs and on the combined application of covalent binding measurements with transcriptomic, metabonomic, and proteomic technologies in an effort to discern (and thereby predict) the characteristics of a toxic response. Until we develop a better understanding of the risk of toxicity arising from the formation of reactive metabolites, the advancement of potent (low-dose) drug candidates with only a limited propensity to form reactive intermediates would appear to be the most favored strategy in an ideal world.

REFERENCES

1. Kramer JA, Sagartz JE, Morris DL. The application of discovery toxicology and pathology towards the design of safer pharmaceutical lead candidates. *Nat Rev Drug Discov.* 2007;6(8):636–649.
2. Lasser KE, Allen PD, Woolhandler SJ, et al. Timing of new black box warnings and withdrawals for prescription medications. *JAMA.* 2002;287(17):2215–2220.

3. Olson H, Betton G, Robinson D, et al. Concordance of the toxicity of pharmaceuticals in humans and in animals. *Regul Toxicol Pharmacol.* 2000;32(1):56–67.
4. Miller EC, Miller JA. Mechanisms of chemical carcinogenesis: nature of proximate carcinogens and interactions with macromolecules. *Pharmacol Rev.* 1966;18(1):805–838.
5. Mitchell JR, Jollow DJ, Potter WZ, et al. Acetaminophen-induced hepatic necrosis. I. Role of drug metabolism. *J Pharmacol Exp Ther.* 1973;187(1):185–194.
6. Jollow DJ, Mitchell JR, Potter WZ, et al . Acetaminophen-induced hepatic necrosis. II. Role of covalent binding in vivo. *J Pharmacol Exp Ther.* 1973;187(1):195–202.
7. Potter WZ, Davis DC, Mitchell JR, et al. Acetaminophen-induced hepatic necrosis. III. Cytochrome P-450-mediated covalent binding in vitro. *J Pharmacol Exp Ther.* 1973;187(1):203–210.
8. Mitchell JR, Jollow D, Potter WZ, et al. Acetaminophen-induced hepatic necrosis. IV. Protective role of glutathione. *J Pharmacol Exp Ther.* 1973;187(1):211–217.
9. Dahlin DC, Miwa GT, Lu AY, et al. N-acetyl-p-benzoquinone imine: A cytochrome P-450-mediated oxidation product of acetaminophen. *Proc Natl Acad Sci USA.* 1984;81(5):1327–1331.
10. Zhao Z, Baldo BA, Rimmer J beta-Lactam allergenic determinants: fine structural recognition of a cross-reacting determinant on benzylpenicillin and cephalothin. *Clin Exp Allergy.* 2002;32(11):1644–1650.
11. Hess DA, Sisson ME, Suria H, et al. Cytotoxicity of sulfonamide reactive metabolites: Apoptosis and selective toxicity of CD8(+) cells by the hydroxylamine of sulfamethoxazole. *FASEB J.* 1999:13(13):1688–1698.
12. Lecoeur S, Andre C, Beaune PH. Tienilic acid-induced autoimmune hepatitis: Anti-liver and-kidney microsomal type 2 autoantibodies recognize a three-site conformational epitope on cytochrome P4502C9. *Mol Pharmacol.* 1996;50(2):326–333.
13. Bourdi M, Gautier, JC, Mircheva J, et al. Anti-liver microsomes autoantibodies and dihydralazine-induced hepatitis: Specificity of autoantibodies and inductive capacity of the drug. *Mol Pharmacol.* 1992;42(2):280–285.
14. Bourdi M, Chen W, Peter RM, et al. Human cytochrome P450 2E1 is a major autoantigen associated with halothane hepatitis. *Chem Res Toxicol.* 1996;9(7):1159–1166.
15. Kalgutkar AS, Soglia JR. Minimising the potential for metabolic activation in drug discovery. *Expert Opin Drug Metab Toxicol.* 2005;1(1):91–142.
16. Kalgutkar AS, Gardner I, Obach RS, et al. A comprehensive listing of bioactivation pathways of organic functional groups. *Curr Drug Metab.* 2005;6(3):161–225.
17. Correia MA, Krowech G, Caldera-Munoz P, et al. Morphine metabolism revisited. II. Isolation and chemical characterization of a glutathionylmorphine adduct from rat liver microsomal preparations. *Chem Biol Interact.* 1984;51(1):13–24.
18. Soglia JR, Harriman SP, Zhao S, et al. The development of a higher throughput reactive intermediate screening assay incorporating micro-bore liquid chromatography-micro-electrospray ionization-tandem mass spectrometry and glutathione ethyl ester as an in vitro conjugating agent. *J Pharm Biomed Anal.* 2004;36(1):105–116.
19. Baillie TA, Davis MR. Mass spectrometry in the analysis of glutathione conjugates. *Biol Mass Spectrom.* 1993;22(6):319–325.
20. Dieckhaus CM, Fernández-Metzler CL, King R, et al. Negative ion tandem mass spectrometry for the detection of glutathione conjugates. *Chem Res Toxicol.* 2005;18(4):630–638.
21. Mutlib A, Lam W, Atherton J, et al. Application of stable isotope labeled glutathione and rapid scanning mass spectrometers in detecting and characterizing reactive metabolites. *Rapid Commun Mass Spectrom.* 2005;19(23):3482–3492.
22. Gan J, Harper TW, Hsueh MM, et al. Dansyl glutathione as a trapping agent for the quantitative estimation and identification of reactive metabolites. *Chem Res Toxicol.* 2005;18(5):896–903.

23. Soglia JR, Contillo LG, Kalgutkar AS, et al. A semiquantitative method for the determination of reactive metabolite conjugate levels in vitro utilizing liquid chromatography-tandem mass spectrometry and novel quaternary ammonium glutathione analogues. *Chem Res Toxicol.* 2006;19(3):480–490.
24. Sahali-Sahly Y, Balani SK, Lin JH, et al. In vitro studies on the metabolic activation of the furanopyridine L-754,394, a highly potent and selective mechanism-based inhibitor of cytochrome P450 3A4. *Chem Res Toxicol.* 1996;9(6):1007–1012.
25. Olsen R, Molander P, Øvrebø S, et al. Reaction of glyoxal with 2′-deoxyguanosine, 2′-deoxyadenosine, 2′-deoxycytidine, cytidine, thymidine, and calf thymus DNA: identification of DNA adducts. *Chem Res Toxicol.* 2005;18(4):730–739.
26. Gorrod JW, Whittlesea CM, Lam SP. Trapping of reactive intermediates by incorporation of 14C-sodium cyanide during microsomal oxidation. *Adv Exp Med Biol.* 1991;283:657–664.
27. Argoti D, Liang L, Conteh A, et al. Cyanide trapping of iminium ion reactive intermediates followed by detection and structure identification using liquid chromatography-tandem mass spectrometry (LC-MS/MS). *Chem Res Toxicol.* 2005;18(10):1537–1544.
28. Walker GS, Atherton J, Bauman J, et al. Determination of degradation pathways and kinetics of acyl glucuronides by NMR spectroscopy. *Chem Res Toxicol.* 2007;20(6):876–886.
29. Johnson CH, Wilson ID, Harding JR, et al. NMR spectroscopic studies on the in vitro acyl glucuronide migration kinetics of Ibuprofen ((+/-)-(R,S)-2-(4-isobutylphenyl) propanoic acid), its metabolites, and analogues. *Anal Chem.* 2007;79(22):8720–8727.
30. Ding A, Ojingwa JC, McDonagh AF, et al. Evidence for covalent binding of acyl glucuronides to serum albumin via an imine mechanism as revealed by tandem mass spectrometry. *Proc Natl Acad Sci USA.* 1993;90(9):3797–3801.
31. Benet LZ, Spahn-Langguth H, Iwakawa S, et al. Predictability of the covalent binding of acidic drugs in man. *Life Sci.* 1993;53(8):PL141–146.
32. Evans DC, Watt AP, Nicoll-Griffith DA, et al. Drug-protein adducts: an industry perspective on minimizing the potential for drug bioactivation in drug discovery and development. *Chem Res Toxicol.* 2004;17(1):3–16.
33. Zhang D, Ogan M, Gedamke R, et al. Protein covalent binding of maxipost through a cytochrome P450-mediated ortho-quinone methide intermediate in rats. *Drug Metab Dispos.* 2003;31(7):837–845.
34. Zhang D, Krishna R, Wang L, et al. Metabolism, pharmacokinetics, and protein covalent binding of radiolabeled MaxiPost (BMS-204352) in humans. *Drug Metab Dispos.* 2005;33(1):83–93.
35. Jurva U, Wikstrom HV, Weidolf L, et al. Comparison between electrochemistry/mass spectrometry and cytochrome P450 catalyzed oxidation reactions. *Rapid Commun Mass Spectrom.* 2003;17(8):800–810.
36. Johansson T, Weidolf L, Jurva U. Mimicry of phase I drug metabolism – Novel methods for metabolite characterization and synthesis. *Rapid Commun Mass Spectrom.* 2007;21(14):2323–2331.
37. Getek TA, Korfmacher WA, McRae TA, et al. Utility of solution electrochemistry mass spectrometry for investigating the formation and detection of biologically important conjugates of acetaminophen. *J Chromatogr.* 1989;474(1):245–256.
38. Jurva U, Holmen A, Gronberg G, et al. Electrochemical generation of electrophilic drug metabolites: Characterization of amodiaquine quinoneimine and cysteinyl conjugates by MS, IR, and NMR. *Chem Res Toxicol.* 2008;21(4):928–935.
39. Smith KS, Smith PL, Heady TN, et al. In vitro metabolism of tolcapone to reactive intermediates: Relevance to tolcapone liver toxicity. *Chem Res Toxicol.* 2003;16(2):123–128.
40. Madsen KG, Skonberg C, Jurva U, et al. Bioactivation of diclofenac in vitro and in vivo: Correlation to electrochemical studies. *Chem Res Toxicol.* 2008;21(5):1107–1119.

41. Madsen KG, Olsen J, Skonberg C, et al. Development and evaluation of an electrochemical method for studying reactive phase-I metabolites: Correlation to in vitro drug metabolism. *Chem Res Toxicol.* 2007;20(5):821–831.
42. Madsen KG, Gronberg G, Skonberg C, et al. Electrochemical oxidation of troglitazone: Identification and characterization of the major reactive metabolite in liver microsomes. *Chem Res Toxicol.* 2008;21(10):2035–2041.
43. Larrey D, Tinel M, Amouyal G, et al. Genetically determined oxidation polymorphism and drug hepatotoxicity. Study of 51 patients. *J Hepatol.* 1989;8(2):158–164.
44. Olanow CW. Tolcapone and hepatotoxic effects. Tasmar advisory panel. *Arch Neurol.* 2000;57(2)263–267.
45. Aithal GP. Diclofenac-induced liver injury: A paradigm of idiosyncratic drug toxicity. *Expert Opin Drug Saf.* 2004;3(6):519–523.
46. Schulte PF. Risk of clozapine-associated agranulocytosis and mandatory white blood cell monitoring. *Ann Pharmacother.* 2006;40(4):683–688.
47. Burt RA. Review of adverse reactions associated with cinoxacin and other drugs used to treat urinary tract infections. *Urology.* 1984;23(1):101–107.
48. Faich GA, Moseley RH. Troglitazone (Rezulin) and hepatic injury. *Pharmacoepidemiol Drug Saf.* 2001;30(2):155–160.
49. O'Neill PM, Harrison AC, Storr RC, et al. The effect of fluorine substitution on the metabolism and antimalarial activity of amodiaquine. *J Med Chem.* 1994;37(9): 1362–1370.
50. Tang W. The metabolism of diclofenac – Enzymology and toxicology perspectives. *Curr Drug Metab.* 2003;4(4):319–329.
51. Liu ZC, Uetrecht JP. Clozapine is oxidized by activated human neutrophils to a reactive nitrenium ion that irreversibly binds to the cells. *J Pharmacol Exp Ther.* 1995;275(3):1476–1483.
52. Uetrecht JP. Metabolism of clozapine by neutrophils. Possible implications for clozapine-induced agranulocytosis. *Drug Saf.* 1992;7(Suppl 1):51–56.
53. Lai WG, Zahid N, Uetrecht JP. Metabolism of trimethoprim to a reactive iminoquinone methide by activated human neutrophils and hepatic microsomes. *J Pharmacol Exp Ther.* 1999;291(1):292–299.
54. Kassahun K, Pearson PG, Tang W, et al. Studies on the metabolism of troglitazone to reactive intermediates in vitro and in vivo. Evidence for novel biotransformation pathways involving quinone methide formation and thiazolidinedione ring scission. *Chem Res Toxicol.* 2001;14(1):62–70.
55. Alvarez-Sanchez R, Montavon F, Hartung T, et al. Thiazolidinedione bioactivation: A comparison of the bioactivation potentials of troglitazone, rosiglitazone, and pioglitazone using stable isotope-labeled analogues and liquid chromatography tandem mass spectrometry. *Chem Res Toxicol.* 2006;19(8):1106–1116.
56. Baughman TM, Graham RA, Wells-Knecht K, et al. Metabolic activation of pioglitazone identified from rat and human liver microsomes and freshly isolated hepatocytes. *Drug Metab Dispos.* 2005;33(6):733–738.
57. Cruciani G, Carosati E, De Boeck B, et al. MetaSite: Understanding metabolism in human cytochromes from the perspective of the chemist. *J Med Chem.* 2005;48(22):6970–6979.
58. Trunzer M, Faller B, Zimmerlin A. Metabolic soft spot identification and compound optimization in early discovery phases using MetaSite and LC-MS/MS validation. *J Med Chem.* 2009;52(2):329–335.
59. Ahlström MM, Ridderström M, Zamora I, et al. CYP2C9 structure-metabolism relationships: Optimizing the metabolic stability of COX-2 inhibitors. *J Med Chem.* 2007;50(18):4444–4452.
60. Boyer D, Bauman JN, Walker DP, et al. Utility of *MetaSite* in improving metabolic stability of the neutral indomethacin amide derivative and selective cyclooxygenase-2 (COX-2) inhibitor 2-(1-(4-chlorobenzoyl)-5-methoxy-2-methyl-1*H*-indol-3-yl]-*N*-phenethyl-acetamide. *Drug Metab Dispos.* 2009;37(5):999–1008.

61. Remmel RP, Crews BC, Kozak KR, et al. Studies on the metabolism of the novel, selective cyclooxygenase-2 inhibitor indomethacin phenethylamide in rat, mouse, and human liver microsomes: Identification of active metabolites. *Drug Metab Dispos.* 2004;32(1):113–122.
62. Koymans L, van Lenthe JH, van de Straat R, et al. A theoretical study on the metabolic activation of paracetamol by cytochrome P-450: Indications for a uniform oxidation mechanism. *Chem Res Toxicol.* 1989;2(1):60–66.
63. Koymans L, Van Lenthe JH, Donné-op Den Kelder GM, et al. Mechanisms of activation of phenacetin to reactive metabolites by cytochrome P-450: A theoretical study involving radical intermediates. *Mol Pharmacol.* 1990;37(3):452–460.
64. Erve JC, Svensson MA, von Euler-Chelpin H, et al. Characterization of glutathione conjugates of the remoxipride hydroquinone metabolite NCQ-344 formed in vitro and detection following oxidation by human neutrophils. *Chem Res Toxicol.* 2004;17(4):564–571.
65. Kalgutkar AS, Vaz AD, Lame ME, et al. Bioactivation of the nontricyclic antidepressant nefazodone to a reactive quinone-imine species in human liver microsomes and recombinant cytochrome P450 3A4. *Drug Metab Dispos.* 2005;33(2):243–253.
66. Dearden JC. In silico prediction of drug toxicity. *J Comput Aided Mol Des.* 2003;17(2–4):119–127.
67. Kalgutkar AS, Dalvie DK, Aubrecht J, et al. Genotoxicity of 2-(3-chlorobenzyloxy)-6-(piperazinyl)pyrazine, a novel 5-hydroxytryptamine2c receptor agonist for the treatment of obesity: Role of metabolic activation. *Drug Metab Dispos.* 2007;35(6):848–858.
68. Singh R, Silva Elipe MV, Pearson PG, et al. Metabolic activation of a pyrazinone-containing thrombin inhibitor. Evidence for novel biotransformation involving pyrazinone ring oxidation, rearrangement, and covalent binding to proteins. *Chem Res Toxicol.* 2003;16(2):198–207.
69. Amos HE, Lake BG, Artis J. Possible role of antibody specific for a practolol metabolite in the pathogenesis of oculomucocutaneous syndrome. *Br Med J.* 1978;1(6110):402–404.
70. Orton C, Lowery C. Practolol metabolism. III. Irreversible binding of [14C] practolol metabolite(s) to mammalian liver microsomes. *J Pharmacol Exp Ther.* 1981;219(1):207–212.
71. Borchard U. Pharmacokinetics of beta-adrenoceptor blocking agents: Clinical significance of hepatic and/or renal clearance. *Clin Physiol Biochem.* 1990;8(Suppl 2):28–34.
72. Gardner I, Leeder JS, Chin T, et al. A comparison of the covalent binding of clozapine and olanzapine to human neutrophils in vitro and in vivo. *Mol Pharmacol.* 1998;53(6):999–1008.
73. Uetrecht J, Zahid N, Tehim A, et al. Structural features associated with reactive metabolite formation in clozapine analogues. *Chem Biol Interact.* 1997;104(2–3)117–129.
74. Goldkind L, Laine L. A systematic review of NSAIDs withdrawn from the market due to hepatotoxicity: Lessons learned from the bromfenac experience. *Pharmacoepidemiol Drug Saf.* 2006;15(4):213–220.
75. Wang J, Davis M, Li F, et al. A novel approach for predicting acyl glucuronide reactivity via Schiff base formation: Development of rapidly formed peptide adducts for LC/MS/MS measurements. *Chem Res Toxicol.* 2004;17(9):1206–1216.
76. Yardley-Jones A, Anderson D, Parke DV. The toxicity of benzene and its metabolism and molecular pathology in human risk assessment. *Br J Ind Med.* 1991;48(7):437–444.
77. Rietjens IM, den Besten C, Hanzlik RP, et al. Cytochrome P450-catalyzed oxidation of halobenzene derivatives. *Chem Res Toxicol.* 1997;10(6):629–635.
78. Jacobsen W, Kuhn B, Soldner A, et al. Lactonization is the critical first step in the disposition of the 3-hydroxy-3-methylglutaryl-CoA reductase inhibitor atorvastatin. *Drug Metab Dispos.* 2000;28(11):1369–1378.

79. Prueksaritanont T, Subramanian R, Fang X, et al. Glucuronidation of statins in animals and humans: A novel mechanism of statin lactonization. *Drug Metab Dispos.* 2002;30(5):505–512.
80. Savi P, Pereillo JM, Uzabiaga MF, et al. Identification and biological activity of the active metabolite of clopidogrel. *Thromb Haemost.* 2000;84(5):891–896.
81. Savi P, Zachayus JL, Delesque-Touchard N, et al. The active metabolite of Clopidogrel disrupts P2Y12 receptor oligomers and partitions them out of lipid rafts. *Proc Natl Acad Sci USA.* 2006;103(29):11069–11074.
82. Herbert JM, Savi P. P2Y12, a new platelet ADP receptor, target of clopidogrel. *Semin Vasc Med.* 2003;3(2):113–122.
83. Olbe L, Carlsson E, Lindberg P. A proton-pump inhibitor expedition: The case histories of omeprazole and esomeprazole. *Nat Rev Drug Discov.* 2003;2(2):132–139.
84. Fellenius E, Berglindh T, Sachs G, et al. Substituted benzimidazoles inhibit gastric acid secretion by blocking (H+ + K+)ATPase. *Nature.* 1981;290(5802):159–161.
85. Durand A, Thenot JP, Bianchetti G, et al. Comparative pharmacokinetic profile of two imidazopyridine drugs: Zolpidem and alpidem. *Drug Metab Rev.* 1992;24(2):239–266.
86. Chen Q, Ngui JS, Doss GA, et al. Cytochrome P450 3A4-mediated bioactivation of raloxifene: Irreversible enzyme inhibition and thiol adduct formation. *Chem Res Toxicol.* 2002;15(7):907–914.
87. Kemp DC, Fan PW, Stevens JC. Characterization of raloxifene glucuronidation in vitro: Contribution of intestinal metabolism to presystemic clearance. *Drug Metab Dispos.* 2002;30(6):694–700.
88. Rashed MS, Streeter AJ, Nelson SD. Investigations of the N-hydroxylation of 3′-hydroxyacetanilide, a non-hepatotoxic potential isomer of acetaminophen. *Drug Metab Dispos.* 1989;17(4):355–359.
89. Masubuchi N, Makino C, Murayama N. Prediction of in vivo potential for metabolic activation of drugs into chemically reactive intermediate: Correlation of in vitro and in vivo generation of reactive intermediates and in vitro glutathione conjugate formation in rats and humans. *Chem Res Toxicol.* 2007;20(3):455–464.
90. Obach RS, Kalgutkar AS, Soglia JR, et al. Can in vitro metabolism-dependent covalent binding data in liver microsomes distinguish hepatotoxic from nonhepatotoxic drugs? An analysis of 18 drugs with consideration of intrinsic clearance and daily dose. *Chem Res Toxicol.* 2008;21(9):1814–1822.
91. Bauman JN, Kelly JM, Tripathy S, et al. Can in vitro metabolism-dependent covalent binding data distinguish hepatotoxic from nonhepatotoxic drugs? An analysis using human hepatocytes and liver S-9 fraction. *Chem Res Toxicol.* 2009;22(2):332–340.
92. Zhao SX, Dalvie DK, Kelly JM, et al. NADPH-dependent covalent binding of [3H] paroxetine to human liver microsomes and S-9 fractions: Identification of an electrophilic quinone metabolite of paroxetine. *Chem Res Toxicol.* 2007;20(11):1649–1657.
93. Ring BJ, Patterson BE, Mitchell MI, et al. Effect of tadalafil on cytochrome P450 3A4-mediated clearance: Studies in vitro and in vivo. *Clin Pharmacol Ther.* 2005;77(1):63–75.
94. Erve JC, Vashishtha SC, DeMaio W, et al. Metabolism of prazosin in rat, dog, and human liver microsomes and cryopreserved rat and human hepatocytes and characterization of metabolites by liquid chromatography/tandem mass spectrometry. *Drug Metab Dispos.* 2007;35(6):908–916.
95. Hughes AR, Brothers CH, Mosteller M, et al. Genetic association studies to detect adverse drug reactions: Abacavir hypersensitivity as an example. *Pharmacogenomics.* 2009;10(2):225–233.

7 **Immunotoxicity**

Technologies for predicting immune stimulation, a focus on nucleic acids and haptens

Jörg Vollmer

7.1 ADVERSE DRUG REACTIONS MEDIATED BY THE ADAPTIVE IMMUNE SYSTEM

The adaptive immune system is responsible for the occurrence of drug allergies after applying certain chemicals for example to the skin. Symptoms of such allergic hypersensitivities are observed only in the elicitation phase and not in the preceding sensitization phase, as only the second exposure to the causative drug results in T cell- or antibody-mediated adverse effects.

In 1935, Karl Landsteiner introduced for the first time low molecular reactive chemicals as haptens,[1] which after covalent coupling to proteins induce hapten-specific antibodies, or stimulate specific T cell responses. Hapten recognition by T cells requires covalent attachment of the hapten to major histocompatibility complex (MHC)-associated peptides on antigen-presenting cells (APCs), for example with trinitrophenyl (TNP).[2,3] However, nonreactive drugs also can result in T and B cell-mediated allergic hyperreactivities. Such so-called prohaptens upon cellular metabolism are transformed into reactive metabolites that are able to bind to MHC-binding self peptides. One of the best studied examples for prohaptens is urushiol from the North American poison ivy.[4] In addition to haptens and prohaptens, transition metals such as chromium, beryllium, or nickel are important contact allergens in the industrialized world.[5] In rare cases, topical antibiotics such as beta-lactams can result in allergic contact dermatitis, a well-documented side effect of such antibiotics (e.g., penicillin).[6,7] In addition, animal or plant proteins as well may induce allergic skin reactions and contact hypersensitivities.[8]

In vivo, drug-protein (hapten-carrier) complexes can be taken up by APCs, are transported into local draining lymph nodes, and are processed and/or presented to naïve T cells by MHCs on APCs. T cells with the appropriate specificity recognize these complexes and are induced to proliferate and expand as primed T cells. In addition, hapten-carrier complexes can be antigenic for B cells. Such hapten-carrier complex-specific B cells, in the presence of T cell help, proliferate and differentiate into plasma cells that produce different antibody isotypes.

Haptens or prohaptens can induce type I to IV immune reactions (Gell and Coombs classification)[9]: IgE-mediated drug hypersensitivity (type I), IgG-mediated cytotoxicity (type II), immune complex deposition (type III), and T cell-mediated hypersensitivity (type IV). The IgE-mediated hypersensitivity is one of the two most frequently observed drug allergies (which are of type I and IV). The first contact with the drug results in the formation of drug-specific IgE antibodies, which upon secondary contact lead to activation of mast cells, release of inflammatory factors (e.g., histamines, leukotrienes, or cytokines), and symptoms such as vasodilation, increased vascular permeability, or bronchoconstriction.

The second most frequent drug allergy is the T cell-mediated hypersensitivity. Chemicals that come in contact with the skin can induce contact hypersensitivity reactions. Hapten-specific T cells are guided to the site of allergen contact, most probably due to continued or subsequent exposure of the site to the allergen,[10] and result in immune-mediated skin reactions through the release of, for example, cytokines or chemokines.

7.2 NICKEL-MEDIATED CONTACT HYPERSENSITIVITY

Nickel is the most prevalent contact allergen in the industrialized world, and studies on the induction of T cell-mediated immune responses to nickel help to better understand allergic reactions to contact allergens.[11]

T cells can respond to Ni-MHC-peptide complexes similar to normal haptens covalently bound to self peptides in the MHC-binding groove of APCs (Figure 7.1). For example, Lu et al.[12] demonstrated that nickel can form a complex with a self peptide and a MHC Class II (MHC-DR) protein, and specific T cell responses were dependent on a certain amino acid residue in the MHC beta chain presenting the peptide to the T cell receptor. It is possible that nickel complexed to the MHC-bound peptide interacts with some portion of the T cell receptor alpha chain. Indeed, a certain amino acid position in the T cell receptor alpha CDR2 region of a nickel-specific T cell receptor was suggested to participate in the nickel-mediated T cell activation.[13] Moreover, on the site of the T cell receptor, it was shown that strongly sensitized nickel allergic individuals over-represented the T cell receptor Vbeta17 element.[14,15] In such nickel-specific T cell receptors an Arg-Asp motif in the T cell receptor beta CDR3 region was suggested as another contact site of the T cell receptor to the nickel-peptide-MHC complex.[16]

Gamerdinger et al.[17] described nickel that behaved different from classical haptens (Figure 7.1). Nickel-mediated T cell receptor stimulation can be totally independent of the nature of the peptide associated with the restricting HLA Class II (HLA-DR) molecule, and antigen contacts localize solely to the T cell receptor alpha chain. Such a stimulation is reminiscent of superantigen-mediated activation, bridging suitable T cell receptor alpha chain elements with MHC molecules independent of the kind of associated peptide and of the specificity of the T cell receptor.[18] Besides these hapten-like or -unlike nickel reactions, interference of nickel with the processing of self proteins, and the exposure of reactive T cells to modified, cryptic self peptides was suggested to be responsible for nickel contact hypersensitivities[19] (Figure 7.1).

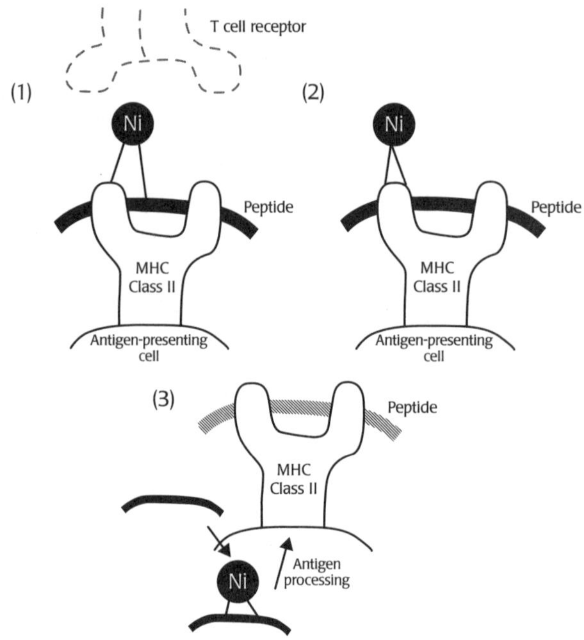

Figure 7-1: Activation of T cells by metal ions. Nickel and other metal ions appear to activate specific T cells by several different molecular mechanisms. (1) T cells with their T cell receptor respond to complexes of nickel with MHC-peptide similar to other hapten–peptide complexes. (2) Nickel forms a direct linker between MHC and the T cell receptor independent of the peptide with some similarities to superantigen-mediated T cell stimulation. (3) The processing of self peptides is disturbed by nickel resulting in cryptic self peptides presented to a T cell receptor.

7.3 TECHNOLOGIES TO PREDICT CONTACT SENSITIZATION

Patients with suspected allergic contact hypersensitivities usually are skin patch tested with a number of the most common contact allergens.[20] Simple identification of potential sensitizing chemicals can be performed *in vivo* or *in vitro*. A small number of guinea pig tests used for the assessment of skin sensitization exist.[21] Such tests as the Buehler occluded patch test and the guinea pig maximization test use protocols including an induction phase of contact hypersensitivity, an elicitation (or "challenge") phase, and a final subjective visual assessment of potential skin reactions. In contrast, in the local lymph node assay, the immune response during the induction phase and not elicitation phase is measured by the ability of a potential allergen to stimulate proliferative responses in draining lymph nodes following repeated topical exposure.[21]

Predictive *in vitro* test methods are as well developed as nonanimal test alternatives, including specific cell-based assays.[22] Such cellular assays include the culture of keratinocytes that represent very often the first cells in the skin to encounter potential reactive chemicals. Purified keratinocytes are cultured with a specific test chemical, and the production of proinflammatory cytokines or chemokines are then measured. Another cell population that can be used to test for chemicals inducing contact allergy are Langerhans cells (LCs). LCs are the antigen-presenting cells of the skin and play a critical role in the development of skin hypersensitivities.[23,24] However, only small populations of LCs can be isolated from the skin so that the use of LCs is hampered.[25] If LCs are used, it is possible to measure upon contact with a potential hapten or prohapten: changes in cell surface marker expression, internalization of MHC class II molecules from the cell surface, tyrosine phosphorylation, or induction of LC migration.[25] Instead of LCs, (dermal) dendritic cells (DCs) either generated *in vitro* or purified from peripheral blood mononuclear cells (PBMC) or from skin can be used.[25,26] DCs are antigen-presenting cells, and culture with contact allergens can result in phenotypic alterations, changes in cell surface marker expression, internalization of MHC class II molecules, or cytokine production.

In addition to these simpler cell-based assays, more complex assays can be employed to measure the induction of specific T cell responses to haptens. It is possible to stimulate naïve T cells to proliferate *in vitro* in the presence of antigen-presenting cells such as LCs.[27,28] In addition, effector T cells (T cell clones) can be used to investigate T cell stimulation induced by haptens in the presence of the appropriate antigen-presenting cells.[29,30] Another complex, but easy to use assay is based on the culture of purified human PBMC in the presence of potential reactive chemicals, and the measurement of proliferation or cytokine production.[31–33]

7.4 ADVERSE DRUG REACTIONS MEDIATED BY THE INNATE IMMUNE SYSTEM

7.4.1 Nucleic acids stimulating Toll-like receptor 9

One of the best understood pathways to induce innate immune activation is the family of Toll-like receptors (TLRs). TLRs detect highly conserved components of pathogens that are not present in our own cells. The TLRs appear to have evolved as a warning system to detect infections, and in some cases they can be triggered by synthetic nucleic acid therapeutics or accidentally by self molecules.[34]

Therapeutic targeting strategies using nucleic acids have the potential to impact a broad array of human diseases. For example, antisense oligodeoxynucleotides (AS ODNs) are short synthetic single-stranded DNA oligonucleotides designed to target specific mRNAs to eliminate a subsequent event like mRNA splicing or translation. Certain phosphorothioate (PS) AS ODNs of the first generation were found to induce strong and unexpected immune stimulatory effects.[35–37] Specific sequence motifs can be found in such AS ODNs that contain a central deoxycytidyl-deoxyguanosin CpG dinucleotide, in which the cytosine nucleobase is unmethylated.[38] The receptor responsible for CpG-mediated immune effects, TLR9,[39] detects a subtle difference in vertebrate DNA compared to that of pathogens.[40] Genomic DNAs in vertebrates in contrast to bacterial and viral DNAs are mostly methylated at cytosines that are followed by

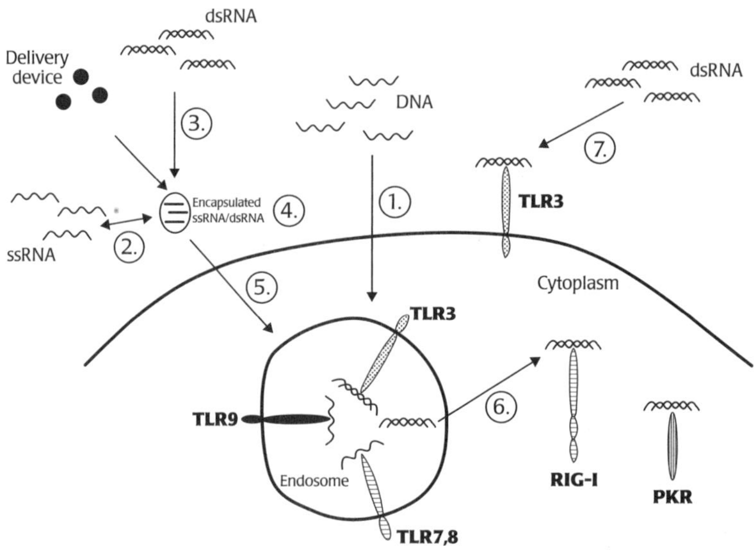

Figure 7-2: Activation of nucleic acid receptors by RNA or DNA. The innate immune system expresses a variety of different receptors responding to foreign but also synthetic nucleic acids. Single-stranded DNA oligonucleotides such as PS AS ODNs enter the cell and localize to endosomes (1) where they are recognized by TLR9. Signaling induced via TLR9 results in a variety of immune effects such as IFN-alpha production from pDCs. Single-stranded immune stimulatory RNA oligonucleotides (2), or double-stranded siRNAs (3), upon encapsulation in specific delivery systems (4) can be transported to the cytoplasm via endosomes (5) where they can stimulate TLR7,8 or TLR3 resulting in cytokine production. Release of double-stranded RNA into the cytoplasm can result in the stimulation of the cytoplasmic receptors RIG-I or PKR (6). In contrast, naked double-stranded RNA not encapsulated into a delivery system may stimulate TLR3 that also is expressed on the cell surface (7).

guanosines. The presence of a CpG dinucleotide, surrounded by certain flanking bases on the 5′ and 3′ sides, which have become known as "CpG motifs," are responsible for the strong innate immune effects observed *in vitro* and *in vivo* with AS ODNs containing such sequences.[41] Human TLR9 is expressed rather exclusively in intracellular endolysosomal compartments of B cells and plasmacytoid dendritic cells (pDCs) (Figure 7.2). Stimulation of human immune cells with CpG ODNs results in a variety of effects, characterized amongst others by the stimulation of Th1 and Th1-like cytokines.[40] For example, TLR9 expressing pDCs are unique in their ability to respond to TLR9 activation by producing large amounts of type I interferons. Moreover, stimulation of B cells leads to additional immune effects such as B cell proliferation and Ig secretion.

Such effects can be seen as adverse events when developing nucleic acid therapeutics such as AS ODNs, although therapeutic CpG ODNs containing optimized CpG motifs to induce strongest human innate immune responses are currently under development in different human diseases. CpG ODNs due to their specific immune effects are attractive drugs to trigger Th1 effects and stimulate efficient DC stimulation and antigen-specific B and T cell responses. Animal models in infectious diseases, cancer, and asthma/allergy have proven the ability of CpG ODNs to eradicate tumors, elicit efficient antiviral responses, or prevent and reverse allergen-induced changes of acute inflammation.[42–45]

7.4.2 Nucleic acids stimulating Toll-like receptors 7 and 8

RNA interference (RNAi) is a natural regulatory mechanism observed in eukaryotic cells.[46,47] Synthetic double-stranded small interfering RNAs (siRNAs) containing a "sense" and an "antisense" strand with sequence identity to a specific target mRNA are bound by the RNA-induced silencing complex (RISC) that cleaves the target mRNA between bases 10 and 11 relative to the 5′ end of the antisense RNA strand. Due to the ability of siRNAs to silence disease-associated genes, these molecules are currently under development for several clinical applications. Many of the same issues observed at the beginning of the development of AS ODNs are reemerging with the use of siRNAs, including efficient delivery to the target, metabolic stability, and nonspecific or off-target effects.[48] Recently, single-stranded viral RNA was found to induce an immune response via TLR7 and TLR8 that are expressed in endolysosomal compartments similar to TLR9 (Figure 7.2).[49] The immune stimulation mediated by viral RNA can be mimicked by synthetic single- or double-stranded oligoribonucleotides (ORNs) or siRNAs containing uracil and guanosine, and RNA motifs rich in these nucleotides function as ligands for these nucleic acid receptors.[49,50] In addition, TLR3 that can be also expressed on the surface of cells such as endothelial cells is stimulated by siRNAs that are not formulated with a delivery system (Figure 7.2).[51] Additional receptors exist, such as RIG-I-like receptors (RLRs) or the double-stranded RNA-activated protein kinase (PKR),[49,50,52,53] that in principle can also be stimulated by synthetic double-stranded RNAs, and these ubiquitous receptors are expressed in the cytoplasm of a variety of different cells, not only immune cells (Figure 7.2).

In contrast to human TLR9 and TLR7, which have a very similar cellular expression pattern, TLR8 has a different cell-type specific expression, including cells of the myeloid compartment such as monocytes.[54] Stimulation of immune cells with single-stranded ORNs or double-stranded siRNAs can result in the production of Th1, Th1-like and proinflammatory cytokines including IFN-alpha from pDCs, and TNF-alpha from monocytes or myeloid DCs (mDCs).[55–60] Injection of ORNs or siRNAs encapsulated in specific delivery systems in mice can also result in a strong production of Th1 and proinflammatory cytokines.

Due to their strong and specific immunological activities, several therapeutic preclinical approaches employ single-stranded immune stimulatory ORNs. Similar to CpG ODNs, the addition of antigens to lipid-encapsulated ORNs induces enhanced levels of antigen-specific antibodies, as well as increased numbers of antigen-specific IFN-gamma-producing T cells and stronger antigen-specific CTL responses compared to mice immunized with lipid-encapsulated antigen alone.[57,61–63] Such single-stranded ORNs also can have antitumor effects when applied alone or together with chemotherapy in mouse tumor models (unpublished observation).

7.5 TECHNOLOGIES TO PREDICT IMMUNE ACTIVATION BY NUCLEIC ACIDS

AS ODNs can have sequence-dependent and -independent adverse effects. Sequence-independent toxicities are suggested to be mainly due to class-specific effects. Especially PS AS ODNs are known to bind proteins with different affinities, and at high doses a distinctive pattern of toxicities can be observed common to all PS ODNs, although toxicities usually do not occur at the pharmacologically relevant doses.[64] A sequence-dependent characteristic toxicity of AS ODNs is their activation of the innate immune system. Upon exposure to immune stimulatory (CpG) ODNs, specific signaling pathways in B cells and pDCs are stimulated, and, as a consequence of TLR9-mediated activation, a multiplicity of secondary effects that can be measured *in vitro* and *in vivo* are stimulated. TLR9 signaling in purified pDCs in *in vitro* culture results most prominently in the production of Th1 and Th1-like cytokines such as type I IFN, or to the upregulation of cell surface activation markers.[65–67] Additional effects that can be measured *in vitro* involve maturation of purified pDCs to potent APCs, transition of purified monocytes into functional DCs, or natural killer (NK) cell stimulation.[66,68,69] B cells in PBMC or upon purification are stimulated upon TLR9 ligation to proliferate, enhance costimulatory molecule expression, produce cytokines, secrete antibodies, or gain apoptosis resistance.[39,70]

Stimulation of human PBMC with immune stimulatory single-stranded ORNs or double-stranded siRNAs *in vitro* results in the production of Th1, Th1-like, and proinflammatory cytokines including IFN-alpha from pDCs, TNF-alpha, or IL-12 from monocytes and/or mDCs, as well as IL-6 or IFN-gamma.[34,54] Due to the expression of TLR7 and TLR8 in different cell types and their strongest stimulation by different RNA sequence motifs,[71] it is highly recommended to measure at least the production of IFN-alpha from pDCs (TLR7) as well as the production of TNF-alpha from monocytes (TLR8) upon culture of human PBMC. Stimulation with such immune stimulatory oligonucleotides also results in enhanced expression of cell surface molecules on murine and human APCs (e.g., the expression of the early-activation marker CD69 on T cells, NK cells, or NKT cells or the enhanced proliferation of alloreactive T cells[49,71–73]).

7.6 SUMMARY

Adverse drug reactions can be induced by drugs of very diverse nature, including antibiotics, low molecular chemicals, or nucleic acids. Such reactions can be induced directly or indirectly in various ways. Direct effects on the immune system can result in immunosuppression, or in immune stimulation such as with some nucleic acid therapeutics: siRNAs or AS ODNs. In contrast, indirect immune effects are caused by immune responses to a chemical or to self-determinants altered by a chemical such as with low molecular small molecules.

Such compounds usually are too small to be immunogenic, and they are thought to act as a hapten or prohapten. Testing of immune system adverse events can include *in vivo* assays, but *in vitro* assays are also to be considered when analyzing potential immunotoxicological effects of nucleic acids or haptens.

ACKNOWLEDGMENTS

I want to thank Dr. Corinne Moulon for stimulating discussions throughout our work on haptens, and Silke Fähndrich for outstanding assistance in manuscript preparation.

REFERENCES

1. Landsteiner K, Jacobs JL. Studies on the sensitization of animals with simple chemical compounds. *J Exp Med.* 1935;61:643.
2. Ortmann B, Martin S, von Bonin A, et al. Synthetic peptides anchor T cell-specific TNP epitopes to MHC antigens. *J Immunol.* 1992;148:1445–1450.
3. von Bonin A, Ortmann B, Martin S, et al. Peptide-conjugated hapten groups are the major antigenic determinants for trinitrophenyl-specific cytotoxic T cells. *Int Immunol.* 1992;4:869–874.
4. Kalish RS, Wood JA, LaPorte A. Processing of urushiol (poison ivy) hapten by both endogenous and exogenous pathways for presentation to T cells in vitro. *J Clin Invest.* 1994;93:2039–2047.
5. Thierse HJ, Gamerdinger K, Junkes C, et al. T cell receptor (TCR) interaction with haptens: Metal ions as non-classical haptens. *Toxicology.* 2005;209:101–7.
6. Padovan E, Mauri-Hellweg D, Pichler WJ, et al. T cell recognition of penicillin G: Structural features determining antigenic specificity. *Eur J Immunol.* 1996;26:42–48.
7. Gehrig KA, Warshaw EM. Allergic contact dermatitis to topical antibiotics: Epidemiology, responsible allergens, and management. *J Am Acad Dermatol.* 2008;58:1–21.
8. Levin C, Warshaw E. Protein contact dermatitis: allergens, pathogenesis, and management. *Dermatitis.* 2008;19:241–251.
9. Ryan CA, Hulette BC, Gerberick GF. Approaches for the development of cell-based in vitro methods for contact sensitization. *Toxicol In Vitro.* 2001;15:43–55.
10. Khan FD, Roychowdhury S, Gaspari AA, et al. Immune response to xenobiotics in the skin: From contact sensitivity to drug allergy. *Expert Opin Drug Metab Toxicol.* 2006;2:261–272.
11. Thierse HJ, Gamerdinger K, Junkes C, et al. T cell receptor (TCR) interaction with haptens: metal ions as non-classical haptens. *Toxicology.* 2005;209:101–7.
12. Lu L, Vollmer J, Moulon C, et al. Components of the ligand for a Ni++ reactive human T cell clone. *J Exp Med.* 2003;197:567–574.
13. Vollmer J, Weltzien HU, Gamerdinger K, et al. Antigen contacts by Ni-reactive TCR: Typical alphas chain cooperation versus alpha chain-dominated specificity. *Int Immunol.* 2000;12:1723–1731.
14. Vollmer J, Fritz M, Dormoy A, et al. Dominance of the BV17 element in nickel-specific human T cell receptors relates to severity of contact sensitivity. *Eur J Immunol.* 1997;27:1865–1874.
15. Budinger L, Neuser N, Totzke U, et al. Preferential usage of TCR-Vbeta17 by peripheral and cutaneous T cells in nickel-induced contact dermatitis. *J Immunol.* 2001;167:6038–44.

16. Vollmer J, Weltzien HU, Moulon C. TCR reactivity in human nickel allergy indicates contacts with complementarity-determining region 3 but excludes superantigen-like recognition. *J Immunol.* 1999;163:2723–2731.
17. Gamerdinger K, Moulon C, Karp DR, et al. A new type of metal recognition by human T cells: contact residues for peptide-independent bridging of T cell receptor and major histocompatibility complex by nickel. *J Exp Med.* 2003;197:1345–53.
18. Thierse HJ, Gamerdinger K, Junkes C, et al. T cell receptor (TCR) interaction with haptens: metal ions as non-classical haptens. *Toxicology.* 2005;209:101–7.
19. Griem P, von Vultee C, Panthel K, et al. T cell cross-reactivity to heavy metals: identical cryptic peptides may be presented from protein exposed to different metals. *Eur J Immunol.* 1998;28:1941–7.
20. Jakobson E, Masjedi K, Ahlborg N, et al. Cytokine production in nickel-sensitized individuals analysed with enzyme-linked immunospot assay: Possible implication for diagnosis. *Br J Dermatol.* 2002;147:442–449.
21. Basketter D, Darlenski R, Fluhr JW. Skin irritation and sensitization: mechanisms and new approaches for risk assessment. *Skin Pharmacol Physiol.* 2008;21:191–202.
22. Ryan CA, Hulette BC, Gerberick GF. Approaches for the development of cell-based in vitro methods for contact sensitization. *Toxicol In Vitro.* 2001;15:43–55.
23. Enk AH, Katz SI. Contact sensitivity as a model for T-cell activation in skin. *J Invest Dermatol.* 1995;105:80S–83S.
24. Toebak MJ, Gibbs S, Bruynzeel DP, et al. Dendritic cells: Biology of the skin. *Contact Dermatitis.* 2009;60:2–20.
25. Ryan CA, Hulette BC, Gerberick GF. Approaches for the development of cell-based in vitro methods for contact sensitization. *Toxicol In Vitro.* 2001;15:43–55.
26. Toebak MJ, Gibbs S, Bruynzeel DP, et al. Dendritic cells: Biology of the skin. *Contact Dermatitis.* 2009;60:2–20.
27. Hauser C, Katz SI. Activation and expansion of hapten- and protein-specific T helper cells from nonsensitized mice. *Proc Natl Acad Sci USA.* 1988;85:5625–5628.
28. Moulon C, Peguet-Navarro J, Courtellemont P, et al. In vitro primary sensitization and restimulation of hapten-specific T cells by fresh and cultured human epidermal Langerhans' cells. *Immunology.* 1993;80:373–379.
29. Moulon C, Vollmer J, Weltzien HU. Characterization of processing requirements and metal cross-reactivities in T cell clones from patients with allergic contact dermatitis to nickel. *Eur J Immunol.* 1995;25:3308–3315.
30. Kohler J, Martin S, Pflugfelder U, et al. Cross-reactive trinitrophenylated peptides as antigens for class II major histocompatibility complex-restricted T cells and inducers of contact sensitivity in mice. Limited T cell receptor repertoire. *Eur J Immunol.* 1995;25:92–101.
31. Moulon C, Vollmer J, Weltzien HU. Characterization of processing requirements and metal cross-reactivities in T cell clones from patients with allergic contact dermatitis to nickel. *Eur J Immunol.* 1995;25:3308–3315.
32. Spiewak R, Moed H, von Blomberg BM, et al. Allergic contact dermatitis to nickel: modified in vitro test protocols for better detection of allergen-specific response. *Contact Dermatitis.* 2007;56:63–69.
33. Vollmer J, Fritz M, Dormoy A, et al. Dominance of the BV17 element in nickel-specific human T cell receptors relates to severity of contact sensitivity. *Eur J Immunol.* 1997;27:1865–1874.
34. Krieg AM, Vollmer J. Toll-like receptors 7, 8, and 9: Linking innate immunity to autoimmunity. *Immunol Rev.* 2007;220:251–269.
35. Jahrsdorfer B, Jox R, Muhlenhoff L, et al. Modulation of malignant B cell activation and apoptosis by bcl-2 antisense ODN and immunostimulatory CpG ODN. *J Leukoc Biol.* 2002;72:83–92.
36. Leaman DW. Recent progress in oligonucleotide therapeutics: Antisense to aptamers. *Expert Opinion Drug Discov.* 2008;3:997–1009.

37. Vollmer J, Jepsen JS, Uhlmann E, et al. Modulation of CpG oligodeoxynucleotide-mediated immune stimulation by locked nucleic acid (LNA). *Oligonucleotides.* 2004;14:23–31.
38. Krieg AM, Yi AK, Matson S, et al. CpG motifs in bacterial DNA trigger direct B-cell activation. *Nature* 1995;374:546–549.
39. Vollmer J. TLR9 in Health and Disease. *Int Rev Immunol.* 2006;25:155–181.
40. Krieg AM. CpG motifs in bacterial DNA and their immune effects. *Annu Rev Immunol.* 2002;20:709–760.
41. Vollmer J. Editorial: CpG motifs to modulate innate and adaptive immune responses. *Int Rev Immunol.* 2006;25:125–134.
42. Klinman DM. Use of CpG oligodeoxynucleotides as immunoprotective agents. *Expert Opin Biol Ther.* 2004;4:937–946.
43. Hussain I, Kline JN. CpG oligodeoxynucleotides: A novel therapeutic approach for atopic disorders. *Curr Drug Targets Inflamm Allergy.* 2003;2:199–205.
44. Uhlmann E, Vollmer J. Recent advances in the development of immunostimulatory oligonucleotides. *Curr Opin Drug Discov Devel.* 2003;6:204–217.
45. Krieg AM. Antitumor applications of stimulating toll-like receptor 9 with CpG oligodeoxynucleotides. *Curr Oncol Rep.* 2004;6:88–95.
46. Leung RK, Whittaker PA. RNA interference: From gene silencing to gene-specific therapeutics. *Pharmacol Ther.* 2005;107:222–239.
47. Aagaard L, Rossi JJ. RNAi therapeutics: Principles, prospects and challenges. *Adv Drug Deliv Rev.* 2007;59:75–86.
48. Agrawal S, Kandimalla ER. Antisense and siRNA as agonists of Toll-like receptors. *Nat Biotechnol.* 2004;22:1533–7.
49. Heil F, Hemmi H, Hochrein H, et al. Species-specific recognition of single-stranded RNA via toll-like receptor 7 and 8. *Science.* 2004;303:1526–1529.
50. Sioud M. Induction of inflammatory cytokines and interferon responses by double-stranded and single-stranded siRNAs is sequence-dependent and requires endosomal localization. *J Mol Biol.* 2005;348:1079–1090.
51. Kleinman ME, Yamada K, Takeda A, et al. Sequence- and target-independent angiogenesis suppression by siRNA via TLR3. *Nature.* 2008;452(7187):591–597.
52. Puthenveetil S, Whitby L, Ren J, et al. Controlling activation of the RNA-dependent protein kinase by siRNAs using site-specific chemical modification. *Nucleic Acids Res.* 2006;34:4900–4911.
53. de Veer MJ, Sledz CA, Williams BR. Detection of foreign RNA: Implications for RNAi. *Immunol Cell Biol.* 2005;83:224–228.
54. Vollmer J, Krieg A. Mechanisms and therapeutic applications of immune modulatory oligodeoxynucleotide and oligoribonucleotide ligands for toll-like receptors. In: Crooke ST, ed., *Antisense Drug Technology,* Boca Raton: Taylor & Francis; 2007:747–772.
55. Scheel B, Braedel S, Probst J, et al. Immunostimulating capacities of stabilized RNA molecules. *Eur J Immunol.* 2004;34:537–547.
56. Vollmer J, Tluk S, Schmitz C, et al. Immune stimulation mediated by autoantigen binding sites within small nuclear RNAs involves Toll-like receptors 7 and 8. *J Exp Med.* 2005;202:1575–1585.
57. Nemorin JG, Lampron C, McCluskie M, et al. Adjuvant activity of ssRNA in Hepatitis B vaccine. First Meeting of the Oligonucleotide Therapeutics Society; New York, 2005.
58. Bekeredjian-Ding I, Roth SI, Gilles S, et al. T cell-independent, TLR-induced IL-12p70 production in primary human monocytes. *J Immunol.* 2006;176:7438–7446.
59. Sioud M. Single-stranded small interfering RNA are more immunostimulatory than their double-stranded counterparts: a central role for 2′-hydroxyl uridines in immune responses. *Eur J Immunol.* 2006;36:1222–1230.
60. Diebold SS, Kaisho T, Hemmi H, et al. Innate antiviral responses by means of TLR7-mediated recognition of single-stranded RNA. *Science.* 2004;303:1529–1531.

61. Riedl P, Stober D, Oehninger C, et al. Priming Th1 immunity to viral core particles is facilitated by trace amounts of RNA bound to its arginine-rich domain. *J Immunol.* 2002;168:4951–4959.
62. Westwood A, Elvin SJ, Healey GD, et al. Immunological responses after immunisation of mice with microparticles containing antigen and single stranded RNA (polyuridylic acid). *Vaccine.* 2006;24:1736–1743.
63. Scheel B, Braedel S, Probst J, et al. Immunostimulating capacities of stabilized RNA molecules. *Eur J Immunol.* 2004;34:537–547.
64. Levin AA, Monteith JM, Leeds JM, et al. Toxicity of oligodeoxynucleotide therapeutics. In: Crooke ST, ed. *Antisense Research and Application.* Springer-Verlag, Berlin; 1998: 169–216.
65. Gursel M, Verthelyi D, Gursel I, et al. Differential and competitive activation of human immune cells by distinct classes of CpG oligodeoxynucleotide. *J Leukoc Biol.* 2002;71:813–20.
66. Krug A, Rothenfusser S, Hornung V, et al. Identification of CpG oligonucleotide sequences with high induction of IFN-alpha/beta in plasmacytoid dendritic cells. *Eur J Immunol.* 2001;31:2154–1263.
67. Vollmer J, Weeratna R, Payette P, et al. Characterization of three CpG oligodeoxynucleotide classes with distinct immunostimulatory activities. *Eur J Immunol.* 2004;34:251–262.
68. Gursel M, Verthelyi D, Klinman DM. CpG oligodeoxynucleotides induce human monocytes to mature into functional dendritic cells. *Eur J Immunol.* 2002;32:2617–2622.
69. Ballas ZK, Rasmussen WL, Krieg AM. Induction of NK activity in murine and human cells by CpG motifs in oligodeoxynucleotides and bacterial DNA. *J Immunol.* 1996;157:1840–1845.
70. Hartmann G, Krieg AM. Mechanism and function of a newly identified CpG DNA motif in human primary B cells. *J Immunol.* 2000;164:944–953.
71. Forsbach A, Nemorin JG, Montino C, et al. Identification of RNA sequence motifs stimulating sequence-specific TLR8-dependent immune responses. *J Immunol.* 2008;180:3729–3738.
72. Forsbach A, Nemorin J, Völp K, et al. Characterization of conserved viral leader RNA sequences that stimulate innate immunity through TLRs. *Oligonucleotides.* 2007;17:405–417.
73. Hornung V, Guenthner-Biller M, Bourquin C, et al. Sequence-specific potent induction of IFN-alpha by short interfering RNA in plasmacytoid dendritic cells through TLR7. *Nat Med.* 2005;11:263–270.

8 Predictive models for neurotoxicity assessment

Lucio G. Costa, Gennaro Giordano, and Marina Guizzetti

8.1 INTRODUCTION

The human nervous system is one of the most complex organ systems in terms of both structure and function. It contains billions of neurons, each forming thousands of synapses leading to a very large number of connections. It also contains perhaps ten times more glial cells (astrocytes, oligodendrocytes, microglia) than neurons, which play important roles in the overall development and functioning of the nervous system.[1] Anatomically, the nervous system is composed of a central (CNS) and a peripheral (PNS) component, whose basic functions are to detect and relay sensory information inside and outside the body, to direct motor functions, and to integrate thought processes, learning, and memory. Such functions and their complexity, together with some intrinsic characteristics (e.g., mature neurons do not divide, they are highly dependent upon oxygen and glucose) make the nervous system particularly vulnerable to toxic insults.

Neurotoxicity can be defined as any adverse effect on the chemistry, structure, or function of the nervous system, during development or at maturity, induced by chemical or physical influences.[2] A first issue is what constitutes an adverse effect. A proposed definition of an adverse effect is "any treatment related change which interferes with normal function and compromises adaptation to the environment."[3] Thus, most morphological changes such as neuronopathy (a loss of neurons), axonopathy (a degeneration of the neuronal axon), or myelinopathy (a loss of the glial cells surrounding the axon), or other gliopathies, would be considered adverse, even if structural and/or functional changes were mild or transitory. Neurochemical changes, even in the absence of structural damage should also be considered adverse, even if they are reversible. For example, exposure to organophosphorus insecticides or to certain solvents may cause only transient nervous system effects, but these should be considered neurotoxic, as they lead to impaired function.

A large number of compounds are known to be neurotoxic. Grandjean and Landrigan[4] list 201 chemicals known to be neurotoxic to humans. This list includes metals, organic solvents, pesticides, and other organic substances, but does not include drugs and natural neurotoxins. In their authoritative book

Experimental and Clinical Neurotoxicology, Spencer et al.[5] list 372 substances for which evidence of neurotoxicity, provided by animal studies or by observations in humans, exists. Table 8.1 lists thirty chemicals, among the most thoroughly studied, known to be neurotoxic in humans.

The definition of neurotoxicity also indicates a potential difference between the developing and the mature nervous system, to underscore the fact that developmental neurotoxicity is an important aspect of neurotoxicology. Most known human neurotoxicants are indeed developmental neurotoxicants.[4] In most, but not all cases, the developing nervous system is more sensitive to adverse effects than the adult nervous system, as indicated, for example, by the most deleterious effects of ethanol, methylmercury, or lead when exposure occurs *in utero* or during childhood. Furthermore, the blood–brain barrier (BBB), which protects the mature nervous system from the entry of a number of substances, appears to be poorly developed at birth and during the first few years of life.[6]

Neurotoxicity can also occur as a result of indirect effects. For example, damage to hepatic, renal, circulatory, or pancreatic structures may result in secondary effects on the function and structure of the nervous system, such as encephalopathy or polyneuropathy. Secondary effects would not cause a substance to be considered neurotoxic, though at high enough doses, neurotoxicity could be evident. Thus, for the purpose of this review, a substance is defined as neurotoxic when it or its metabolites produce adverse effects as a result of direct interactions with the nervous system. It should be noted, nevertheless, that some chemicals may have multiple modes of action and affect the nervous system directly and indirectly. For example, several halogenated compounds (e.g., polychlorinated biphenyls (PCB), polybrominated diphenyl ethers (PBDE)) may interact directly with brain cells, and also affect the development of the nervous system by altering thyroid hormone homeostasis.[7,8]

8.2 *IN VIVO* TESTING FOR NEUROTOXICITY AND DEVELOPMENTAL NEUROTOXICITY

Neurotoxic effects can be detected in the course of standard toxicity testing (acute, subacute, subchronic, chronic, developmental/reproductive toxicity) required by regulatory agencies worldwide. However, specific guidelines exist to further probe the potential neurotoxicity of chemicals.[9,10] Such tests are performed in rodents and are meant to assess specific effects of the tested chemical on the nervous system. The U.S. Environmental Protection Agency (USEPA) guidelines focus on a functional observational battery, on measurements of motor activity, and on neuropathological examinations.[9] The Organization for Economic Co-operation and Development (OECD) guidelines similarly focus on clinical observations, functional tests (e.g., motor activity, sensory reactivity to stimuli), and neuropathology.[10] These batteries are not meant to provide a complete evaluation of neurotoxicity, but to act as a Tier 1 screening for potential neurotoxicity. If no effects are seen at the appropriate dose level, and if

Table 8-1. Examples of chemicals known to be neurotoxic in humans

Chemical class	Compound	Neurotoxic effect
Metals	Manganese	Extrapyramidal syndrome
	Methylmercury	Cerebellar syndrome, visual dysfunction, encephalopathy, CNS teratogenicity
	Lead	Peripheral neuropathy, encephalopathy
	Organotin compounds	Encephalopathy, neuronopathy (trimethyltin); leukoencephalopathy, vacuolar myelinopathy (triethyltin)
	Thallium	Peripheral neuropathy, optic neuropathy
Organic solvents	Carbon disulfide	Peripheral neuropathy
	Ethanol	Acute, chronic encephalopathy, CNS teratogenicity (fetal alcohol syndrome)
	n-Hexane	Peripheral neuropathy
	Methanol	Optical neuropathy
	Toluene	Encephalopathy, CNS teratogenicity (fetal solvent syndrome)
Pesticides	Carbamates	Cholinergic syndrome
	Chlordecone	Cerebellar syndrome, tremors
	Chlorinated cyclodienes	Seizures
	Methyl bromide	Acute encephalopathy, peripheral neuropathy, optic neuropathy
	Organophosphates	Cholinergic syndrome, delayed peripheral neuropathy (some)
Other organic substances	Acrylamide	Peripheral neuropathy
	Cyanide	Seizures
	Hydrogen sulfide	Acute encephalopathy
	Polychlorinated biphenyls	Behavioral developmental neurotoxicity
	Tri-*o*-tolyl phosphate	Peripheral neuropathy
Drugs	Cisplatin	Peripheral neuropathy
	Chlorpromazine	Extrapyramidal disorders, seizures
	Doxorubicin	Ganglioneuropathy
	Thalidomide	Peripheral neuropathy, teratogenicity
	Valproic acid	Acute encephalopathy, CNS teratogenicity
Natural compounds	Botulinum toxin	Neuromuscular transmission syndrome
	Ciguatoxin	Ion channel syndrome (Na+ channels)
	Domoic acid	Encephalopathy, neuronopathy, seizures
	Ricin	Neuronopathy
	Tetrodotoxin	Ion channel syndrome (Na+ channels)

Source: Selected from Spencer et al.[5]

the chemical structure of the substance and/or its metabolites does not suggest concern for potential neurotoxicity, the substance may be considered as not neurotoxic. On the other hand, positive findings can be followed up by further testing (Tier 2) in case of commonly existing substances with commercial value or wide exposure; for new chemical entities, development of the molecule may instead be abandoned. The decision to carry out additional studies should be thus made on a case-by-case approach and may depend upon factors such as the intended use of the chemical, the potential of human exposure, and its potential to accumulate in biological systems. Such Tier 2 studies may include specialized behavioral tests, electrophysiological and neurochemical measurements, and additional morphologic studies. Examples are tests for measuring learning and memory, measurements of nerve conduction velocity, and biochemical parameters related to neurotransmission or to indices of cell integrity and functions.[2]

The nervous system undergoes gradual development that continues well after birth in both animals and humans. On one hand, the developing nervous system may more readily adapt to, or compensate for, functional losses as a result of a toxic insult; however, on the other hand, damage to the nervous system during key periods of brain development may result in long-term, irreversible damage.[2] Evidence that developmental exposure to chemicals and drugs may alter behavioral functions in young animals began to emerge in the early 1970s. The field of developmental neurotoxicology thus evolved from the disciplines of neurotoxicology, developmental toxicology, and experimental psychology.[11] In response to this issue, developmental neurotoxicity (DNT) testing guidelines were developed both in the United States and in Europe.[12,13] The mother is exposed to the test chemicals from gestational day 6 to postnatal day 10 or 21, thus ensuring exposure *in utero* and through maternal milk. Tests involve measurements of developmental landmarks and reflexes, motor activity, auditory startle test, learning and memory tests, and neuropathology.[12,13] As for neurotoxicity testing, DNT testing has been proven to be useful and effective in identifying compounds with developmental neurotoxicity potential.[11] This is not to say that current DNT testing guidelines cannot be improved; indeed, it has been pointed out that they may be overly sensitive and produce a high rate of false positives,[14] or, in contrast, that they may be too insensitive and not comprehensive enough.[15]

In the past several years, the need to develop acceptable alternatives to conventional animal testing has been increasingly recognized by toxicologists, to address problems related to the escalating costs and time required for toxicity assessments, the increasing number of chemicals being developed and commercialized, the need to respond to recent legislations (e.g., REACH (Registration Evaluation and Authorization of Chemicals) and the Cosmetics Directive (76/768/EEC) in the E.U.), and efforts aimed at reducing the number of animals used for toxicity testing.[2,16–19] Hence, efforts have been directed toward the development of alternative models, utilizing either mammalian cells *in vitro* or nonmammalian model systems, which could serve as tools

Table 8-2. Some general advantages and disadvantages of *in vitro* neurotoxicity testing

Advantages	Disadvantages
chemical and physical environment is uniform	Integrated functions are unavailable
Exposure parameters are strictly controlled	Blood–brain barrier is unavailable
Small amount of chemical are needed	Target concentration is not known
Systemic (e.g., hepatic) effects are bypassed	Compensatory mechanisms cannot be determined
Range of donor species are available, including human	Single test cannot cover all targets and mechanisms
Testing is potentially adaptable to high throughput	
Number of animals is reduced	
Costs are decreased	

for neurotoxicity and developmental neurotoxicity testing, particularly for screening purposes.

8.3 *IN VITRO* NEUROTOXICITY TESTING IN MAMMALIAN CELLS

In vitro testing procedures utilizing mammalian cells have two main purposes: (a) investigate mode and/or mechanism of action of chemicals, particularly related to early, upstream events in the neurotoxic process and (b) screen chemicals of unknown toxicity to flag compounds for further *in vitro* and *in vivo* studies. There are a number of general advantages and disadvantages involved in the use of *in vitro* methods for neurotoxicity testing, as shown in Table 8.2. Several issues need to be considered when exploring potential *in vitro* models for neurotoxicity and developmental neurotoxicity. First, the nervous system comprises several types of cells (neurons, astrocytes, oligodendrocytes, Schwann cells, microglia, and neural stem (progenitor) cells).[20,21] Different models also can be used; in increasing level of complexity they are immortalized cell lines, primary cells, cells in coculture, aggregating cell cultures, and brain slices (Figure 8.1). Each model has its own advantages and disadvantages. For example a cell line provides a defined and homogenous population of cells (usually clonal) derived from tumors or using oncogene-containing retroviruses. Cell lines are easy to grow, divide rapidly, are available from various animal species including humans, and can be induced to differentiate. On the other hand, transformed cell lines may not exhibit the same phenotype of primary cells or may represent a specific cell subpopulation. There is also increased genetic instability with increased number of passages; neurites may not represent true axons or dendrites, and cell–cell interactions are missing.

A more complex system, such as aggregating brain cell cultures, has the advantage of providing a three-dimensional cell system containing all cell types and allowing cell–cell interactions and permits testing of multiple endpoints in

	In vivo-like complexity	Reduction of animals	Neuro behavior	Neuro pathology	Neuro physiology	Neuro chemistry	Handling reproducibility
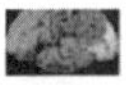 *In vivo*	+++++	–	+++++	+++++	+++++	+++++	++
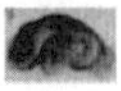 Slices	++++	+(+)	–	++++	+++	+++++	+++
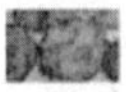 Aggregates	+++(+)	+++	–	+++	+++	+++++	+++
 Mixed primary cultures	++(+)	+++	–	++	++	+++++	++++
 Primary cells	+(+)	+++	–	+	+	+++	++++
 Human cell lines	+	+++++	–	+	+	++	+++++
 Other cell lines	–	+++++	–	+	+	++	+++++

Figure 8-1: Characteristics of *in vitro* models vs. *in vivo* neurotoxicity testing. Reprinted from *Environmental Toxicology and Pharmocology*, vol. 22/2, Coecke et al., "The Value of Alternative Testing for Neurotoxicity in the Context of Regulatory Needs," 15, 2006, with permission from Elsevier.

different cell types, including, for example, inflammatory responses.[22] However, such cultures are difficult to prepare and maintain, there is a notable degree of variability between aggregates, and the anatomical organization of the tissue is missing. Similar considerations on advantages and disadvantages can be made for other *in vitro* system using mammalian cells (Figure 8.1).

A number of additional questions may also be posed. For example, is it better to use human or animal cell lines? Are primary cells a better model than cell lines? Do they provide a higher sensitivity? Which cell type/brain area should I choose? There are no clear answers to these questions. For instance, though the use of human cell lines may be preferred, there is no compelling evidence that they would be more sensitive or predictive of neurotoxicity.[23,24] In most cases, human and animal cell lines appear to respond similarly to neurotoxicants; however, in a few cases, opposite effects have been found (e.g., lead and neurite initiation[25]). There is also a general belief that cells in primary culture may be more sensitive to the effects of neurotoxicants. Though this is true at times, it is not always the case,[18,24] and differences are often due to different culturing conditions. In contrast, cell type and brain area may represent an important determinant in the response to neurotoxicants. For example, cocaine was shown to inhibit neurite outgrowth in neurons from the locus coeruleus, but not of the substantia nigra.[25] Rodent neural stem cells were found to be two orders of magnitude more sensitive than hippocampal neurons to the toxicity of methylmercury.[26] Cerebellar Purkinje neurons were eightfold more susceptible to the toxicity of PCB126 (a dioxin-like PCB) than cerebellar granule neurons.[24] Astrocytes, which have higher glutathione content than neurons, are normally more resistant to the toxicity of chemicals that cause oxidative stress.[27] Thus, while selection of the appropriate cell model can be driven by specific knowledge or hypotheses in case of mechanistic studies, it remains a primary concern for applications to screening.

8.3.1 *In vitro* systems for mechanistic studies

In vitro systems are amenable and very useful for mechanistic studies at the cellular and molecular level. As such, they have been used extensively in neurobiology in neurotoxicology. Because of the complexity of the nervous system, no single *in vitro* preparation can be relied on to detect all possible endpoints. However, depending on the knowledge on the neurotoxicity of a certain compound, and of the specific questions that are being asked, different cellular systems or preparations can be used, and a tiered approach can be applied in this context as well. There are indeed hundreds of examples in which different cell culture models have been successfully utilized to investigate specific mechanisms of action of neurotoxicants. *In vitro* test systems are amenable to biochemical, molecular, electrophysiologic, and morphologic examinations. In the context of mechanistic *in vitro* neurotoxicology, one can point out studies investigating mechanisms of neurotoxicant-induced neuronal cell death,[28] inhibition of cell proliferation,[29] alteration of signal transduction pathways,[30] modulation of neurotoxicity by cell–cell interactions,[31,32] alterations of inhibitory or excitatory circuitries,[33] and many others. While extrapolation of *in vitro* findings to *in vivo* effects still requires important considerations, related for instance to dose selection,[34] role of metabolism and pharmacokinetics,[19,21] BBB permeability,[19] and so on, there is no doubt that *in vitro* systems play the most relevant role in mechanistic neurotoxicology.

In some cases, even limited mechanistic knowledge may lead to the use of *in vitro* methods to screen for a particular neurotoxicity. Organophosphorus (OP) compounds are a major class of insecticides. Their acute neurotoxicity is the result of inhibition of the enzyme acetylcholinesterase (AChE) and accumulation of acetylcholine at cholinergic synapses, causing a cholinergic syndrome. Some OPs can also cause a delayed polyneuropathy, which is unrelated to their inhibition of AChE, and is attributed instead to irreversible inhibition of another esterase, NTE (neuropathy target esterase).[35] Knowledge of the two targets for acute toxicity (AChE) and delayed neurotoxicity (NTE) has allowed the use of an *in vitro* system, utilizing human neuroblastoma cells, to screen OPs for their potential in inducing delayed polyneuropathy.[36] As shown in Table 8.3, the test can provide the ratio of relative inhibitory potency toward AChE and NTE. Indeed, paraoxon and malaoxon do not cause delayed polyneuropathy *in vivo*, while the other two compounds do (Table 8.3). Though a correlation between relative *in vitro* potency toward AChE and NTE and *in vivo* delayed neurotoxicity has been shown for a few additional compounds, this *in vitro* test has not been fully validated. As such, this approach has not been accepted by regulatory agencies, which still require an *in vivo* test.

Another example is that of the use of cerebellar granule neurons from transgenic mice to investigate neurotoxicant-induced oxidative stress. Mice lacking GCLM (the modifier subunit of glutamate cysteine ligase, the first and rate-limiting enzyme in the synthesis of glutathione) have very low glutathione content, and as such, are more susceptible to the toxic effects of chemicals that

Table 8-3. AChE and NTE inhibition by organophosphates in human neuroblastoma cells

		IC_{50} (μM)		Ratio
OP	AChE	NTE	Cytotoxicity	NTE/AChE
Paraoxon	0.0023	1,600	2,600	700,000
Malaoxon	0.0097	740	3,600	76,000
DBVP	0.00094	0.0076	520	0.81
DOVP	0.72	0.40	380	0.56

Notes: Human SH-SY5Y neuroblastoma cells were incubated for 1 h with different concentrations of each organophosphate (OP). Cytotoxicity was measured by the neutral red assay. Results represent the IC_{50} values for inhibition of AChE and NTE activities and for cytotoxicity. DBVP = O,O-dibutyl O-(2,2-dichlorovinyl) phosphate; DOVP = O,O-dioctyl O-(2,2-dichlorovinyl) phosphate. A high ratio of NTE IC_{50}/AChE IC_{50} indicates that the OP is likely to cause acute rather than delayed neurotoxic effects *in vivo*.

Source: Adapted from Ehrich et al.[36]

Table 8-4. Toxicity of various compounds in mouse cerebellar granule neurons

Compound	*Gclm* (+/+)	*Gclm* (–/–)	Ratio
H_2O_2	5.8	0.2	29.0
DMNQ	9.0	0.5	18.0
Domoic acid	3.4	0.4	8.5
BDE-153	19.9	2.3	8.6
$PbCl_2$	2.1	0.6	3.5
MeHg	2.9	0.9	3.2
Ouabain	70.6	73.2	0.9
Acrylamide	74.5	50.5	1.5
Colchicine	1.0	0.8	1.2

Notes: Values are IC_{50} (μM) in the MTT cytotoxicity assay. Neurons from *Gclm* (–/–) mice, which lack the modifier subunit of glutamate cysteine ligase have very low glutathione levels. DMNQ = dimethoxy-1,4-naphtoquinone.

Source: Giordano and Costa (unpublished results).

cause oxidative stress. Table 8.4 shows that this simple *in vitro* system may be exploited to screen neurotoxic chemicals for their ability to induce oxidative stress. Preliminary evidence indicates that *Gclm* (–/–) mice are more susceptible than their wild type counterparts to the *in vivo* acute neurotoxicity of a polybrominated diphenyl ether (BDE-47). Indeed, a single administration of BDE-47 in 10-day-old mice causes a significant higher degree of oxidative stress and of apoptotic neuronal death in cerebellum of *Gclm* (–/–) mice than in *Gclm* (+/+) mice (Giordano and Costa, unpublished observations). Thus, *in vitro* findings appear to be predictive of *in vivo* observations.

8.3.2 *In vitro* systems for neurotoxicity screening

As said, a second primary objective of *in vitro* systems is that of providing a rapid, relatively inexpensive, and reliable way for screening chemicals for potential neurotoxicity and/or developmental neurotoxicity. Screening is by definition a Tier 1 evaluation of chemicals that will be followed by more specific and complex tests, both *in vitro* and *in vivo*. The same general criteria for *in vitro* screening approaches for other endpoints of toxicity also apply to the neurotoxicity screening: (a) low incidence of false positives and false negatives; (b) high correlation with *in vivo* data (i.e., good predictive value); (c) sensitive, relatively simple, rapid (amenable for medium- to high-throughput screening), economical, and versatile.[2]

The choice of one or more *in vitro* models for neurotoxicity screening poses a number of problems, as one has to decide which cell type to use, the degree of model complexity, and particularly, which endpoints are to be measured. A common belief is that for screening purposes one should examine general cellular processes such as cell viability or proliferation, differentiation of precursors, or elaboration of axon or dendrites. However, each possibility requires careful considerations. For example, basic tests of cytotoxicity and viability are common to most cell types and include measurements of cell death, membrane permeability, mitochondrial function, cell growth and reproduction, energy regulation, and synthesis of macromolecules. If these endpoints are affected by a chemical in neuronal/glial cells, one cannot conclude that a chemical is neurotoxic but only that it displays cytotoxicity in these cells.[2] For example, Gartlon et al.[18] examined thirteen neurotoxic compounds and two nonneurotoxic compounds in undifferentiated or differentiated PC12 cells and in rat cerebellar granule neurons. Though various endpoints were utilized in this study, such as cell viability, ATP depletion, production of reactive oxygen species, and cytoskeletal modifications, the system did not provide distinction between cytotoxicity and neurotoxicity. Breier et al.[37] utilized ReNcell CX (an immortalized neuroprogenitor cell line from 14-week human fetal cortex) to study the neurotoxicity of sixteen chemicals (half of which are known neurotoxicants), utilizing cell viability and cell proliferation as endpoints. The assay, which was adapted to high throughput, revealed 2/8 false negatives and 2/8 false positives. It should be noted that both false negatives (valproic acid and 5,5-diphenylhydantoin) and both false positives (diphenhydramine and omeprazole) are pharmaceutical compounds. The reason(s) for such false positive/negative results are not apparent, so far.

The use of nonneuronal cell types may provide initial information on whether a chemical may have differential effects, or display different potencies, in neuronal versus nonneuronal cells. For example, a battery of seventeen different cell types, including cell lines and primary cells (both neuronal and glial), human and rat cells, and nervous system and nonnervous system cells, was utilized to assess the toxicity of known developmental neurotoxicants, such as methylmercury and polychlorinated biphenyls (PCBs).[24] Endpoints were cell viability and cell proliferation, and a summary of results for methylmercury and PCB-153 is shown in Table 8.5. This simple approach would flag methylmercury as a potential neurotoxicant, as toxicity was greater in neuronal cells than in other cell types. PCB-153 would also be flagged as a potential neurotoxicant, though

Table 8-5. Effect of methylmercury and PCB-153 on cell viability

	MeHg	PCB-153
	IC_{50} (μM)	
Neuronal cells	0.5–3.6	16.7–52.4
Astroglial cells	3.8–8.1	26.7–64.8
Non-nervous-system cells	13.5–18.9*	70.3–147.0**

Notes: Cell viability was determined with the MTT assay. Neuronal cells: PC12 (rat pheocromocytoma), SH-SY5Y (human neuroblastoma), rat hippocampal neurons, cortical neurons, mixed cerebellar neurons, cerebellar granule neurons, cerebellar Purkinje neurons. Astroglial cells: C6 (rat glioma), 1321N1 (human astrocytoma), rat astrocytes from cortex, hippocampus, cerebellum, brainstem. Non-nervous-system cells: 3T3 (mouse fibroblasts), TT (human thyroid cells), Pz-HPV-7 (human prostate cells), LNCaP (human prostate carcinoma cells).

* In TT cells IC_{50} was 4.2 μM. ** In Pz-HPV-7 cells IC_{50} was 11.6 μM.

Source: Adapted from Costa et al.[24]

not specific for neurons, as glial cells were similarly affected (Table 8.5). This study, which is discussed as an example of possible *in vitro* approaches, has a number of limitations. Indeed, only three compounds (the third being PCB-126) were utilized; all are known neurotoxicants, and no negative control was included. Furthermore, for both methylmercury and PCB-153, nonneuronal cell lines (thyroid and prostate cells, respectively), displayed high sensitivity to their toxicity, which may, nevertheless, provide evidence for other possible targets of toxicity.[24]

When the objective is that of screening potential developmental neurotoxicants, neurite outgrowth has been proposed as an important endpoint.[25] This can be measured in cell lines induced to differentiate by various factors, or in primary cultures or neural stem cells. In a recent study, a subclone of PC12 cells (Neuroscreen-1 cells), induced to differentiate with nerve growth factor, was used to examine the ability of twenty-one compounds to inhibit neurite outgrowth, as a model to screen for potential developmental neurotoxicants (Table 8.6).[38] Five chemicals, already known to inhibit neurite outgrowth, tested positive at concentrations devoid of any cytotoxicity. Among nonneurotoxic compounds, 6/8 had no effect on neurite outgrowth, while two increased neurite outgrowth at subcytotoxic concentrations. Among neurotoxic compounds, only two (*trans*-retinoic acid and methylmercury) inhibited neurite outgrowth at subcytotoxic concentrations; two compounds (dexamethasone and cadmium) equally affected cell viability, while one increased neurite outgrowth (amphetamine), and three (lead, valproic acid, and diphenylhydantoin) were devoid of effects. If one considers alteration of neurite outgrowth (either inhibition or augmentation) and index of potential neurotoxicity, this study would provide 2/8 false positives and 3/8 false negatives. Thus, even though this approach may be promising, as it is amenable to high-throughput screening, it still requires further validation.

Using the more complex model of aggregating cell cultures, van Vliet et al.[39] investigated an *in vitro* metabolomics approach for neurotoxicity testing. A neurotoxic compound, methylmercury, at subcytotoxic concentrations, caused

Table 8-6. *In vitro* screening of chemicals for effects on neurite outgrowth

Compound	Use	Effect on neurite outgrowth	Effect on cell viability
Positive controls			
Bis-I	PKC inhibitor	**Inhibition**	No effect
UO1261	MAPK inhibitor	**Inhibition**	No effect
Okaidic acid	Phosphatase inhibitor	**Inhibition**	No effect
Vincristine	Microtubule depolarizing agent	**Inhibition**	No effect
K252a	Tyrosine kinase inhibitor	**Inhibition**	No effect
Nonneurotoxic compounds			
Amoxicillin	Drug (antibiotic)	No effect	No effect
Sorbitol	Sweetener	No effect	No effect
Saccharin	Artificial sweetener	No effect	No effect
Acetominophen	Drug (antipyretic)	No effect	No effect
Dimethyl phthalate	Plasticizer	**Increase**	No effect
Diphenylhydramine	Drug (antihistamine)	No effect	No effect
Omeprazole	Drug (antiulcer)	**Increase**	No effect
Glyphosate	Herbicide	No effect	No effect
Developmentally neurotoxic compounds			
Diphenylhydantoin	Drug (anticonvulsant)	No effect	No effect
Trans-retinoic acid	Vitamin (antiacne)	**Inhibition**	No effect
Valproic acid	Drug (anticonvulsant)	No effect	No effect
Dexamethasone	Synthetic gluccocorticoid	**Inhibition**	**Decrease**
Amphetamine	Drug (stimulant)	**Increase**	No effect
Cadmium	Metal	**Inhibition**	**Decrease**
Lead	Metal	No effect	No effect
Methylmercury	Organometal	**Inhibition**	No effect

Source: Adapted from Radio et al.[38]

significant changes in the levels of GABA, choline, glutamine, spermine, and creatine, while the brain stimulant caffeine altered levels of spermine and creatine only. This profile was mimicked by three other known neurotoxicants (trimethyltin, methylmercury, paraquat), while a series of five nonneurotoxic compounds elicited a metabolomic profile similar to that observed in control cultures. This interesting and novel approach should be further pursued using a larger battery of known neurotoxic and nonneurotoxic compounds, as well as known neuropharmacological agents. These investigators, using the same *in vitro* system, also explored the possibility of electrophysiological measurements by means of a multielectrode array system.[40] Initial experiments indicated that electrophysiological recordings of evoked field potentials in reaggregating brain cell cultures involve glutamatergic and GABAergic synaptic transmission. Electrophysiological changes in neural activity can be detected before any morphological change occurs, and may thus represent a promising and sensitive approach to detect early effects of chemicals. As expected, however, the test method cannot distinguish between pharmacological actions (e.g., interactions with neurotransmitters or their receptors) and neurotoxicity. Nevertheless, it was found that trimethyltin and methylmercury caused a decrease in field potential amplitude, and an irreversible loss of neuronal electric activity at high concentrations. In contrast, the effects of ethanol were fully reversible upon wash-out. Thus, the simple observation of loss/recovery of electrical function may allow differentiation between neurotoxic or acute pharmacological effects.[40]

The few examples provided in this section suggest that there may be several mammalian *in vitro* systems of different complexity that may be utilized to screen for potential neurotoxicants and/or developmental neurotoxicants. However, the current situation is far from satisfactory. The main issue relates to the very limited progress that has been made in the validation process. Over a decade ago, we wrote that "the validation process should require the testing, under standardized conditions, of a large number of chemicals, some of which are neurotoxic... and others that are known not to affect the nervous system."[2] A decade later, one can find an almost identical statement "in order to make meaningful comparisons between model systems, a standard set of chemicals should be tested in all models. This reference set should include compounds known to inhibit neurite outgrowth, as well as compounds that are non-toxic."[25] Indeed, despite the development of several models and tests of potential usefulness, the lack of validation to determine the rate of false positives/false negatives, and the degree of inter-laboratory variability has hampered the further use of such alternative approaches.

8.4 NONMAMMALIAN MODELS FOR NEUROTOXICITY TESTING

In the not so distant past, animals other than mammals, with few exceptions such as certain birds or fish, were not considered ideal for the study of biomedical sciences, because of their phylogenic distance from humans. Yet, several organisms have proven to be of great similitude to humans and have provided great insights into fundamental biological processes, two excellent examples being the marine snail *Aplysia* and the fly *Drosophila*. A number of alternative nonmammalian models are starting to be investigated also in the context of screening for neurotoxic chemicals.[41] Zebrafish and *Caenorhabditis elegans* will be briefly considered here, but others (e.g., sea urchin) have also been proposed and utilized to a limited extent.[42,43]

Zebrafish has been used historically to assess environmental toxicity and is an approved model for aquatic toxicity testing. The small size, chemical permeability, and optical transparency of the zebrafish embryo are also inducive to small molecule screening, and the zebrafish embryo has found application in the area of cardiac toxicity.[44] The zebrafish is providing an excellent model to study the development of the nervous system,[45] as it presents many similarities to the mammalian counterpart, including the presence of a BBB.[46] More recently, zebrafish have also been proposed as a model for neurotoxicity and developmental neurotoxicity studies that combine cellular, molecular, behavioral, and genetic approaches.[47,48] A few known neurotoxic compounds have been investigated in zebrafish, leading to a proof of concept; for example, 6-hydroxydopamine and MPTP have been shown to cause a loss of dopaminergic neurons, as seen in mammals.[48,49] However, these studies examined only a limited number of chemicals and did not include any negative controls; thus, validation studies are still required to exploit the full potential of this model.

An even simpler model is represented by the nematode *C. elegans*. It has a very small size (~1 mm), is transparent, has a short life span, has simple measurable behaviors, and is easily amenable to genetic manipulations. Homologues for 60–80 percent of human genes have been found in *C. elegans*.[50] The acute toxicities of several chemicals in worms correlate with those found in rats and mice.[51] The structure, metabolism, and bioenergetics of *C. elegans* mitochondria are very similar to those of humans, contributing to its potential usefulness in investigating various mechanisms of oxidative stress-mediated toxicity. Its nervous system contains only a few hundreds neurons and fewer than 7,000 synapses,[52] as well as most neurotransmitters and signaling systems found in humans. The conservation of neuroanatomic, neurochemical, and neurophysiological components from nematodes to humans has allowed the study of basic mechanisms of neuronal fate, differentiation, and migration; of axon guidance; and of synaptogenesis and of axon degeneration.[53] Mechanistic elucidation of the apoptotic pathways have also been carried out extensively in *C. elegans*.[54] *C. elegans* has been used over the years to study effects and mechanisms of a number of neurotoxic metals and pesticides and as a model for studying neurodegenerative diseases.[53] *C. elegans* has also been recently proposed as a model for high-throughput neurotoxicity screening.[51,53,55] A series of eight compounds has been tested utilizing four endpoints (growth, feeding, reproduction, and locomotion), but the data are too preliminary to allow any conclusion.[55] Nevertheless, evidence accumulated so far suggests that changes in *C. elegans* following chemical exposure appear to be predictive of developmental shifts and/or neurological damage in rodents, highlighting the promise of this worm as an alternative screening model for neurotoxicity and developmental neurotoxicity.

8.5 CONCLUSIONS

Neurotoxicity is an important adverse health effect not only of hundreds of environmental contaminants and occupational chemicals but also of several pharmaceutical drugs. Indeed, several drugs are known to induce neurological complications such as cognitive impairment, cerebellar syndromes, or neuromuscular disorders.[5,56] Most chemotherapeutic drugs induce neuropathies,[57] while a wide array of pharmaceuticals have been associated with headaches.[58]

Some of these side effects may be impossible to detect either *in vivo* or using alternative model systems; nevertheless, the availability of models that would be predictive of neurotoxic effect is of great relevance for the risk assessment of existing chemicals and of new molecular entities. *In vivo* testing guidelines for neurotoxicity and developmental neurotoxicity have been developed, implemented, and validated. Though there is still room for improvements and refinements, these *in vivo* tests have been shown, so far, to provide reliable indications on the potential neurotoxicity of chemical substances. However, such *in vivo* tests are time consuming and expensive and require the use of a substantial number of animals.

Hence, there is a great need to develop alternative models, utilizing mammalian cell preparations of different complexity and/or nonmammalian animal system, as indicated earlier. These alternative tests should serve as Tier 1 tests to allow the screening of compounds whose potential neurotoxicity is unknown. Given the complexity of the nervous system and the multiple facets of possible neurotoxic effects, it is highly unlikely that a single test (as the Ames test for mutagenicity) will cover the spectrum of neurotoxicity. Rather, a battery of tests that may include some *in vitro* tests with mammalian cells and one or two tests with nonmammalian models should be considered. This may be complemented by quantitative structure-activity relationship (QSAR)-based computational approaches.[59] Novel approaches, part of the "omics" technologies, may also find a role in such endeavor. Genomics, proteomics, and metabolomics each offer the potential of fingerprinting potential neurotoxic compounds and thus find application to neurotoxicity screening. However, such approaches in this context still need to be developed.

Whatever approach is chosen, it needs to undergo a rigorous validation process with the testing of several known neurotoxicants and nonneurotoxicants to determine the sensitivity and specificity of the battery, in addition to providing information on reproducibility and interlaboratory variability. Key elements of the validation process are the choice of neurotoxic compounds (which ones and how many) and their concentrations to be used in *in vitro* tests. This is particularly challenging for neurotoxicity, as multiple cell types and cellular mechanisms can be targeted by neurotoxicants. As indicated earlier, neurons and various types of glial cells can be affected by neurotoxicants. A chemical may cause a neuronopathy, provoke an axonopathy, or affect synaptic transmission; it may alter astrocyte or oligodendrocyte/Schwann cell functions, or act by other mechanisms that may lead to neuro-inflammation. Alternative models for neurotoxicity should thus attempt to mimic several processes that may occur *in vivo*. Similarly, chemicals to be used as positive controls in validation studies should cover most, if not all, of these processes and would thus need to be several dozens. So far, only between ten and twenty chemicals have been used in limited validation experiments. The concentration of chemical to be used in these studies is also most relevant. One has to consider whether to rely on plasma levels, if known, or on cerebrospinal fluid levels,[60] which are most often unknown. In this respect, additional *in vitro* test systems may be used to assess the permeability of chemicals through the BBB.[61–63] The scenario for neurotoxicity is thus much more complex than that for other target organs of toxicity. For example, it has been shown that hepatotoxicity can be predicted by a few specific features (e.g., mitochondrial damage, oxidative stress, intracellular glutathione), which has allowed the development of potentially highly predictive screening approaches.[64]

Finally, a battery of alternative testing models for neurotoxicity is not expected to fully replace current *in vivo* animal testing, but it would limit such testing only to those compounds for which, for different reasons, additional information on neurotoxicity is deemed important. Without concerted efforts by regulatory agencies, institutions, foundations, and private entities worldwide, it is doubtful that such a validation process will take place. If so, ten years from now, we will still be discussing perhaps new, sophisticated models, that have the potential to serve as screening tool for neurotoxicity, but that would leave this potential still unfulfilled.

REFERENCES

1. Barres BA. The mystery and magic of glia: A perspective on their roles in health and disease. *Neuron*. 2008;60:430–440.
2. Costa LG. Neurotoxicity testing: A discussion of in vitro alternatives. *Environ Health Perspect*. 1998;106(Suppl. 2) 505–510.
3. ECETOC. *Evaluation of the Neurotoxic Potential of Chemicals*. Brussels: European Center for Ecotoxicology and Toxicology of Chemicals; 1992.
4. Grandjean P, Landrigan PJ. Developmental neurotoxicity of industrial chemicals. *Lancet*. 2006; 368: 2167–2178.
5. Spencer PS, Schaumburg HH, Ludolph AC, eds. *Experimental and Clinical Neurotoxicology*. Oxford: Oxford University Press: 2000:1310.
6. Jensen KF, Catalano SM. Brain morphogenesis and developmental neurotoxicology. In: Slikker W, Chang LW, eds., *Handbook of Developmental Neurotoxicology*. San Diego: Academic Press; 1998:3–41.
7. Costa LG, Giordano G. Developmental neurotoxicity of polybrominated diphenyl ether (PBDE) flame retardants. *Neurotoxicology*. 2007;28:1047–1067.
8. Crofton KM. Thyroid disrupting chemicals: mechanisms and mixtures. *Int. J. Androl*. 2008;31:209–223.
9. USEPA (U.S. Environmental Protection Agency). Health Effects Test Guidelines. OPPTS 870.6200. Neurotoxicity screening battery. Washington, DC: USEPA; 1998.
10. OECD (Organization for Economic Co-operation and Development). Test Guideline 424. OECD Guideline for Testing of Chemicals. Neurotoxicity study in rodents. Paris: OECD; 1997.
11. Makris SL, Raffaele K, Allen S, et al. A retrospective performance assessment of the developmental neurotoxicity study in support of OECD test guideline 426. *Environ. Health Perspect*. 2009;117:17–25.
12. USEPA (U.S. Environmental Protection Agency). Health Effects Test Guidelines. OPPTS 870.6300. Developmental neurotoxicity study. Washington, DC: USEPA; 1998.
13. OECD (Organization for Economic Co-operation and Development). Test Guideline 426. OECD Guideline for Testing of Chemicals. Developmental neurotoxicity study. Paris: OECD; 2007.
14. Claudio L, Kwa WC, Russell AL, et al. Testing methods for developmental neurotoxicity of environmental chemicals. *Toxicol Appl Pharmacol*. 2000;164:1–14.

15. Cory-Slechta DA, Crofton KM, Foran JA, et al. Methods to identify and characterize developmental neurotoxicity for human health risk assessment. I: Behavioral effects. *Environ Health Perspect.* 109(Suppl. 1):79–91.
16. Harry GJ, Billingsley M, Bruinink A, et al. In vitro techniques for the assessment of neurotoxicity. *Environ Health Perspect.* 1998;106(Suppl. 1):131–158.
17. Sunol C, Babot Z, Fonfria E, et al. Studies with neuronal cells: From basic studies of mechanisms of neurotoxicity to the prediction of chemical toxicity. *Toxicol In Vitro.* 2008;22:1350–1355.
18. Gartlon J, Kinsner A, Bal-Price A, et al. Evaluation of a proposed in vitro test strategy using neuronal and non-neuronal cell systems for detecting neurotoxicity. *Toxicol In Vitro.* 2006;20:1569–1581.
19. Bal-Price AK, Hogberg HT, Buzanska L, et al. Relevance of in vitro neurotoxicity testing for regulatory requirements: Challenges to be considered. *Neurotoxicol. Teratol.* 2010;32:36–41.
20. Silva RFM, Falcao AS, Fernandes A, et al. Dissociated primary nerve cell cultures as models for assessment of neurotoxicity. *Toxicol Lett.* 2006;163:1–9.
21. Coecke S, Eskes C, Gartlon J, et al. The value of alternative testing for neurotoxicity in the context of regulatory needs. *Environ Toxicol Pharmacol.* 2006;21:153–167.
22. Honegger P, Monnet-Tschudi F. Aggregating neural cell cultures. In: (Fedoroff S, Richardson A, eds. *Protocols for Neural Cell Cultures.* Ottawa: Humana Press: 2001:199–218.
23. McLean WG, Holme AD, Janneh O, et al. The effect of benomyl on neurite outgrowth in mouse NB2A and human SH-SY5Y neuroblastoma cells in vitro. *Neurotoxicology.* 1998;19:629–632.
24. Costa LG, Fattori V, Giordano G, et al. An in vitro approach to assess the toxicity of certain food contaminants: Methylmercury and polychlorinated biphenyls. *Toxicology.* 2007;237:65–76.
25. Dey S, Mactutus CF, Booze RM, et al. Specificity of prenatal cocaine on inhibition of locus coeruleus neurite outgrowth. *Neuroscience.* 2006;139:899–907.
25. Radio NM, Mundy WR. Developmental neurotoxicity testing in vitro: Models for assessing chemical effects on neurite outgrowth. *Neurotoxicology.* 2008;29:361–376.
26. Tamm C, Duckworth J, Hemanson O, et al. High susceptibility of neural stem cells to methylmercury toxic effects on cell survival and neuronal differentiation. *J Neurochem.* 2006; 7:69–78.
27. Giordano G, Kavanagh TJ, Costa LG. Neurotoxicity of a polybrominated diphenyl ether mixture (DE-71) in mouse neurons and astrocytes is modulated by intracellular glutathione levels. *Toxicol Appl Pharmacol.* 2008;232:161–168.
28. Giordano G, White CC, Mohar I, et al. Glutathione levels modulate domoic acid-induced apoptosis in mouse cerebellar granule cells. *Toxicol. Sci.* 2007;100: 433–444.
29. Guizzetti M, Thompson BD, Kim Y, et al. Role of phospholipase D signaling in ethanol induced inhibition of carbachol-stimulated DNA synthesis of 1321N1 astrocytoma cells. *J Neurochem.* 2004;90:646–653.
30. Kodavanti PR, Ward TR. Differential effects of commercial polybrominated diphenyl ether and polychlorinated biphenyl mixtures on intracellular signaling in rat brain in vitro. *Toxicol Sci.* 2005;85:952–962.
31. Zurich MG, Honegger P, Schilter B, et al. Involvement of glial cells in the neurotoxicity of parathion and chlorpyrifos. *Toxico. Sci.* 2004;201:97–104.
32. Giordano G, Kavanagh TJ, Costa LG. Mouse cerebellar astrocytes protect cerebellar granule neurons against toxicity of the polybrominated diphenyl ether (PBDE) mixture DE-71. *Neurotoxicology.* 2009;30:326–329.
33. Janigro D, Costa LG. Effects of trimethyltin on granule cells excitability in the in vitro rat dentate gyrus. *Neurotoxicol Teratol.* 1987;9:33–38.
34. Goldoni M, Vettori MV, Alinovi R, et al. Models of neurotoxicity: Extrapolation of threshold doses in vitro. *Risk Anal.* 2003;23:505–514.

35. Lotti M, Moretto A. Organophosphate-induced delayed polyneuropathy. *Toxicol Rev.* 2005;24:37–49.
36. Ehrich M, Correll L, Veronesi B. Acetylcholinesterase and neuropathy target esterase inhibitions in neuroblastoma cells to distinguish organophosphorus compounds causing acute and delayed neurotoxicity. *Fund Appl Toxicol.* 1997;38:55–63.
37. Breier JM, Radio NM, Mundy WR, et al. Development of a high-throughput screening assay for chemical effects on proliferation and viability of immortalized human neural progenitor cells. *Toxicol Sci.* 2008;105:119–133.
38. Radio NM, Breier JM, Shafer TJ, et al. Assessment of chemical effects on neurite outgrowth in PC12 cells using high content screening. *Toxicol Sci.* 2008;105:106–118.
39. Van Vliet E, Morath S, Eskes C, et al. A novel metabolomics approach for neurotoxicity testing, proof of principle for methylmercury chloride and caffeine. *Neurotoxicology.* 2008;29:1–12.
40. Van Vliet E, Stoppini L, Balestrino M, et al. Electrophysiological recording of re-aggregating brain cell cultures on multi-electrode arrays to detect acute neurotoxic effects. *Neurotoxicology.* 2007;28:1136–1146.
41. Peterson RT, Nass R, Boyd WA, et al. Use of non-mammalian alternative models for neurotoxicological study. *Neurotoxicology.* 2008;29:546–555.
42. Buznikov GA, Nikitina LA, Bezuglov VV, et al. An invertebrate model of the developmental neurotoxicity of insecticides: Effects of chlorpyrifos and dieldrin in sea urchin embryos and larvae. *Environ Health Perspect.* 2001;109:651–661.
43. Falugi C, Lammerding-Koppel M, Aluigi MG. Sea urchin development: An alternative model for mechanistic understanding of neurodevelopment and neurotoxicity. *Birth Defects Res (Pt C).* 2008;84:188–2003.
44. Zon LJ, Peterson RT. In vivo drug discovery in the zebrafish. *Nature Rev Drug Discov.* 2005;4:35–44.
45. Blader P, Strahle U. Zebrafish developmental genetics and central nervous system development. *Hum Mol Genet.* 2000;9:945–951.
46. Jeong JY, Kwon HB, Ahn JC, et al. Functional and developmental analysis of the blood–brain barrier in zebrafish. *Brain Res Bull.* 2008;75:619–628.
47. Ton C, Lin Y, Willett C. Zebrafish as a model for developmental neurotoxicity testing. *Birth Defects Res (Pt. A.)* 2006;76:553–567.
48. Parng C, Roy NM, Ton C, et al. Neurotoxicity assessment using zebrafish. *J. Pharmacol Toxicol Meth.* 2007;55:103–112.
49. McKinley ET, Baranowski TC, Blavo DO, et al. Neuroprotection of MPTP-induced toxicity in zebrafish dopaminergic neurons. *Brain Res Mol. Brain Res.* 2005;141:128–137.
50. Kaletta T, Hengartner MO. Finding function in novel targets: *C. elegans* as a model organism. *Nat Rev Drug Discovery.* 2006;5:387–398.
51. Helmke KJ, Avila DS, Aschner M. Utility of *Caenorhabditis elegans* in high throughput neurotoxicological research. *Neurotoxicol. Teratol.* 2010;32:62–67.
52. White JG, Southgate J, Thomson JN, et al. The structure of the nervous system of the nematode *Caenorhabditis elegans. Philos Trans R Soc Lond, B Bio. Sci.* 1986; 314:1–340.
53. Leung MCK, Williams PL, Benedetto A, et al. *Caenorhabditis elegans*: An emerging model in biomedical and environmental toxicology. *Toxicol Sci.* 2008;106:5–28.
54. Hengartner MO, Horvitz HR. Programmed cell death in *Caenorhabditis elegans. Curr Op Genet Dev.* 1994;4:581–586.
55. Boyd WA, Smith MV, Kissling G, et al. Medium- and high-throughput screening of neurotoxicants using *C. elegans. Neurotoxicol Teratol.* 2010;32:68–73.
56. Grosset KA, Grosset DG. Prescribed drugs and neurological complications. *J Neurol Neurosurg Psychi.* 2004;75:2–8.
57. Windebank AJ, Grisold W. Chemotherapy-induced neuropathy. *J Periph Nervous Sys.* 2008;13:27–46.
58. Ferrari A. Headache: One of the most common and troublesome adverse reactions to drugs. *Curr Drug Saf.* 2006;1:43–58.

59. Piotrowski PL, Sumter BG, Malling HV, et al. A toxicity evaluation and predictive system based on neural networks and wavelets. *J Chem Inf Model*. 2007;47:676–685.
60. Lin JH. CSF as a surrogate for assessing CNS exposure: An industrial perspective. *Curr Drug Metab*. 2008;9: 6–59.
61. Abbott NJ, Dolman DE, Patabendige AK. Assays to predict drug permeation across the blood–brain barrier, and distribution to brain. *Curr Drug Metab*. 2008;9:901–910.
62. Vastag M, Keseru GM. Current in vitro and in silico models of blood–brain barrier penetration: A practical view. *Curr Opin Drug Discov Devel*. 2009;12:115–124.
63. Hallier-Vanuxeem D, Prieto P, Culot M, et al. New strategy for alerting central nervous system toxicity: integration of blood–brain barrier toxicity and permeability in neurotoxicity assessment. *Toxicol In Vitro*. 2009;23:447–453.
64. Xu JJ, Henstock PV, Dunn MC, et al. Cellular imaging predictions of clinical drug-induced liver injury. *Toxicol Sci*. 2008;105:97–105.

9 De-risking developmental toxicity-mediated drug attrition in the pharmaceutical industry

Terence R. S. Ozolinš

9.1 INTRODUCTION: THE BUSINESS NEED FOR *IN VITRO* TESTS

Each year, the pharmaceutical industry synthesizes thousands of novel chemical entities with an array of biological activities; however, only a small fraction will make it to market due to poor efficacy or toxicity concerns.[1] Although the drug candidate attrition rate will always be high, the key determinant of its economic consequence is whether it occurs early or late in product development.[1] This point is particularly poignant with respect to developmental toxicity because the first indication of teratogenicity is at the time of the regulatory compliant embryo/fetal toxicity study, which is generally conducted relatively late in drug development, at the transition from Phase II to Phase III. So even though it has been estimated that only about 7 percent of pharmaceutical attrition is due to reproductive and developmental toxicity concerns (about 3.5 percent to developmental toxicity alone), the significant investment of time and money to this point makes such failures catastrophic. Thus, a key challenge is the early identification and management of developmental toxicity risks prior to the conduct of pivotal *in vivo* embryo/fetal toxicity studies. For the purposes of this chapter, there are three aspects to meeting this challenge. The first is the assessment of the inherent risk of the therapeutic target. How important is the target during embryogenesis and what are the consequences of modulating its activity? The second relates to *in silico* structure activity relationship (SAR) approaches that may identify chemical-specific effects, occurring either as pharmacologically mediated events, or as "off-target" effects. The third component is the use of *in vitro* screening models for lead optimization. Each of the three approaches has some inherent value, but it is their strategic integration that synergistically mitigates developmental toxicity risk. Thus, a generic strategy is discussed, and adherence to it or a similar strategy will significantly reduce the possibility of failure at the pivotal preclinical safety study. The reality is that no strategy is perfect, and therefore efforts continue toward improving the way one assesses (a) the role of a target during gestation, (b) *in silico* SAR, and (c) *in vitro* embryotoxicity. Together, these improvements, which are discussed in the final section, will shape the future of developmental toxicity risk management.

9.2 ASSESSING THE RISK OF MODULATING THE THERAPEUTIC TARGET

9.2.1 Target-mediated versus chemotype-mediated teratogenesis

From the pharmaceutical perspective, there are two fundamental causes of teratogenicity, each with different implications for drug development strategies. The first, relates to the inherent embryo/fetal toxicity risk of the therapeutic target. That is, the therapeutic target plays such a critical role during embryogenesis that any pharmacologic interference results in teratogenesis, as manifest by malformations, fetal death, or intrauterine growth retardation (IUGR). If such effects are mediated by the intended pharmacology of a drug, strategies that provide knowledge about species-specific expression or gestational function of the target should facilitate an understanding of the developmental toxicity risk. The second cause of teratogenicity is unrelated to the intended pharmacology but, instead, is a result of unintended off-target interactions that are chemotype-dependent. These may include, for example, reversible receptor-mediated interactions with related receptor subtypes, unexpected pharmacologic effects with unrelated proteins, or more generalized irreversible toxicological reactions such as adduct formation or oxidative stress. From a pharmaceutical perspective, the earlier one is able to discriminate between intended pharmacology and off-target events, the sooner one is able to assess the possible risk of a therapeutic campaign and make an appropriate business decision

9.2.2 Does one need a developmental toxicity risk management strategy?

Inherent developmental toxicity risk does not necessarily preclude a cellular molecule from being a viable therapeutic target. For example, therapeutic areas such as cancer or Alzheimer's disease may tolerate such risk because these therapies are, respectively, life-saving or in a demographic situation where women of child-bearing potential are not a concern. Another consideration is whether risk tolerance for a disease may change over time. Due to the long duration from idea to clinic, the risks that may have been acceptable when the drug program was initiated may no longer be appropriate as it enters the market. A clear example of this is AIDS therapy. Initially HIV infection was considered a terminal condition, with little regard for embryo/fetal safety; however, more recently with the advent of sero-positive mothers giving birth to sero-negative offspring, the absence of teratogenicity is a critical aspect of market success. Thus, the disease indication and the intended patient demographic together determine whether the absence of teratogenicity is important and whether a developmental toxicity risk management strategy is even warranted.

9.2.3 What targets need to be assessed?

The completion of the human genome with high-quality annotation revealed approximately 30,000 genes,[2,3] and with it, much exuberance about the potential for thousands of novel drug targets;[4] however, it also presents the daunting challenge of devising ways to predict the developmental role of these gene products. But do we really need to know the developmental role of all 30,000 genes?[5] Probably not because of the idea known as the "druggable genome." The concept of the druggable genome is that only about 3,000 proteins favor interactions with drug-like chemicals.[4] Proteins lacking such features may be of biological importance, but they are unlikely to be amenable to pharmacologic intervention.[4,6] Moreover, not all druggable targets are disease modifying, and it has been proposed that these represent only about 10 percent of the genome.[7] The intersection of the druggable and disease-modifying genes reveal about 600–1,500 viable therapeutic targets,[4] suggesting that to predict the embryo toxicity risk one need "only" investigate about 1,500 targets and not the entire genome.

With the druggable genome in mind, the author's institution has developed a "Fetal Map" database.[8] Briefly, it describes the mRNA expression levels of 4,000 potentially druggable genes in early and late organogenesis-stage embryos and extra-embryonic membranes from humans and toxicologically relevant animal test species (mouse, rat, and rabbit). This database provides at least two valuable pieces of information. First, it identifies whether a gene is present or absent during organogenesis, the period most susceptible to teratogenic insult. If present, this may trigger the need for investigative work to localize the expression domains or to use genetically modified animal models to understand the potential consequences of its over- or underexpression (see discussion that follows). The absence or very low expression of a target protein suggests a low risk for pharmacologically mediated developmental toxicity, although indirect maternally mediated effects are still possible, as are off-target toxicities. Second, Fetal Map also identifies whether there are quantitative or localization differences in gene expression between humans and the test species that may require further investigation and that, importantly, may impact species selection for preclinical safety studies. For example, in contrast to the rodent, the yolk sac does not have as significant a nutritional role in nonrodents, such as primates and lagomorphs (reviewed in Reference 9), suggesting rodents may not reflect the human risk associated with such targets. Fetal Map may soon become publicly available.

9.2.4 Genetically modified animal models

Having identified that a target is expressed during a susceptible window of embryogenesis, one may need to understand its developmental role to determine if its pharmacological modulation may pose a risk. A conceptually simple way of assessing this is to remove the gene and examine the developmental effects. Owing to their fecundity and fully annotated genome, the mutant mouse is the most popular genetically modified vertebrate animal model. Loss and gain of function models and other genetic manipulations have become an integral part of evidence-based therapeutic target selection (reviewed in References 10, 11), and are a maturing resource for toxicologic research. These animal models and clinical observations have also increased our understanding about the functionality of gene products during embryogenesis and provide clues as to the consequences of altering these targets pharmacologically. The down-side of this approach is that small molecules are considered efficacious when they inhibit the function of their target by ≈50 percent. A knockout mouse, with no functional target protein, is a poor model for a reduction in function of 40–60 percent.

The biological consequences of genetically modifying a potential therapeutic target are available from a variety of sources. If the protein is not novel, there may be considerable information in the public literature as well as searchable databases belonging to a variety of research institutes (e.g., Jackson Labs). Although freely available, these sources are widely dispersed and time consuming to search. To be cost-effective, this resource requires the development of robust search engines to facilitate quick and thorough access of all pertinent public data. These specific search algorithms are not publicly available and must therefore be developed in-house.

Information about the phenotypes of many modified mouse models is not publicly available, and therefore there may be a need to develop the model. This may be done in-house or as a fee for service. With about a one year development time and a cost of approximately $100,000/gene target, Taconic, for example, will deliver several founder animals from which a colony can be derived and maintained. The resource requirement for a comprehensive knockout program directed at the full druggable genome is prohibitive, even for a large multinational pharmaceutical company. A viable alternative is the outsourcing to obtain phenotypic information as a fee for service.[11]

In this regard, at Pfizer a program called Phenotype Pfinder has been used since 2000 to systematically interrogate the phenotypes of genetically modified mice.[12] Here, a battery of clinically relevant tests with about 250 endpoints is used to describe the changing health status of these animals for a period of about 17 weeks. If, after heterozygous matings, either malformed pups or non-Mendelian ratios of the anticipated genotypes are encountered, it triggers the investigation of the embryo/fetal phenotype by the Developmental and Reproductive Toxicology group. To date, unusual or lethal mutant phenotypes have not been used to terminate a therapeutic program, but rather, these data have been used to influence the drug development strategy.[12] For example, a different therapeutic indication may be found for a target, one in which women of child-bearing potential are a less likely patient population. It may trigger higher-throughput screening initiatives to identify structures that are less apt to enter into the embryo/fetal compartment. If the program appears to be very compelling, pivotal toxicity studies may be "front-loaded" to get an earlier indication of developmental toxicity risks. In addition, certain biological processes occurring *in utero* also occur in the adult animal and therefore embryo/fetal phenotypes may be valuable portents to the consequences of pharmacological inhibition in the adult. One example of this at Pfizer was an embryolethal mutant that died *in utero* due to impaired vasculogenesis.[12] Although the heterozygous mutant adult animals did not display a related pathology, a variety of chemically distinct antagonists directed against this target all caused vascular pathology similar to the homozygous null embryotoxicity, confirming this class or target-related effect. Thus, embryonic phenotypes may provide valuable clues about the consequences of modulating a therapeutic target both during gestation and in the adult.

With the advent of interference RNA technologies, more cost- and time-effective approaches may be used to knock down, rather than knock out targets. In the author's facility, lentiviral delivery systems[13] containing short hairpin (sh) RNA directed at a gene of interest, have been injected into single-cell murine zygotes, and re-implanted into surrogate females.[14,15] Using this technique we reproduced the embryo/fetal phenotype seen in knockouts generated through homologous recombination, and the phenotype was correlated with the degree of knockdown of the target gene.[13] Theoretically, this may more accurately reflect the pharmacologic inhibition of a target, in which the biologic activity has been partially, rather than completely, inhibited, with the added advantage of requiring only a few months to generate the model.

In summary, gene expression databases like Fetal Map can provide important information about the presence and localization of gene products in the conceptus, and their functionality may be interrogated by genetically reducing the activity of the intended target gene during gestation. It should be noted that there may be some discordance between the phenotypes of animal mutant models and human mutant models, and in addition, 50 percent of the knockouts have no discernable phenotype, which may, in part, be due to compensatory increases in the gene expression of related gene family members.[10] Nevertheless, mutant models provide valuable insights that help to paint a more complete picture of a drug target's liabilities, not only *in utero* but also in the adult animals.

9.3 OFF-TARGET EFFECTS

Many drug-induced fetal anomalies are the result of unintended interactions with biological targets. These may be classical receptor-mediated pharmacologic effects due to poor specificity (intended or unintended) or toxicological mechanisms that initiate irreversible adduct formation, reactive oxygen species and so on. Despite a dominant philosophy in drug design having been the generation of chemicals with maximal selectivity, it is clear that many effective pharmaceuticals modulate several targets simultaneously.[16] Such molecules are described as having a "rich pharmacology." Targeted polypharmacology is a logical extension of this observation.[17,18] In a further step forward, the advent of systems biology has produced another drug discovery paradigm, namely "network pharmacology," in which multiple members of a signaling cascade are targeted to elicit a desired clinical biological change.[18] The bi- or multitargeted approach to target therapy is double-edged sword. Whereas the intended therapeutic effects may be superior owing to several modifications within a receptor family or a common biologic pathway, there is also the increased risk of unanticipated unfavorable interactions. In theory, the most cost-effective approach to avoid this issue would be to build structure activity databases in which developmental toxicity may be queried before the chemist attempts a synthesis.[19]

9.3.1 *In silico* approaches

As described elsewhere in this book, SARs of increasing sophistication have been used for some time to make toxicity predictions for a variety of organ systems, including the developing embryo/fetus.[20] *In silico* or computer-based analyses are of two primary kinds: knowledge or "rule-based" systems and correlative or "statistically based" systems. The details of the different prediction systems have been reviewed in detail elsewhere,[21,22] but for the purposes of developmental toxicity prediction two models are discussed briefly here.

The first is a rule-based system, which makes predictions for untested agents by drawing upon the human interpretation of toxicity data and biological information. That is, it captures, organizes, and applies scientific expertise that relates chemical structures with developmental toxicity. Examples of commercially available rule-based approaches include HazardExpert,[23] Deductive Estimation of Risk from Existing Knowledge (DEREK),[24]

The second example, is a statistically based SAR system, in which only statistical or mathematical analyses are used to discriminate between the presence or absence of developmental toxicity in the training set. Analogous to the rule-based approach, predictions cannot be made with novel structures. Commercially available predictive systems include Toxicity Predictions by Komputer Assisted Technology (TOPKAT)[25] and a series of products by MultiCASE[26]: Computer Automated Structure Evaluation (CASE), MultiCASE, CASETOX, and MultiCASE-Expert System. The latter three may be considered to be hybrids because through the statistical analysis of experimental data, they can determine specific fragment rules, which, when combined with literature data may be incorporated into rule-based programs such as DEREK. An important consideration is that the CASETOX system supplies a nonmodifiable training set, whereas MultiCASE allows users to modify the modules or supply their own.

Unfortunately, in spite of several comprehensive catalogs documenting thousands of teratogenic agents (reviewed in References 27–29) and despite the compelling logical appeal of these approaches, efforts to use these data sets to create robust SAR predictions for developmental toxicity have been largely unsuccessful.[22] This has been attributed to a number of factors. Although reviewed in detail elsewhere,[22] some points are worth noting here. First, in contrast to other SAR approaches to predict single-organ toxicity, a developmental SAR must predict toxicity in every organ of the embryo/fetus, which depending upon the gestational period, may approach adult-like complexity; imagine creating a SAR database that predicts simultaneously hepato-, neuro-, photo- and ocular toxicity. Moreover, unlike adult organ systems that are relatively static, and hence theoretically easier to model, the conceptus is highly dynamic with cellular migration, differentiation, carefully orchestrated apoptotic programs, and osmotic gradient fluxes all happening simultaneously, all of which are used to create three-dimensional structures that change throughout gestation.

With respect to developmental toxicity, there is a critical difference between rule-based and statistically based SAR approaches. The rule-based approach requires some biological or biochemical knowledge about the toxicity of interest, and therefore is not particularly useful when the toxicity has not been characterized. Unfortunately, with the exception of a few specific chemical classes (retinoids, phenols, glycol ethers, and steroids), by and large developmental toxicity endpoints are poorly understood.[22] Given the dearth of information concerning teratogenesis endpoints, statistically based approaches may be more fruitful in the near term than those using rule-based systems.

Although some SAR models have claimed reasonable success,[20] due to the factors described previously, we have not found SAR approaches particularly useful; however, in the one instance DEREK identified a "hit," the chemical in question did test positive for embryotoxicity *in vitro* (whole embryo culture and the embryonic stem cell test).

9.4 *IN VITRO* TESTS

Due to the limited applicability of *in silico* SAR approaches for developmental toxicity, there is more reliance on *in vitro* screening. From what has been publicly disclosed, it is evident that the four *in vitro* tests used for industrial screening are chick embryonic neural retina (CENR) micromass culture, whole embryo culture (WEC, rodent or rabbit), and mouse embryonic stem cells (EST). Recently, there has been significant interest within the pharmaceutical industry in the use of zebrafish for developmental toxicity testing,[30] but because this aspect is in its infancy, there is little that has been publicly disclosed except limited abstracts and slide decks at several workshops.[31] Although reviewed in considerable detail elsewhere,[30,32–36] each test will be briefly compared and contrasted here.

All screening tests share several limitations. The first is that these models only assess the potential consequences if the test system is exposed to the test article. Thus, they make no assessment about maternal-embryo/fetal partition coefficients, which often determine *in vivo* embryonic exposure and teratogenic risk.[37,38] In addition, many drugs are proteratogens. That is, that they require biotransformation, often in the maternal or placental compartment,[39] to mediate developmental toxicity. As a result of the low or absent biotransformation capacity of these test systems, the consequences of downstream metabolites cannot be tested unless specifically synthesized by the chemist. For broad screening programs, this may be a disadvantage,[40] but for specific investigative efforts this facilitates the separation of parent versus metabolite-mediated developmental toxicity, something that is almost impossible to do *in vivo*. Indeed, at Pfizer, by engaging the chemists, we have used this approach with whole embryo culture

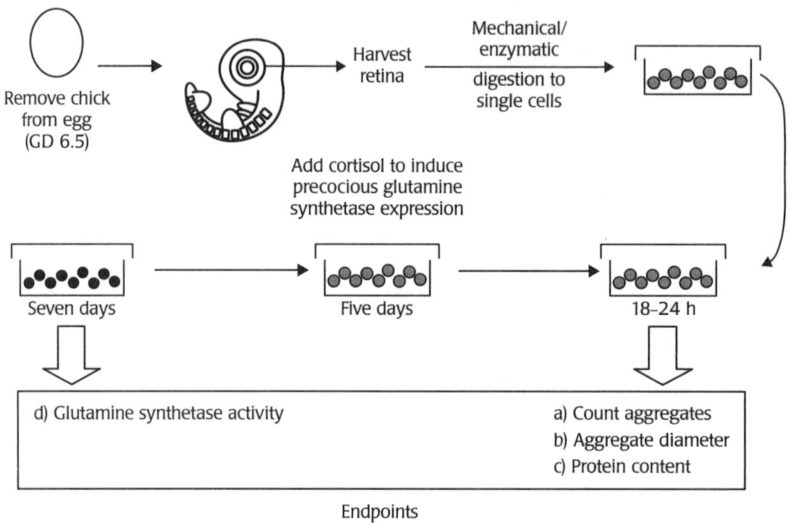

Figure 9-1: The highlights of the chick embryonic neural retina micromass cultures are depicted. The tissue is harvested and digested to a single-cell suspension. These are placed into culture, and after 24 h three parameters are measured: (a) the number of aggregates that are produced, (b) the size of the aggregates, and (c) their protein content. After five days cortisol is added to precociously induce glutamine synthetase activity. This is measured two days later, after a total of seven days of culture. Each parameter is uniquely sensitive to different agents, but a decrease in any one parameter is considered to be toxicologically relevant.

to help direct programs toward chemical backbones that do not produce specific metabolite moieties.[41] In specific non-screening-related cases, exogenous drug metabolizing systems have been added to stem cells,[42] whole embryos,[43–46] and zebrafish[47] to look at the effect of metabolites on developmental toxicity, but such strategies have not been incorporated into industrial screening efforts.

9.4.1 Chick embryo neural retina cell culture model

The chick embryo neural retina cell culture model is a micromass test, developed and used at Proctor and Gamble. Its appeal is the technical simplicity and low cost, in which the intact embryonic organ, in this case the chick eye, is harvested and dissociated into a single-cell suspension *via* mechanical forces and enzymatic digestion. These cells are placed into culture where they are allowed to replicate, migrate, reaggregate, and differentiate into specific multicellular aggregates that eventually express a histologic and biochemical phenotype similar to the *in situ* retina.[36] The capacity of a test article to interfere with these processes reflects, at least in theory, its *in vivo* teratogenic potential. A schematic representation of the chick neural cell culture method is depicted in Figure 9.1.

9.4.2 Embryonic stem cells

Recent advances in embryonic stem cell technology have made these cells available for a variety of toxicity models.[48–50] The use of murine embryonic stem cells for developmental toxicity testing is based upon the observation that, in culture, these pluripotent cells, derived from the inner cell mass of a blastocyst, may be induced to differentiate into cell types from the three primary germ layers. The gene expression patterns also reflect a rough concordance with the gene expression patterns observed during the differentiation of early, preimplantation embryos *in vivo*,[51] suggesting that *in vitro* embryonic stem cell differentiation may recapitulate many aspects of early *in vivo* embryogenesis and therefore may be an appropriate surrogate for the embryo with respect to developmental toxicity testing. As a result of these properties and the fact that stem cells are a self-renewing cell line, the European Committee for the Validation of Alternative Methods (ECVAM) provided both administrative and financial support for the development and international validation of a stem-cell-based *in vitro* toxicity test.[32]

Stem cells are grown under specific conditions[52] (Figure 9.2) that produce a variety of cell types, but most importantly beating cardiomyocytes. The formation of contracting cardiomyocytes is relatively complex, dependant upon a variety of fundamental processes such as cellular differentiation, migration, cell–cell recognition, and ultimately the communication of synchronized electric impulses across a large surface area (as these cells tend to beat in unison). In principle, developmental toxicants reduce the frequency of wells (within a 24-well plate) that contain beating cells, whereas nontoxicants do not.

9.4.3 Whole embryo culture

The reader is referred to several excellent reviews on rodent whole embryo culture and its use as a tool for *in vitro* toxicity screening.[33,34] The procedure is based upon the explantation of presomitic or early somitic rodent embryos with intact visceral yolk sacs. If rat embryos are explanted on gestation day 10 and grown for about 48 h, they will develop a beating heart, functional circulation, closed neural tubes, and limb buds and will possess many of the *anlagen* for major organs such as eyes, ears, maxilla, and mandible. When terminated at the 30–32 somite stage, the *in vitro* growth and development of embryos are virtually indistinguishable from *in vivo*, save a small decrease total embryonic protein,[53] and a transient induction of immediate/early response genes.[54] Lastly, similar to an *in vivo* embryo/fetal toxicity study, the presence and frequency of deformities can also be determined, and in many cases, the phenotype of chemically induced malformations *in vitro* correlate with those found following *in vivo* administration.[55] Taken together, these endpoints make whole embryo culture very data- rich and *in vivo*-like, and because animal use is reduced relative to animal experiments, ECVAM also supported the development and validation of an *in vitro* test based on rat whole embryos[56] (Figure 9.3). The rabbit is the most frequently used nonrodent developmental toxicity test species, and *in vitro* culture techniques have been described. Dow Chemical Co. generally favors the use of rabbit embryo

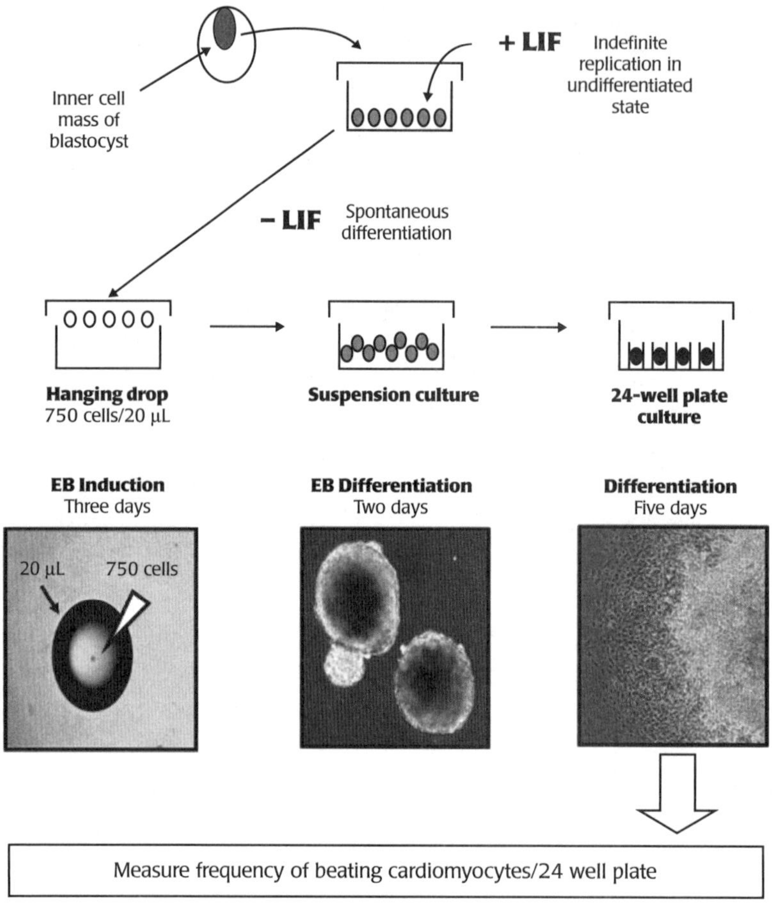

Figure 9-2: The notable points of stem culture are depicted. Embryonic stem cells are isolated from the inner cell mass of a blastocyst. When placed into culture in the presence of Leukemia Inhibitory Factor (LIF) they will maintain their pleuripotency and replicate indefinitely. The ECVAM stem cell model begins with the removal of LIF, from a permanent stem cell line, which induces stem cells to differentiate. During 3 days of hanging drop cultures, gravity forces stem cells into close proximity resulting in the induction of spheroidal aggregates, termed embryoid bodies (EB). Two days of suspension culture permit EB to further differentiate. A single EB is then placed into each well of a 24-well plate to differentiate a further five days. Although a variety of factors may be added to the media to drive stem cell differentiation down specific pathways, the ECVAM protocol allows stem cells to spontaneously produce a variety of cell types including beating cardiomyocytes. A decrease in the number of wells that contain beating cardiomyocytes is a measure of developmental toxicity. Photographs graciously provided by Donald B. Stedman.

culture to rat culture in its *in vitro* studies (E. Carney (EWCarney@dow.com), personal communication).

9.4.4 Zebrafish

The developmental highlights of the zebrafish are depicted in Figure 9.4 and are the subject of several excellent reviews.[30,57] A zebrafish-based toxicity model

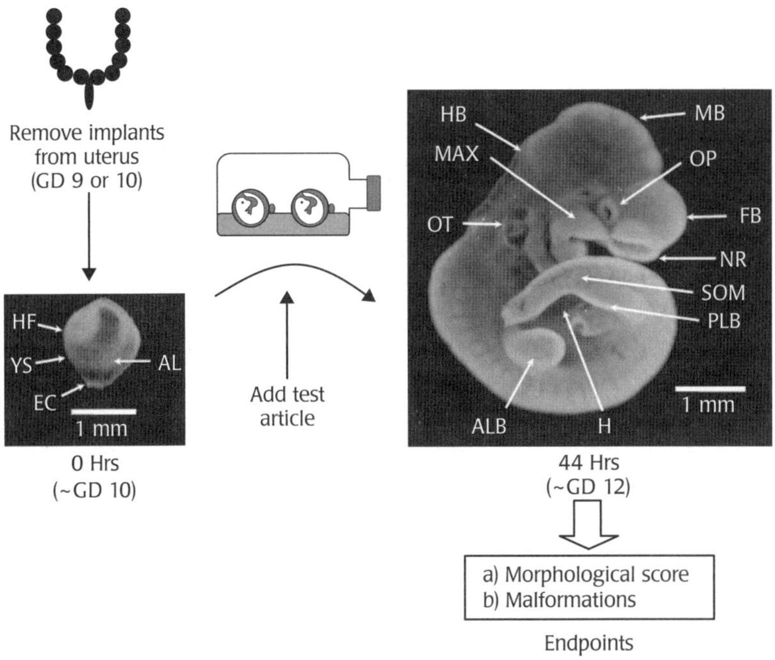

Figure 9-3: The highlights of rat whole embryo culture. The implants are removed from the gestation day (GD) 10 uterus and microdissected to yield an embryo of about 0–6 somites with intact visceral yolk sac. These are grown in a rat serum-based medium with intermittent exposure to increasing oxygen levels. After approximately 44–48 hours, the embryo is virtually indistinguishable from an *in vivo* grown GD 12 embryo. A number of *anlagen* have developed at this time including: hind brain (HB), midbrain (MB), optic region (OP), forebrain (FB), nasal ridge (NR), somites (SOM), posterior limb buds (PLB), anterior limb buds (ALB), otic region (OT), and maxillary process (MAX). Although many endpoints may be measured, for the purposes of the ECVAM prediction model, two endpoints are evaluated; (a) the speed of development as assessed by the Total Morphological Score, which is the sum total development of 17 *anlagen* and (b) abnormal development (~26 malformations),

has been proposed as a test for environment contaminants, and although some teratogens have been studied in zebrafish, their use for industrial developmental toxicity screening is relatively new. Consequently, the protocols currently in use are diverse, and not surprisingly each has distinct advantages and shortcomings, which have been previously reviewed.[30,57] Important considerations include when to initiate exposure and for what duration. The route of exposure is also an important consideration because most pharmaceutical agents are not highly water soluble, and therefore the fish may not be amenable to exposure via the water. There is evidence to suggest that the chorion surrounding the embryo may reduce exposure to agents, and therefore some researchers remove it prior to drug exposure. In view of these considerations it has also been proposed that test articles be injected directly into the yolk. In addition, the relevant endpoints and how they ought to be assessed have not been determined. With more pharmaceutical users and consortia using zebrafish, more standardized procedures are expected to appear shortly.

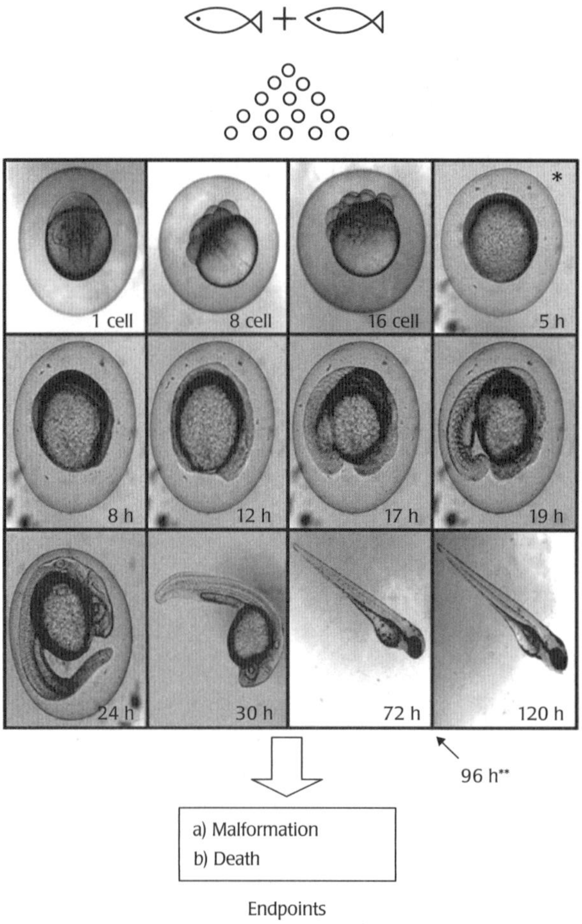

Figure 9-4: The highlights of zebrafish development. Following breeding, eggs are harvested through a grated bottom fish tank and placed into culture dishes containing "fish water," and grown for up to 5 days (120 h). The points measured are malformations and death in response to increasing concentrations of test article. Of note, 5 h (*) corresponds roughly to the time of implantation; GD 6 in rat and rabbit and 7–8 in humans. This is when dosing starts in preclinical developmental toxicity studies. 96 h (**) approximates the time of palatal shelf closure; GD 16 rat, GD 18 rabbit, and GD 56 in humans. This is the termination of dosing in regulatory studies.

9.5 INTERPRETATION OF *IN VIVO* AND *IN VITRO* EMBRYOTOXICITY DATA

9.5.1 *In vivo*

In vitro screening models all represent an embryonic target, surrogate or real, against which to directly test chemically mediated developmental toxicity without confounding maternal influences. However, in their simplicity, these models also pose a challenge because the "dose" that may be administered is limited only by the solubility of the test article, and therefore, with sufficient concentration, virtually any agent can induce embryotoxicity. Thus, these *in vitro* assays differ from the regulatory compliant *in vivo* fetal toxicity testing, where maternal toxicity will be dose limiting. In fact, the teratogenic risk of chemical agents in preclinical toxicity studies is assessed by benchmarking doses that induce malformations against doses causing maternal or embryo/fetal toxicity (Table 9.1). For example, there is little concern if an agent only produces structural malformations at doses that cause maternal toxicity and overt embryotoxicity such as intrauterine growth retardation or *in utero* death. In contrast, there is unease if malformations occur in the absence of maternal toxicity, and added concern if they occur in the absence of embryotoxicity.

9.5.2 *In vitro*

In the chick embryo neural retinal model, three endpoints are measured: the number of aggregates formed, their protein content, and glutamine synthetase activity, which reflect the capacity for cell–cell interactions, growth, and differentiation, respectively.[36] Although none of these parameters represent maternal toxicity *per se*, the number of formed aggregates and protein content may be views as a surrogate for embryotoxicity (*in utero* death or growth retardation). A given test article may affect each of the three endpoints to different extents, but in this assay only one endpoint needs to be affected for it to be considered at risk for developmental toxicity.[35]

The two ECVAM-validated assays, the embryonic stem cell test and whole embryo culture have *in vitro* surrogates identified for each of maternal toxicity, embryotoxicity, and frank malformations[32] (Table 9.1). Shared by both the EST and WEC is the cytotoxicity of the test article in terminally differentiated 3T3 fibroblasts, representing maternal toxicity. The correlate to *in vivo* malformations is the inhibition of beating cardiomyocyte formation and dysmorphogenesis in the EST and WEC, respectively. Frank embryotoxicity is represented by standard cytotoxicity (cell death) in the stem cells and a decrease in embryonic growth as assessed by declines in the total morphological score. The morphological score ascribes numerical scores, in a fairly unbiased way, to various developmental landmarks in seventeen distinct organ/*anlagen* systems.[60] Their sum yields a total morphological score that increases linearly with advancing age during the middle window of organogenesis, thereby providing a reasonable measure of the speed of development. The most widely used scoring system was developed for rat by Brown and Fabro,[60] but others for mouse[61] and rabbit have also been reported.[62,63]

There are at least four competing efforts to use zebrafish as a platform for a developmental toxicity test, and the strategies used in all but one are closely guarded. In a Phylonix/Bristol-Myers Squibb collaboration, there is no surrogate for maternal toxicity, but frank embryotoxicity is one endpoint as is evidence of malformed fish.[59]

9.5.3 Interpretation of *in vitro* developmental toxicity data

The endpoints of the *in vitro* assays have been described, but how does one use this data to make assessments about developmental toxicity risk? In the past,

Table 9-1. Comparison of *in vivo* and *in vitro* determinants of developmental toxicity

In vivo	Maternal toxicity	Embryo toxicity	Structural/ functional deficits	Determination of developmental hazard
	- Exaggerated pharmacology of test article (e.g., convulsion) - ↓ absolute body weight - > 10% in body weight gain - Death	- IUGR (intrauterine growth retardation) - ↓ fetal viability - ↑ postimplantation loss - ↓ litter size	- ↑ variations - External gross malformations - Skeletal malformations - Visceral malformations - Behavioral effects	- Consensus meeting to determine whether structural/ functional deficits occur the absence of maternal or embryo toxicity
In vitro	**Surrogate**	**Surrogate**	**Surrogate**	**Surrogate**
CENR	- None	- Cell aggregate count - Aggregate size - Aggregate protein content	- Glutamine synthetase activity	- Perturbation of any endpoint
ECVAM EST	- 3T3 cytotoxicity	Embryonic stem cell cytotoxicity	- ↓ frequency of wells with beating cardiomyocytes	- Biostatistical prediction model
ECVAM WEC	- 3T3 cytotoxicity	- ↓ TMS	- ↑ dysmorphogenesis	- Biostatistical prediction model
Zebrafish	- None	- Death	- Malformations	- Teratogencity quotient

Notes: The relationship between the various determinants of developmental toxicity risk is compared between *in vivo* and *in vivo* tests. The risk of *in vivo* developmental toxicity is low if neither embryotoxicity nor structural deficits occur in the face of maternal toxicity. Conversely, the risk is high if embryotoxicity or structural/functional deficits are observed in the absence of maternal toxicity. In real life, the distinction is never this clear requiring "consensus" meetings with multiple "experts" to make the determination, although consensus is seldom achieved. The *in vitro* surrogates for maternal toxicity, embryotoxicity and structural/functional deficits are described. In the chick embryo neural retinal test (CENR) has no surrogate for maternal toxicity.[36] The embryonic stem cell test (EST) and whole embryo culture (WEC) have surrogates for all three *in vivo* toxicities and the determination of developmental risk through a biostatistical prediction model.[32] The zebrafish has no maternal toxicity surrogate, and it uses a teratogenicity quotient to assesses teratogenic risk; several approaches have been described for the calculation of a teratogenicity quotient.[30,58,59] with WEC, the *in vitro* concentration needed to induce malformations was correlated to the predicted maternal serum concentrations. This works retrospectively, but for a pharmaceutical screening program, *in silico* absorption, distribution, metabolism and excretion (ADME) predictions of therapeutic concentrations must be used, but these predictions still need improvement.[64]

As indicated previously, in the chick embryonic neural retina assay inhibition of any endpoint indicates a developmental toxicity risk. In contrast, the ECVAM assays rely on biostatistical prediction models. As a first step in model development twenty chemicals that represented three classes of embryotoxicity (non, weak or strong) were identified.[65] These test articles were applied to the respective models, and toxicity curves were generated for each of the surrogate measures of maternal toxicity, embryo/fetal toxicity and malformations. Like the *in vivo* situation in which there is a different relationship between maternal toxicity, fetal toxicity, and fetal malformations for teratogens and nonteratogens, it was assumed that a relationship also existed between the *in vitro* surrogate measures of these same toxicities for non, weak, and strong embryotoxicants; however, under *in vitro* conditions this relationship would be described biostatistically using linear discriminate function analysis rather than through expert consensus.[32] In this way unknowns could be applied to the test system, without knowing its therapeutic concentration and the *in vivo* developmental toxicity risk predicted from *in vitro* data. Currently it is debated how universally applicable these models are for "all chemical space."[31,66,67]

For the only publicly disclosed zebrafish model, it is clear that a maternal toxicity component is not used, but rather normalization is against frank embryotoxicity (death). Briefly, a ratio of the LC_{50} and a malformation concentration are calculated, and depending upon the value of this ratio a test article is described as none, weak, or potent.[59]

9.5.4 Comparison of all four tests: advantages/disadvantages

Each of the four tests has inherent advantages and disadvantages, which are summarized in Table 9.2. One point that does require some elaboration relates to the complexity of the model systems. The chick embryonic neural retina assay and the embryonic stem cell test are each based upon the development of a single organ, retinal cell generation and beating cardiomyocytes, respectively. In contrast, the entire embryo and all of its *anlagen* are represented in whole embryo culture rendering it very data rich. Although more life-like than the aforementioned assays, whole embryo culture is also the shortest, which raises an important question: What is the practical utility of a two-day assay spanning but 10 percent of rodent gestation? As illustrated in Figure 9.5, the sensitivity to teratogenic insult varies during gestation, with organogenesis being the most sensitive. Thus, the critical determinant of teratogenicity is the window, not the duration, of exposure. Serendipitously, the time period during which the whole embryo culture is conducted (gestation day 9–11 or 10–12 in the rat) is the most sensitive window of organogenesis. In fact, the developmental events that are

Table 9-2. Summary of the characteristics of the developmental toxicity assays used in pharmaceutical industry

Characteristic	CENR	EST	WEC	Zebrafish
Duration of the *in vitro* test	Seven days	Ten days	Two days	Five days
Gestational days (GD) represented[a]	10–13	~ 5–10	10–12	Entire gestational window
Approximate gestational processes represented	Eye formation	Mammalian blastocyst formation to beating heart tube	Early/mid organogenesis of entire mammalian embryogenesis	All processes in fish
Approximate location on the teratogen sensitivity curve (Figure 9.4)	Near peak (high sensitivity)	Near peak (higher sensitivity)	Near peak (higher sensitivity)	Entire curve (highest sensitivity)
Endpoint measured	1. Malformations 2. Death	1. Frequency of wells containing beating cardiomyocytes	1. Speed of development (total morphological score of 17 organ *anlagen*) 2. ~ 26 discrete malformations	1. Malformation 2. Death
Technical difficulty				
- Experimental conduct	+	+++++	++++	+
- Endpoint assessment	+	+	+++++	+++++
Cost				
- Set up	+++	+++	++++	+++++
- Conduct	++	++++	+++	+
Animal requirements:				
- Tissue donors	Yes	No	Yes	Yes
- Serum in Media	Yes	Yes	Yes	No
Current species used	Chicken	Mouse	Rat	Zebrafish
Other possible species		Rabbit Human	Mouse Rabbit Hamster	N/A
Validated	No	ECVAM validation	ECVAM validation	Not currently, but possible validation through Consortia

Notes: The various characteristics of the developmental toxicity assays are summarized. Technical difficulty and costs are rated as high (+++++) or low (+).
[a] The gestation days are equivalent to rat.

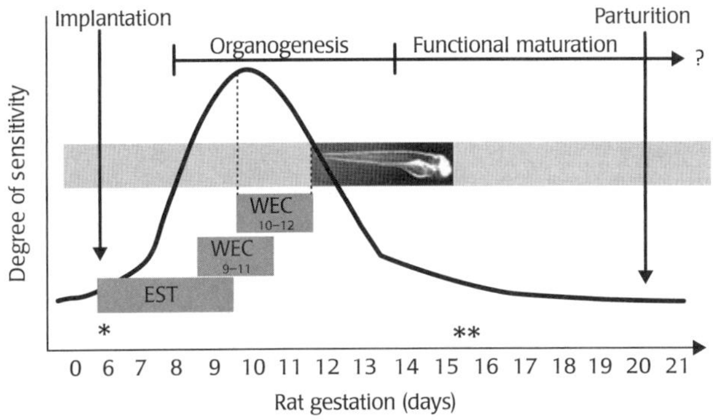

Figure 9-5: The sensitivity of the conceptus to a theoretical teratogen during rat gestation (modified from 161). The most susceptible window is organogenesis with low levels of vulnerability at the time of implantation and the period of functional maturation. Superimposed are the approximations of when the developmental landmarks that are represented in the four *in vitro* tests occur. The chick embryo neural retina model (CENR) represents events around GD 10–13. The mouse embryonic stem cell test (EST) corresponds roughly to the period of GD 6–10 in the rat, near the peak of sensitivity. Whole embryo culture (WEC) recapitulates the window at the peak of sensitivity, between GD 9–11 or GD 10–12 depending upon the window within which the culture is conducted. Rabbit cultures are also done between GD 10–12. Represented by the single (*) and double asterisk (**), respectively, are the initiation and termination of the dosing period in regulatory compliant preclinical embryo/fetal toxicity studies. Thus, the zebrafish is the only model that permits exposure to test article during this important period.

represented in the CNER, stem cell test, and whole embryo culture occur at, or near, the peak of sensitivity, an ideal scenario for a short-term *in vitro* toxicity test. The advantages of the zebrafish are that the intact animal is exposed and evaluated (allowing for tissue interactions in a way not captured by the other assays) and that the entire period of development can be exposed, reflecting more closely the developmental windows of the regulatory compliant studies. Thus, in theory, the fish model may provide the greatest potential to assess chemical interactions across the entire period of gestation.

9.5.5 Performance

The performance of the four developmental toxicity tests considered in this chapter is summarized in Table 9.3 using the ECVAM definition of predicitivity and precision (Table 9.4). In the publicly disclosed validation studies, all appear to have a reported accuracy of about 70–80 percent, which approximates the ability of *in vivo* animal studies to correctly predict human teratogens.[68] The chemical test set used in the ECVAM validation of stem cells and whole embryos was an equal mix of older pharmaceutical agents and industrial chemicals because the strategy was to develop prediction models capable of discriminating broad classes of chemicals.[65] Thus, it was unclear how well these models would work when challenged with novel pharmaceuticals based on current chemotype strategies. Surprisingly, the performance approximates that initially reported in the validation studies. The data for the use of zebrafish and pharmaceutical agents is not yet published in peer-reviewed journals and comes from abstracts and slide

Table 9-3. Features of the 3 × 3 contingency table

	In vitro predicted embryotoxicity		
"True" *in vivo* toxicity	Nonembryotoxic	Weakly embryotoxic	Strongly embryotoxic
Non-embryotoxic	***a***	b	c
Weakly Embryotoxic	d	***e***	f
Strongly Embryotoxic	g	h	***i***
Predictivity for nonembryotoxic chemicals		a / (a + d + g) × 100	
Predictivity for weakly embryotoxic chemicals		e / (b + e + h) × 100	
Predictivity for strongly embryotoxic chemicals		i / (c + f + i) × 100	
Precision for nonembryotoxic chemicals		a / (a + b+ c) × 100	
Precision for weakly embryotoxic chemicals		e / (d + e + f) × 100	
Precision for strongly embryotoxic chemicals		i / (g + h + i) × 100	
Accuracy		(a + e + i) / n × 100	

Notes: Contingency tables (3 × 3) permit analysis of *in vitro* predicted embryotoxicity class relative to the "true" *in vivo* embrytoxicity class as previously described.[32] In this format, precision is defined as the proportion of correctly classified strong (weakly or non)embryotoxic compounds from the *in vitro* test that are truly strongly (weakly or non)embryotoxic *in vivo*.Predictivity for strongly (weakly or non)embryotoxicants is the likelihood that a positive prediction in the test correctly identifies the strongly (weakly or non)embryotoxicant. Accuracy is the mean overall predictivity and precision.

decks presented at various workshops. Here, using different test sets and prediction models, the accuracy ranges from 60 to 90 percent. It should be noted that in data reported from the Phylonix/Bristol-Myers Squibb collaboration one-third of the test chemicals were retinoid derivatives, which are well discriminated by virtually all *in vitro* tests; therefore, the data are not likely to be a good indication of the model's true performance with pharmaceutical agents.

9.6 INDUSTRIAL APPLICATION OF *IN VITRO* SCREENS

Due to proprietary concerns, precise details about how these tests have been employed are not publicly available. Therefore, the author can only provide insights from personal experiences at Pfizer, and not the pharmaceutical industry at large. In our facility, with a staffing strategy that favors the stem cell test over whole embryo culture, the annual test article throughput is about sixty and forty chemicals, respectively. Thus, these tests are decidedly low throughput, necessitating their judicious application for specific situations. We use these tests in two circumstances: (a) when there is a theoretical concern about the target based on known biology or a literature precedent or (b) if the first lead produced unanticipated developmental toxicity. These assays are relatively new, and it is unclear what the inherent advantages of each test are; as a result, we use both, with the intention of gathering sufficient data to make this determination in the future.

Table 9-4. Summary of *in vitro* embryotoxicity test performance

	EST					WEC		Zebrafish				CENR
Parameter[a]	ECVAM Validation[b]	Pfizer[c]	Pfizer[d]	Hoffmann La Roche[e]	Pfizer[f]	ECVAM Validation[g]	Pfizer[h]	Danio (Pfizer)[i]	Phylonix (BMS)[j]	DarT[k]	Zf EU Consortium[l]	Proctor & Gamble[m]
Predictivity for nonembryotoxic (%)	72	50	100	86	88	70	100	71				
Predictivity for weakly embryotoxic (%)	70	63	63	67	59	76	67	50	83 True +ve	90 True +ve	78 True +ve	81 True +ve
Predictivity for strongly embryotoxic (%)	100	86	100	83	71	100	53	50				
Precision for nonembryotoxic (%)	70	50	57	100	70	80	64	92				
Precision for weakly embryotoxic (%)	83	79	100	67	77	65	75	57	83 True –ve	97 True –ve	100 True –ve	86 True –ve
Precision for strongly embryotoxic (%)	81	100	100	71	83	100	100	22				

(continued)

Table 9-4 (*continued*)

	EST					WEC		Zebrafish				CENR
Parameter[a]	ECVAM Validation[b]	Pfizer[c]	Pfizer[d]	Hoffmann La Roche[e]	Pfizer[f]	ECVAM Validation[g]	Pfizer[h]	Danio (Pfizer)[i]	Phylonix (BMS)[j]	DarT[k]	Zf EU Consortium[l]	Proctor & Gamble[m]
Accuracy (%)	**78**	**73**	**87**	**81**	**75**	**80**	**77**	**62**	**83**	**93**	**89**	**82**
Number of chemicals	*20*	*18*	*18*	*16*	*53*	*20*	*40*	*29*	*12n*	*41*	*25*	*44*

[a] Contingency tables (3 × 3) permit analysis of *in vitro* predicted embryotoxicity class relative to the "true" *in vivo* embryotoxicity class. The definition of predictivity, precision, and accuracy are defined in Table 9.4

[b] EST as conducted in the ECVAM validation test[32] with the Brown 20 chemical test set.[42]

[c] EST conducted at Pfizer in compliance with the ECVAM protocol on chemicals that were mostly part of the Brown chemical set.[69]

[d] Same experiment as in[3], except instead of using beating cardiomyocytes, the changes in gene expression using a Mahalanobis distance model was used.[69]

[e] EST conducted at Hoffmann La Roche in compliance with the ECVAM protocol using a mix of Brown chemicals and proprietary agents.[70]

[f] EST conducted at Pfizer in compliance with the ECVAM protocol using a mix of Brown chemicals and proprietary agents.[71]

[g] WEC as conducted in the ECVAM validation test.[32]

[h] WEC conducted at Pfizer in accordance with the ECVAM WEC. A mix of Brown compounds and proprietary agents were used.[41]

[i] The zebrafish assay by Danio Ltd. with a mix of pharmaceutical agents and the Brown compounds using an undisclosed proprietary prediction model.[58]

[j] Zebrafish assay as collaborated on by Bristol-Myers Squibb (BMS) and Phylonix using a dichotomous classification; therefore, performance is expressed as percent true positive (+) or negative (–).[59]

[k] Zebrafish DarT assay using a mix of chemicals.[72]

[l] Zebrafish assay as conducted by the EU zebrafish consortium.

[m] The CNER assay conducted at Proctor and Gamble with a mix of industrial and pharmaceutical chemicals.[35]

[n] 25% were retinoids and most *in vitro* assays perform well with this class of compounds.

That said, chemicals that have demonstrated or are considered likely to cause specific craniofacial malformations are tested preferentially in whole embryo culture because of its ability to faithfully recapitulate craniofacial development.

The ECVAM models were designed to facilitate the blinded categorization of a broad array of structurally unrelated agents into three categories of embryotoxicity. Thus, the correct embryotoxicity prediction is critical. We do not use the tests in that way; instead, we use them to rank-order the relative developmental toxicity risk within or across chemical series, to identify the agent with the least inherent risk- irrespective of the ECVAM-predicted embryotoxicity class. We are not alone in this approach, as the chick embryo retinal culture is also used for ranking (G. Daston (daston.gp@pg.com), personal communication).

In our experience, many pharmaceutical agents are categorized as "weak" embryotoxicants, raising the issue of how to discriminate among them. Therefore, we use other endpoints such as gene expression,[69] malformation types, or overall toxicologic potency to discriminate among compounds. In this way, even if the predicted embryotoxicity class is incorrect, the development team can still be given useful information. For example, whole embryo culture tends to generate false positives (true nons predicted to be weakly or strongly embryotoxic), and therefore the message is that a specific chemical or backbone is of "least risk," even if it is categorized as "weak." When used in this way, the tests have proven to be useful.

It should also be noted that we do not use these *in vitro* tests as a "kill-shot," but rather as a way to make business decisions about a drug development program. For example, a particular chemical series had an array of highly desirable synthetic and pharmacokinetic characteristics, but an unacceptable "strong" risk of embryotoxicity was predicted with whole embryo culture. Here, rather than having an *in vitro* embryotoxicity test terminate a series, other low-cost *in vitro* toxicity "kill-shot" tests were front-loaded. It was ultimately found that this series was positive in mutagenicity assays, leading to its demise. In another example, whole embryo culture determined that a particular chemical was of low risk for developmental toxicity, but due to the history of this program, there was still the risk of a late-stage developmental toxicity failure. Therefore, in spite of the clean *in vitro* signal, the *in vivo* embryo/fetal toxicity study was conducted earlier (front-loaded) than usual to mitigate the risk of wasting two years of drug development cost on a late-stage failure. In this instance, the *in vitro* prediction was correct. More examples have been described elsewhere.[34] Taken together, these *in vitro* tests help to steer chemists toward less risky backbones, and they allow development strategies that mitigate late-stage product failures to be developed.

9.7 PUTTING IT ALL TOGETHER

A generally applicable strategy for developmental toxicity risk assessment is depicted in Figure 9.6, although it will be modified to a certain extent for each program. It begins by understanding the theoretical risks associated with the

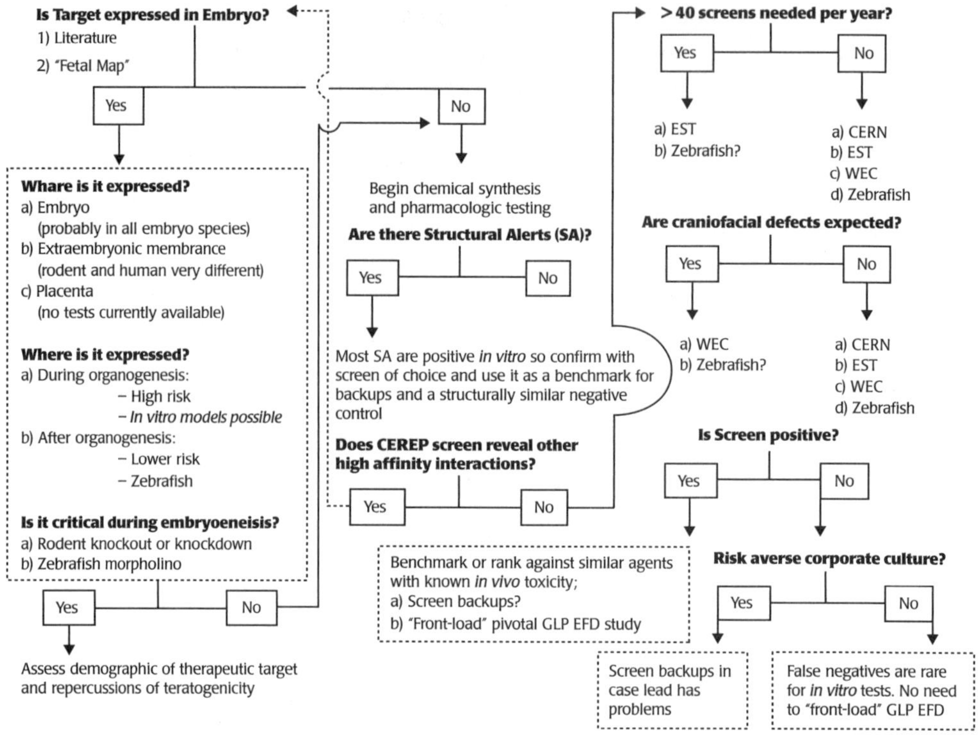

Figure 9-6: A generic strategy integrating the three facets of developmental toxicity risk assessment; namely (a) the risk of pharmacologic modulation of the therapeutic target during gestation, (b) *in silico*, SAR and (c) *in vitro* screening. Abbreviations: The chick embryo neural retina (CENR) embryonic stem cell test (EST), whole embryo culture (WEC), Good Laboratory Practice (GLP), Embryo/Fetal Developmental Toxicity (EFD) study. "Front-loading" is the conduct of the EFD study prior to Phase IIb.

therapeutic target. Most fundamentally, is the gene product present during gestation, where and what is its developmental role? This information may be available from internal or publicly available databases, or it may necessitate the use of mutational models developed in-house or as a fee for service. If the therapeutic target is highly expressed in the embryo during organogenesis the developmental toxicity risk may be high, but several *in vitro* tests are available for low-throughput screening of chemicals that are directed against the target (check that stem cells and chick retina express the therapeutic target first). For targets expressed after organogenesis, pharmacologic modulation of the target is less risky, but there are no *in vitro* models designed to detect late gestational effects. Nevertheless, *in vitro* screening during the organogenesis period may still be useful because it may reveal unanticipated off-target effects. Due to structure/function differences between humans and rodents with respect to extra-embryonic membranes, target expression in this tissue may alert the team to possible future investigative work to determine whether nonrodent test species may be required for the definitive toxicity study. In such instances *ex utero* cultures of yolk sac for example may be adapted for a program-specific toxicity/functional screen.

During chemical synthesis, *in silico* SAR analysis for structural alerts may still be useful because a positive hit, although rare, is very likely to be correct; no comfort can be drawn from a "clean" report. Chemicals of sufficient promise will undergo some kind of receptor interaction screen (e.g., Cerep Laboratories, Redmond WA) to reveal intended and unintended pharmacologic activities; these may require a return to understanding fetal expression and function for a secondary target. Based upon whether a target (primary or secondary) is expressed in the organogenesis embryo, its importance in embryogenesis based upon the analysis of mutants or mutant databases, screening load, and corporate culture, a decision will be made as to whether an *in vitro* screening program is required. The choice of the type of screen to be used will be determined by a variety of factors including the throughput required and the presence or absence of craniofacial malformations. If a screening program reveals no hits, the corporate culture will determine whether to continue screening backups and whether or not to front-load the pivotal study.

9.8 FUTURE PERSPECTIVES

In the future, many of the approaches currently used in the early assessment of developmental toxicity risk will be similar to those used today, but with advancing technologies and collaborations through various consortia, their scope and impact should be greatly enhanced. There may also be a burgeoning of publicly accessible data sets so their efficient access and management will be critical.

9.8.1 Target-specific effects

The ability to determine whether the modulation of a pharmaceutical target may be teratogenic will still be important for many therapeutic indications. To facilitate this determination, both privately funded[8] and publicly funded[8,73,74] embryo/fetal-specific gene expression databases may be more readily available. The International Mouse Knockout Consortium's goal of mutating all protein-coding genes in the mouse will provide invaluable information about their gestational function.[75] It should be recalled that 50 percent of mutant mouse models do not show an embryo/fetal phenotypes.[11] This is in contrast to the fact that a number of structurally diverse pharmacophores against the protein product of those gene targets induce reproducible class-specific anomalies. It has been suggested that in some instances this may be due to compensatory changes in other family members' gene expression that occurs in the generation of knockouts, but not *via* pharmacologic inhibition. With the advent of interfering shRNA used to knock down rather than knock out gene function in embryos,[15] it may more accurately reflect the consequences of the pharmacologic inhibition of a target.

MicroRNAs (mirs) are a novel class of pharmacologic targets. Although the large-scale elucidation of their developmental function may be achieved more quickly and at less expense in the zebrafish than in mammalian species, their conservation across animal species is not as consistent as for gene products. Therefore, the consequences of their disrupted function will be more difficult to predict.

9.8.2 *In silico* SAR mining

To date, the success of the broad application of *in silico* approaches to detect developmental toxicants has not been very productive. Improvements may come with initiatives on several fronts. Although increased computational power will be important, it will only prove useful with better SAR systems. As suggested previously, statistically based SAR systems may hold the most promise because, unlike rule-based systems, they do not require any knowledge about mechanisms of action, an important consideration for the field of teratology because mechanisms of action are rarely known. The statistical models may improve with the use of larger training sets of chemicals that reflect more current pharmaceutical thinking with respect to pharmacologic targets, chemical space, and mechanism of action. For example, many older antineoplastic agents were highly cytotoxic, irreversibly binding alkylating agents. whereas current strategies may target kinases and apoptotic pathways in a reversible receptor-mediated approach. At a 2007 Health and Environmental Sciences Institute (HESI meeting, it was recommended that pharmaceutical companies share their *in vivo* developmental toxicity data sets and chemicals for the purpose of building better *in vitro* developmental toxicity models,[31] but to the author's knowledge no advances have been made here. Such sets would be invaluable for SAR modeling as well.

9.8.3 *In vitro* screening

Perhaps the greatest advances will occur in the field of *in vitro* screening. Current models are low throughput, using crude endpoints (e.g., cell beating and morphology), but there have been efforts to use more sensitive markers. These include gene expression[76–79] and reporter constructs,[80,81] which may lead to automation of both the EST[82]and zebrafish assays,[57] There are several efforts underway to use human stem cells for developmental toxicity testing,[83,84] and this has the potential for more accurate predictions of human developmental toxicity. Moreover, unlike the other mammalian- or avian-based screens, the fish may be exposed for the entire gestational period. It is believed that fish will predict human teratogens because of the fact that there are about seventeen signal transduction pathways that are critical for embryogenesis and common to most animals (metazoan). Interference with any pathway should be detrimental in all species, even though the resultant phenotype may be species specific.[85] This approach assumes we know most of or all the relevant mechanisms or pathways to test.

A report by the National Academy of Sciences proposed that future toxicity screens not be organ-based as they are today, but that they instead focus on detecting specific mechanisms of toxicity.[86] Thus, a suite of such assays may be used to determine what toxicity pathways are triggered by exposure to specific chemicals. Similar approaches may be applied to developmental toxicity tests. In this way, we need not know all the relevant developmental biology pathways to test.

Genetically engineered animals are used to reduce the duration of genotoxicity testing. It is also possible that sensitive molecular sensors may be developed; these sensors would identify perturbations in critical developmental signaling pathways under *in vivo* conditions, where biotransformation and distribution kinetics are accounted for. Such circumstances may permit the use of only several litters to ascertain the risk of teratogenicity. In this way, large-scale *in vivo* teratogenicity screening may be conduced with the use of very few animals.

The ECVAM ReProTect initiative may also reap benefits for industry. Its goal is to build toxicity models for the key aspects of the mammalian reproductive and developmental life cycle using a combination of *in vitro* tests and sensor technologies.[87] The theory is that by integrating the results from all the individual *in vitro* tests, including the previously described embryonic stem cell test and whole embryo culture, a chemical's aggregate reproductive and developmental toxicity risk may be predicted. The other tests being developed for ReProTect assess toxicities in processes that occur outside the window of organogenesis (e.g., implantation, ossification, and neural development), as well as modifiers such as placental transfer kinetics, metabolism, and gametogenesis in females and males. If their utility can be demonstrated, a combination of some of the ReProTect models may prove useful to screen against specific activities.

The *in vitro* tests described have been validated using small chemical entities. With renewed interest in "biologics" (antibodies and protein fragments), there is the possibility that these tests may not prove as useful. Whole embryo culture has been used mechanistically to examine the consequences of *in vitro* exposure to anti–yolk sac antibodies;[88] however, a systematic examination of the effects of exposure to current protein-based therapies in *in vitro* developmental toxicity assays has not been conducted.

In summary, drug candidate attrition due to teratogenicity occurs late in product development. Consequently, its negative impact on pharmaceutical development cost may be substantial, even though it only accounts for about 4 percent of program failures. Several strategies may de-risk developmental toxicity concerns. The first is to use *in silico* or wet lab approaches to interrogate the developmental role of a potential therapeutic target. Although *in silico* SAR is not very robust with respect to teratogenic activity, such screening of the lead material may still be useful because a positive hit, although rare, is invariably of concern. Several *in vitro* embryotoxicity prediction models are used for lead optimization in the industrial setting, and there may be others in use that have not been publicly disclosed. *In vitro* embryotoxicity assays have relatively low throughput, and the selection of the appropriate test will depend upon the relative advantages and disadvantages of each test with respect to the screening needs. These three approaches may all be useful on their own, but when integrated into a larger strategy aimed at discriminating between pharmacologically mediated and off-target teratogenic effects, they may synergistically reduce the risk of candidate attrition mediated by teratogenicity concerns.

REFERENCES

1. Kola I, Landis J . Can the pharmaceutical industry reduce attrition rates? *Nat Rev Drug Discov.* 2004;3(8):711–715.
2. Lander ES, Linton LM, Birren B, et al. Initial sequencing and analysis of the human genome. *Nature.* 2001;409(6822):860–921.
3. Venter JC, Adams MD, Myers EW, et al. The sequence of the human genome. *Science.* 2001;291(5507):1304–1351.
4. Hopkins AL, Groom CR. The druggable genome. *Nat Rev Drug Discov.* 2002;1(9):727–730.
5. Overington JP, Al-Lazikani B, Hopkins AL. How many drug targets are there? *Nat Rev Drug Discov.* 2006;5(12):993–996.
6. Sakharkar MK, Sakharkar KR. Targetability of human disease genes. *Curr Drug Discov Technol.* 2007;4(1):48–58.
7. Claverie JM. Gene number. What if there are only 30,000 human genes? *Science.* 2001;291(5507):1255–1257.
8. Hurtt ME, Streck RD, Kumpf SW, et al. Fetal map: A gene expression database for predicting potential involvement in developmental toxicity for all druggable genes. *Birth Defects Res Pt A.* 2007;29:352.
9. Foote RH, Carney EW. The rabbit as a model for reproductive and developmental toxicity studies. *Reprod Toxicol.* 2000;14(6):477–493.
10. Harris S. Transgenic knockouts as part of high-throughput, evidence-based target selection and validation strategies. *Drug Discov Today.* 2001;6(12):628–636.
11. Zambrowicz BP, Sands AT. Knockouts model the 100 best-selling drugs – Will they model the next 100? *Nat Rev Drug Discov.* 2003;2(1):38–51.
12. Engle SJ. Beasts in the Genomic Jungle: Use of Model Organisms in Drug Development. https://www.nyas.org/_membership/memberlogin.asp?redirect_location=http://www.nyas.org/ebriefreps/main.asp?intSubSectionID%3D5257. Accessed May 1, 2009|.
13. Ozolinš TRS, Fisher TS, Nadeau DM, et al. Defects in embryonic development of EGLN1/PHD2 knockdown transgenic mice are associated with the induction of Igfbp in the placenta. *Biochem Biophys Res Commun.* 2009;390:372–376.
14. Lois C, Hong EJ, Pease S, et al. Germline transmission and tissue-specific expression of transgenes delivered by lentiviral vectors. *Science.* 2002;295(5556):868–872.
15. Dann CT, Alvarado AL, Hammer RE, et al. Heritable and stable gene knockdown in rats. *Proc Natl Acad Sci USA.* 2006;103(30):11246–11251.
16. Ni YG, Miledi R. Blockage of 5HT2C serotonin receptors by fluoxetine (Prozac). *Proc Natl Acad Sci USA.* 1997;94(5):2036–2040.
17. Apsel B, Blair JA, Gonzalez B, et al. Targeted polypharmacology: Discovery of dual inhibitors of tyrosine and phosphoinositide kinases. *Nat Chem Biol.* 2008;4(11):691–699.
18. Hopkins AL. Network pharmacology: The next paradigm in drug discovery. *Nat Chem Biol.* 2008;4(11):682–690.
19. Daston GP. The theoretical and empirical case for in vitro developmental toxicity screens, and potential applications. *Teratology.* 1996;53(6):339–344.
20. Arena VC, Sussman NB, Mazumdar S, et al. The utility of structure-activity relationship (SAR) models for prediction and covariate selection in developmental toxicity: Comparative analysis of logistic regression and decision tree models. *SAR QSAR Environ Res.* 2004;15(1):1–18.
21. Greene N. Computer systems for the prediction of toxicity: an update. *Adv Drug Deliv Rev.* 2002;54(3):417–431.
22. Julien E, Willhite CC, Richard AM, et al. Challenges in constructing statistically based structure-activity relationship models for developmental toxicity. *Birth Defects Res A Clin Mol Teratol.* 2004;70(12):902–911.
23. CompuDrug. HazardExpert Pro. http://www.compudrug.com/print.php?id=46. Accessed May 1, 2009.

24. LHASA . DEREK for Windows. http://www.lhasalimited.org/index.php?cat=2&sub_cat=64. Accessed May 1, 2009.
25. Accelrys. TOPKAT Training. http://accelrys.com/services/training/life-science/topkat.html. Accessed May 1, 2009.
26. MultiCASE I. CASETOX. http://www.multicase.com/products/prod03.htm. Accessed May 1, 2009.
27. Schardein JL. *Chemically induced birth defects*. New York: Marcel Dekker; 2000.
28. Scialli AR. *A clinical guide to reproductive and developmental toxicology*. Boca Raton, FL: CRC Press; 1992.
29. Shepard T. *Catalogue of teratogenic agents*. Baltimore: Johns Hopkins University Press; 1992.
30. Brannen KC, Panzica-Kelly JM, Charlap JH, Augustine-Rauch KA. Zebrafish: A non-mammalian model of developmental toxicology. In: Hansen DK, Abbott, BD, eds. *Developmental Toxicology*. Vol 27. New York: Informa Healthcare; 2008:215–241.
31. Chapin R, Augustine-Rauch K, Beyer B, et al. State of the art in developmental toxicity screening methods and a way forward: A meeting report addressing embryonic stem cells, whole embryo culture, and zebrafish. *Birth Defects Res B Dev Reprod Toxicol*. 2008;83(4):446–456.
32. Genschow E, Spielmann H, Scholz G, et al. The ECVAM international validation study on in vitro embryotoxicity tests: Results of the definitive phase and evaluation of prediction models. European Centre for the Validation of Alternative Methods. *Altern Lab Anim*. 2002;30(2):151–176.
33. Flick B, Klug S. Whole embryo culture: An important tool in developmental toxicology today. *Curr Pharm Des*. 2006;12(12):1467–1488.
34. Ozolinš TR. Use of mammalian in vitro systems, including stem cells, in developmental toxicity testing. In: Hansen DK, Abbot BD, eds. *Developmental Toxicology*. Vol 27. 3rd ed. New York: Informa Healthcare; 2008:171–213.
35. Daston GP, Baines D, Elmore E, et al. Evaluation of chick embryo neural retinal cell culture as a screen for developmental toxicants. *Fundam Appl Toxicol*. 1995;26(2):203–210.
36. Daston GP, Baines D, Yonker JE. Chick embryo neural retina cell culture as a screen for developmental toxicity. *Toxicol Appl Pharmacol*. 1991;109(2):352–366.
37. Juchau MR, Faustman-Watts E. Pharmacokinetic considerations in the maternal-placental-fetal unit. *Clin Obstet Gynecol*. 1983;26(2):379–390.
38. Nau H, Scott WJ, Jr. Weak acids may act as teratogens by accumulating in the basic milieu of the early mammalian embryo. *Nature*. 1986;323(6085):276–278.
39. Juchau MR, Boutelet-Bochan H, Huang Y. Cytochrome-P450-dependent biotransformation of xenobiotics in human and rodent embryonic tissues. *Drug Metab Rev*. 1998;30(3):541–568.
40. Coecke S, Ahr H, Blaauboer BJ, et al. Metabolism: A bottleneck in in vitro toxicological test development. The report and recommendations of ECVAM workshop 54. *Altern Lab Anim*. 2006;34(1):49–84.
41. Ozolinš TRS, Thomson JJ. Use of WEC in pharmaceutical screening/testing. *HESI (Health and Environmental Sciences Institute) Workshop on Alternative Assays for Developmental Toxicity Testing* [http://www.hesiglobal.org/Committees/TechnicalCommittees/DART/HESIAltAssayPresentations.htm. Accessed May 1 2009.
42. Bremer S, Pellizzer C, Coecke S, et al. Detection of the embryotoxic potential of cyclophosphamide by using a combined system of metabolic competent cells and embryonic stem cells. *Altern Lab Anim*. 2002;30(1):77–85.
43. Oglesby LA, Ebron MT, Beyer PE, et al. Co-culture of rat embryos and hepatocytes: In vitro detection of a proteratogen. *Teratog Carcinog Mutagen*. 1986;6(2):129–138.
44. Ozolins TR, Oglesby LA, Wiley MJ, et al. In vitro murine embryotoxicity of cyclophosphamide in embryos co-cultured with maternal hepatocytes: development and application of a murine embryo-hepatocyte co-culture model. *Toxicology*. 1995;102(3):259–274.

45. Piersma AH, van Aerts LA, Verhoef A, et al. Biotransformation of cyclophosphamide in post-implantation rat embryo culture using maternal hepatocytes in co-culture. *Pharmacol Toxicol.* 1991;69(1):47–51.
46. Greenaway JC, Fantel AG, Shepard TH, et al. The in vitro teratogenicity of cyclophosphamide in rat embryos. *Teratology.* 1982;25(3):335–343.
47. Busquet F, Nagel R, von Landenberg F, et al. Development of a new screening assay to identify proteratogenic substances using zebrafish *Danio rerio* embryo combined with an exogenous mammalian metabolic activation system (mDarT). *Toxicol Sci.* 2008;104(1):177–188.
48. Davila JC, Cezar GG, Thiede M, et al. Use and application of stem cells in toxicology. *Toxicol Sci.* 2004;79(2):214–223.
49. Laschinski G, Vogel R, Spielmann H. Cytotoxicity test using blastocyst-derived euploid embryonal stem cells: A new approach to in vitro teratogenesis screening. *Reprod Toxicol.* 1991;5(1):57–64.
50. Newall DR, Beedles KE. The stem-cell test: An in vitro assay for teratogenic potential. Results of a blind trial with 25 compounds. *Toxicol In Vitro.* 1996;10:229–240.
51. Guan K, Rohwedel J, Wobus AM. Embryonic stem cell differentiation models: Cardiogenesis, myogenesis, neurogenesis, epithelial and vascular smooth muscle cell differentiation in vitro. *Cytotechnology.* 1999;30(1–3):211–226.
52. Scholz G, Spielmann H. Embryonic Stem Cell Test (EST). *INVITTOX protocol 113.* http://ecvam-dbalm.jrc.ec.europa.eu/. Accessed May 1, 2009.
53. New DA. Whole-embryo culture and the study of mammalian embryos during organogenesis. *Biol Rev Camb Philos Soc.* 1978;53(1):81–122.
54. Ozolinš TR, Hales BF. Oxidative stress regulates the expression and activity of transcription factor activator protein-1 in rat conceptus. *J Pharmacol Exp Ther.* 1997;280(2):1085–1093.
55. Sadler TW, Horton WE, Warner CW. Whole embryo culture: A screening technique for teratogens? *Teratog Carcinog Mutagen.* 1982;2(3–4):243–253.
56. Spézia F. Embryotoxicity testing using a whole embryo culture (W.E.C.) procedure. *INVITTOX protocol 68.* http://ecvam-dbalm.jrc.ec.europa.eu/. Accessed May 1, 2009.
57. Yang L, Ho NY, Alshut R, et al. Zebrafish embryos as models for embryotoxic and teratological effects of chemicals. *Reprod Toxicol.* 2009;28(2):245–253.
58. Marguerie A. DanioLabs model and Pfizer data. *HESI (Health and Environmental Sciences Institute) Workshop on Alternative Assays for Developmental Toxicity Testing.* http://www.hesiglobal.org/Committees/TechnicalCommittees/DART/HESIAltAssay Presentations.htm. Accessed May 1, 2009.
59. Seng WL. Zebrafish: A predictive model for developmental toxicity. *HESI (Health and Environmental Sciences Institute) Workshop on Alternative Assays for Developmental Toxicity Testing Retrieved.* http://www.hesiglobal.org/Committees/TechnicalCommittees/DART/HESIAltAssayPresentations.htm. Accessed May 1, 2009.
60. Brown NA, Fabro S. Quantitation of rat embryonic development in vitro: A morphological scoring system. *Teratology.* 1981;24(1):65–78.
61. van Maele-Fabry G, Delhaise F, Picard JJ. Evolution of the developmental scores of sixteen morphological features in mouse embryos displaying 0 to 30 somites. *Int J Dev Biol.* 1992;36(1):161–167.
62. Pitt JA, Carney EW. Development of a morphologically-based scoring system for postimplantation New Zealand White rabbit embryos. *Teratology.* 1999;59(2):88–101.
63. Carney EW, Tornesi B, Keller C, et al. Refinement of a morphological scoring system for postimplantation rabbit conceptuses. *Birth Defects Res B Dev Reprod Toxicol.* 2007;80(3):213–222.
64. Hou T, Wang J. Structure-ADME relationship: Still a long way to go? *Expert Opin Drug Metab Toxicol.* 2008;4(6):759–770.
65. Brown NA. Selection of test chemicals for the ECVAM international validation study on in vitro embryotoxicity tests. European Centre for the Validation of Alternative Methods. *Altern Lab Anim.* 2002;30(2):177–198.

66. Spielmann H, Seiler A, Bremer S, et al. The practical application of three validated in vitro embryotoxicity tests. The report and recommendations of an ECVAM/ZEBET workshop (ECVAM workshop 57). *Altern Lab Anim.* 2006;34(5):527–538.
67. Spielmann H. Predicting the risk of developmental toxicity from in vitro assays. *Toxicol Appl Pharmacol.* 2005;207(Suppl 2):375–380.
68. Schwetz BA, Harris MW. Developmental toxicology: status of the field and contribution of the National Toxicology Program. *Environ Health Perspect.* Apr 1993;100: 269–282.
69. Chapin R, Stedman D, Paquette J, et al. Struggles for equivalence: in vitro developmental toxicity model evolution in pharmaceuticals in 2006. *Toxicol In Vitro.* 2007;21(8):1545–1551.
70. Whitlow S, Burgin H, Clemann N. The embryonic stem cell test for the early selection of pharmaceutical compounds. *ALTEX.* 2007;24(1):3–7.
71. Paquette JA, Kumpf SW, Streck RD, et al. Assessment of the Embryonic Stem Cell Test and application and use in the pharmaceutical industry. *Birth Defects Res B Dev Reprod Toxicol.* 2008;83(2):104–111.
72. Nagel R. DarT: The embryo test with the Zebrafish *Danio rerio* – A general model in ecotoxicology and toxicology. *ALTEX.* 2002;19(Suppl 1):38–48.
73. Venkataraman S, Stevenson P, Yang Y, et al. EMAGE – Edinburgh Mouse Atlas of Gene Expression: 2008 update. *Nucleic Acids Res.* 2008;36(Database issue):D860–865.
74. The Virtual Embryo Project (v-Embryo). National Center for Computational Toxicology (NCCT). http://www.epa.gov/ncct/v-Embryo/. Accessed May 1, 2009.
75. Collins FS, Rossant J, Wurst W. A mouse for all reasons. *Cell.* Jan 12 2007;128(1):9–13.
76. zur Nieden NI, Kempka G, Ahr HJ. Molecular multiple endpoint embryonic stem cell test – a possible approach to test for the teratogenic potential of compounds. *Toxicol Appl Pharmacol.* Feb 1 2004;194(3):257–269.
77. zur Nieden NI, Ruf LJ, Kempka G, et al. Molecular markers in embryonic stem cells. *Toxicol In Vitro.* 2001;15(4–5):455–461.
78. Seiler A, Visan A, Pohl I, et al. Improving the embryonic stem cell test (EST) by establishing molecular endpoints of tissue specific development using murine embryonic stem cells (D3 cells)]. *ALTEX.* 2002;19(Suppl 1):55–63.
79. Seiler A, Visan A, Buesen R, et al. Improvement of an in vitro stem cell assay for developmental toxicity: The use of molecular endpoints in the embryonic stem cell test. *Reprod Toxicol.* 2004;18(2):231–240.
80. Chen YH, Wang YH, Yu TH, et al. Transgenic zebrafish line with over-expression of Hedgehog on the skin: A useful tool to screen Hedgehog-inhibiting compounds. *Transgenic Res.* 2009; 18(6):855–864.
81. Paparella M, Kolossov E, Fleischmann BK, et al. The use of quantitative image analysis in the assessment of in vitro embryotoxicity endpoints based on a novel embryonic stem cell clone with endoderm-related GFP expression. *Toxicol In Vitro.* 2002;16(5):589–597.
82. Walmod PS, Gravemann U, Nau H, et al . Discriminative power of an assay for automated in vitro screening of teratogens. *Toxicol In Vitro.* 2004;18(4):511–525.
83. Adler S, Lindqvist J, Uddenberg K, et al. Testing potential developmental toxicants with a cytotoxicity assay based on human embryonic stem cells. *Altern Lab Anim.* 2008;36(2):129–140.
84. Anonymous . Cellartis Enters into a Research Collaboration with Pfizer to Develop a Screening System for Detection of Human Toxicity. http://www.drugs.com/news/cellartis-enters-into-research-collaboration-pfizer-develop-screening-detection-human-toxicity-7760.html. Accessed May 1, 2009.
85. NRC. *Scientific Frontiers in Developmental Toxicology and Risk Assessment.* Washington, DC: National Academy Press; 2000.

86. NRC. *Toxicity Testing in the twenty-first Century: A Vision and a Strategy.* Washington, DC: National Research Council of the National Academies; 2007.
87. Hareng L, Pellizzer C, Bremer S, et al. The integrated project ReProTect: A novel approach in reproductive toxicity hazard assessment. *Reprod Toxicol.* 2005;20(3):441–452.
88. New DA, Brent RL. Effect of yolk-sac antibody on rat embryos grown in culture. *J Embryol Exp Morphol.* 1972;27(3):543–553.

II INTEGRATED APPROACHES OF PREDICTIVE TOXICOLOGY

10 **Integrated approaches to lead optimization**

Improving the therapeutic index

Laszlo Urban, Jianling Wang, Dejan Bojanic, and Susan Ward

10.1 INTRODUCTION: RISK AWARENESS, A MAJOR ELEMENT OF MODERN DRUG DISCOVERY

Since the introduction of simple, *in silico*, and *in vitro* tools for the assessment of physicochemical properties in the 1990s.[1] drug discovery has come a long way. The impact of these tools was based on their acceptable predictive value for *in vivo* pharmacokinetic performance and their cost effectiveness for large-scale profiling. During the past decade, we have seen a rapid improvement in the throughput and quality of these assays, accompanied by an impressive development of *in silico* tools based on accumulating experimental knowledge. Today, most if not all, pharmaceutical companies use an arsenal of these assays to fine-tune compound properties prior to clinical testing. This "revolution" has resulted in diminished attrition rate due to ADME-related liabilities.[2]

The significant improvement in ADME (absorption-distribution-metabolism-elimination) properties in the early phases of drug discovery indeed shifted the challenges in lead optimization and candidate selection toward safety and toxicology aspects. This is partly due to the complexity of safety assessment, which is difficult to translate into high-throughput, cost-effective *in vitro* assays with significant predictive value and partly due to the mandatory use of fixed assays required by regulatory authorities. In addition, some toxicities such as reactive metabolite-related hepatotoxicity remain difficult to predict *in vitro*. To date, most safety-related assays have been performed *in vivo* with limited insight into the underlying mechanisms that would define the link between a particular target molecule and the observed toxic or adverse drug reaction (ADR). However, during the past decade, we have seen considerable efforts in this area of drug discovery.

One of the most advanced and developed area of toxicology is cardiac safety. During the 1990s, it became clear that a large number of small molecules had an effect on electrocardiogram (ECG) performance and caused unacceptable high rates of arrhythmia. The Cardiac Arrhythmia Suppression Trial (CAST)[3] identified several drugs with pro-arrhythmic potential, which resulted in withdrawal or black box labelling.[3] However, the underlying mechanism of the arrhythmogenic properties of small molecules was not known until 1998 when

Keating and colleagues linked it to hERG (human ether-a-go-go-related gene) channel inhibition[4]. The importance of hERG in drug discovery comes from two considerations: (a) The hERG current is an essential component of the repolarizing phase of the cardiac action potential. When this current is inhibited, the action potential duration will be prolonged and might generate early afterdepolarizations, a condition for arrhythmogenesis. Blocking the channel for several seconds could be fatal, thus a brief spike of C_{max} can create a major life threatening condition. (b) The hERG pharmacophore is inherent to many drug-like molecules,[5,6] which makes the chemical optimization of drug candidates more challenging. Based on a meta-analysis by Redfern and colleagues[7] the link between the potency of drugs to inhibit the hERG channel and clinical manifestation of Torsades de Pointes (TdP) was established. According to this study, drugs with at least 30 times less IC_{50} at the hERG channel than the therapeutic plasma concentration are likely to be safe in clinical use. Based on this observation, awareness and mitigation of hERG risk has become an integral part of lead selection and lead optimization activities. This example highlights how safety assessment can be employed early, once the target associated with a clinical ADR has been recognized.

Even though the chapters of this book are concerned with various aspects of *in vitro/in vivo* safety testing of primarily small molecules, this one will focus on the principles of early *in vitro* safety assessment and mostly refers to *in vivo* assays described in details in the accompanying chapters.

10.2 OUTLINE OF THE NEED OF INTEGRATED ASSESSMENT OF ADMET DURING LEAD OPTIMIZATION

The average clinical success rate was 11percent between 1991 and 2000.[2] This does not take into account attrition rates during preclinical phases, particularly from the clinical candidate nomination to Phase I clinical trials. As pharmaceutical and biotechnology companies keep a fairly close lid on their early pipeline figures, it is very difficult to determine the real attrition rates at various stages of preclinical drug discovery. However, there is a consensus in published scientific literature on the estimated necessary numbers of compounds to be generated, screened, and optimized to reach a single candidate to be nominated for clinical trials.[8]

Within the current drug discovery process, safety assessment is set to start right at target discovery (Table 10.1) with the evaluation of the therapeutic target. Note that the chemical space of new therapeutic targets for unmet medical needs or for alternative mechanisms or pathways has shifted the molecular properties of new chemical entities (NCEs) toward higher molecular weight, higher lipophilicity, and more promiscuity against nontherapeutic targets and metabolic enzymes,[9,10] posing additional challenges in drug discovery for selecting NCEs with adequate efficacy and drugability. Frequently, adequate ADME properties have become prerequisites for efficacy assessment as erroneous data obtained in

Table 10-1. General aspects of risk assessment considered during drug discovery

Hit to lead phase	Awareness: Identify risks early
Road to lead nomination	Characterize series: What is the risk within a lead series or chemotype? Is the risk linked to the chemotype or pharmacophore? Is there evidence for separation of the SARs?
Lead nomination	Decide: How likely is it to minimize risk within series? Is the risk worth taking?
Lead optimization	Parallel optimization: Determine the risks versus the desired activity.
Clinical candidate	Characterize candidates: Perform initial characterization of TI to aid in candidate selection.

Note: Various phases require different focus of profiling objectives.

biochemical/cellular assays may be derived without the proper understanding of the interplay between potency and ADME properties. Taken into consideration that adverse drug effects depend to the same extent on ADME properties, it has been widely accepted during the past decade that parallel assessment of efficacy, off-target effects, and comprehensive ADME properties of NCEs is imperative in order to optimize pharmacokinetics/pharmacodynamics and for the prediction of adverse, toxic reactions of drug candidates.[10–14] This effort basically created what we call ADMET characteristics, now adding "T" for toxicology. *In vitro* ADMET assays offer first-line experimental tools to rank and prioritize NCEs, as well as to reveal mechanistic pathways in the early phase of drug discovery.[15] Let's briefly consider the priorities safety profiling should focus on during the various phases of drug discovery.

Target selection

Concerning target selection, the main issue is whether the primary target carries undesirable side effects unrelated to the therapeutic potential (on-target or mechanism-based side effects). These effects might be easy to monitor, but difficult to mitigate. This should be considered within the early safety profiling plan. The plan will assess all known liabilities associated with the target and affected pathways, either from prior clinical experience, human hereditary diseases where the gene of the target is mutated or in case of "first-in-class" drugs from *in vivo* animal data. For example, cyclooxygenase-2 (COX-2), a target for the treatment of rheumatoid arthritis, has essential involvement in different physiological mechanisms: COX-2 enzyme inhibitors are excellent anti-inflammatory agents through the interaction with the prostaglandin system; however, their possible pro-thrombotic effect via selective inhibition of prostacyclin-2 (PGI_2) production could be unacceptable.[16] The COX-2 inhibitors that do not inhibit the production of thromboxane A2 (TxA_2) associated with increased platelet aggregation, may still block PGI_2, thereby tipping the homeostatic balance toward aggregation of platelets and increasing the risk for thrombotic events.[17]

Once a drug discovery team for the COX-2 target is aware of this scenario and the risk assessment provides evidence for a possible clear therapeutic index in target patient populations, a profiling plan that focuses on the mitigation of the likely pro-thrombotic effect can be generated.

Recent studies highlighted a further important aspect of on-target safety, namely that a G-protein coupled receptor (GPCR) can couple with various second messengers depending on the site of expression and in some cases on the type of ligand activation. The β2 adrenergic receptor, for example, couples with G protein (Gi) in the heart and contributes to the maintenance of cardiac homeostasis,[18] but it can cause muscle impairment in skeletal muscle via G protein (Gs) coupling. Blocking this latter effect without causing cardiac side effects might be possible by selective blockade or modulation of the GPCR-Gs complex.

In addition, at target selection, one can already consider off-target effects. This is the case if a target has been already considered and it is known that its pharmacophore significantly overlaps with that of off-targets that might generate unacceptable ADRs. One example is the overlap of the pharmacophores of the chemokine receptor (CCR) and the hERG channel. While separation of effects at these two proteins is very difficult, application of quantitative structure-activity relationship (QSAR) analysis can help to design chemical series with improved selectivity.[19]

Hit expansion – increase awareness

Prior to lead nomination, integrated risk assessment can aid the prioritization and selection of the best chemical structure(s). It is crucial to identify possible liabilities associated with certain chemotypes at this stage. A good structure-activity relationship (SAR) for the therapeutic target is imperative; however, if the chemotype is also associated with targets of known safety issues, one has to make sure that these liabilities do not cripple the primary optimization. The important question is, whether a distinct SAR or chemical space exists between the primary and off-target effect(s). To answer this question, one needs to test several compounds from each chemical series for their ADMET characteristics. While this sounds trivial, the task is difficult because (a) the amount of compounds is limited at this stage of drug discovery; (b) ADME characteristics are not optimized; thus the data quality derived from *in vitro* assays at this stage might be compromised, and *in vivo* testing is rarely possible because of poor biopharmaceutical profile, relatively weak efficacy, or both. Also, for a high-quality integrated risk assessment, a large set of primary assays need to be completed at a significant cost. This concentrated early safety profiling effort pays off only if it is linked with risk awareness, and an associated plan for indication-dependent mitigation. An arsenal of *in vitro* profiling assays developed for large-scale screening, aided by *in silico* tools can detect potentially serious safety issues associated with various chemical structures. Identification of genotoxic potential (micro-Ames), hERG inhibition (radioligand binding), high metabolic rate (microsomal stability), drug–drug interactions (DDI), and extreme pharmacological promiscuity

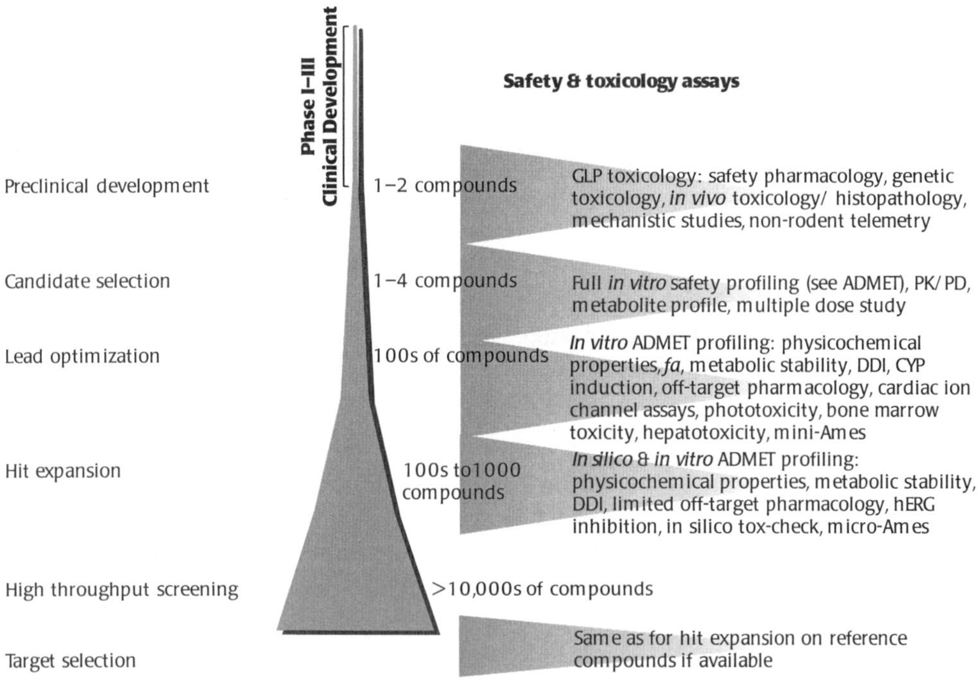

Figure 10-1: Alignment of safety profiling, discovery toxicology, and pathology with the preclinical drug discovery process[8]. Profiling assays are implemented according to requirement of the phase, compound availability, and capacity. The complexity is increasing as projects progress toward clinical candidate selection.

could be detected. At this stage, profiling assays are required to be strongly associated with the chemistry drive (see Figure 10.1). Assays addressing safety risk should avoid false positives, which could be misleading and compromise their impact. The main hurdle at this stage is to deploy the right assays to fulfill these criteria. A diagnostic safety-profiling panel can define what should be looked at and what level of activity one can afford at off-targets. Even though no or only a limited number of complex safety-profiling assays are done at early stages, the number of compounds tested in the less-refined, sentinel assays counterbalance the statistical power. Overall, the generated data set should be comprehensive enough to answer questions for the next decision point, which usually entails the selection of a smaller range of chemotypes for further optimization.

Lead nomination – decision making and hazard identification

How likely can the liability be minimized within a series? What is the confidence to overcome the problem? Strategically, one should consider the balance between observed activity at the therapeutic target (affinity dominance) and perceived liabilities (risk assessment driven). Is "cleaner" or "more potent" the better alternative? As an example, we can refer to the development of antiallergic agents. The first generation of antihistamine drugs had serious central nervous system (CNS) side effects such as somnolence and dizziness caused inconvenience and hazard for the patients, therefore limiting the benefit of these compounds. The second-generation antihistamines (e.g., fexofenadine and cetirizine) overcame these ADRs by focusing on mitigation of the side effects. These later molecules are largely limited to the periphery, at the site of their therapeutic action; they do not cross the blood–brain barrier, and are therefore devoid of the centrally mediated somnolence.[20] The more we know about the SAR of off-target related ADRs, organ-specific distribution, and metabolism-related toxicity, the greater the chance we will be able to mitigate expected ADRs. At lead nomination, this knowledge will largely determine the difficulties that may arise during the optimization phase.

Lead optimization – parallel optimization and elimination loops with continuous risk assessment

This is the most crucial phase for shaping a medicine. During lead optimization, compounds are modified in such a way that as the project advances they will behave more and more as drug-like molecules. Thus, in balance with the desired activity at the primary target, their bioavailability and safety profile will improve. This should include the elimination or mitigation of off-target effect(s) from the desired activity, metabolism and transporter-related drug interactions, and cytotoxicity, genotoxicity, hepatotoxicity, and phototoxicity assays. Typically, a tier-based assay strategy may be required to accommodate the needs at various levels. For instance, high-throughput assays with minimal sample consumption and quick turn-around time can cope with the fast pace and large compound volumes during the lead optimization cycle by flagging potential ADMET risks (e.g., cytochrome P450 (CYP) 3A4 screening and hERG radioligand binding (RLB)). Importantly, follow-up, low-throughput mechanistic assays should be in place to address specific concerns raised in the screening assays (see Figure 10.1). Such hypothesis-based approaches have proved to be powerful and effective in diagnosing and mitigating project-specific or chemotypic issues, in combination with spot-check *in vivo* experiments.

Clinical candidate selection – characterize candidates and assess risk (including regulatory requirements prior to clinical trials) of identified molecules

Selecting a clinical candidate or a maximum of three candidates is the result of a tedious lead optimization process often involving synthesis of 500–1000 molecules.[7] These compounds should match the profile and criteria determined for the clinical application at the start of the project. In general terms, the expected human exposure should provide efficacious concentration at the target site, pharmacokinetics/pharmacodynamics (PK/PD) should be agreeable with the expectations, and side effects should not hinder the clinical benefits. Compounds to move forward should be fully assessed using comprehensive *in vitro* mechanistic assays and *in vivo* models. The candidates selected at this stage should have a favorable ADMET profile and manageable developability against remaining risks. Now the major requirement of the applied profiling assays changes to no or very low tolerance of false negatives. As more and more animal assays are introduced at this stage, questions about species specificity and organ selectivity arise. The choice of the proper animal species is of great importance, as some human equivalent targets do not exist in all toxicology species (e.g., hERG in rodents; metabolic enzymes), molecular and developmental pathways may vary (e.g., differences between hedgehog signaling in mammals and in *Drosophila*), metabolic enzymes could be incompatible (e.g., tamoxifen causes hepatocarcinoma only in rats due to DNA-adduct formation in this species), and receptor distribution could be considerably different even between different strains. Thus, particular care should be taken when analyzing toxicology data obtained from *in vivo* studies. Comparison of *in vivo* observations to *in vitro* pharmacology and gene profiles on human targets is essential. If discrepancies exist, *in vitro* experiments could be repeated using the target from the representative species. The early use of human targets based on *in vitro* profiling assays, recent developments in stem-cell-derived, organ-specific parenchymal cells, and native human primary cells provide a powerful tool to correct or confirm species-specific findings in animal toxicologic studies.

10.3 COMPONENTS OF EARLY ADMET PROFILING

Detailed assessment of drug exposure using *in silico, in vitro*, and *in vivo* tools, albeit not the main focus of this book, is extremely critical from a toxicology point of view. For instance, it is very challenging to determine reasonable therapeutic indices in the absence of adequate solubility. Interpretation of cellular toxicity data also requires an understanding of passive membrane permeability and the involvement of transporters. Poor solubility and low permeability frequently prevent pharmacological and biochemical testing when dealing with less-optimized compounds. Furthermore, some of the toxic pharmacophores are associated with specific physicochemical properties. Also, metabolism is a major source of toxic effects. Metabolites of compounds that belong to scaffolds with known liabilities could revert to the original liability and reduce the therapeutic index (TI) calculated for the parent compound. Several reviews are available to address these matters in more detail.[10,11,,21]

10.3.1 *In vitro* toxicology: The emergence of multiple readout-based approaches

In vitro toxicology and safety models range from biochemical assays to isolated tissue preparations. Figure 10.1 lists a set of *in vitro* safety models/assays that are broadly used for early safety profiling. These assays are designed to accommodate small amounts of test compounds, and their dynamic range is usually broad to measure both high and low level of activities as most of them are designed to estimate safety or therapeutic indices. Those that use single targets, such as assays in the *in vitro* safety pharmacology panels, focus on human proteins associated with clinical ADRs. Others use bacteria or cells (native, stem-cell-derived, or transfected) for phenotypic readouts. More sophisticated assays employ tissue preparations from various organs and small nonmammalian animal models such as zebrafish or *Drosophila*.[22,23] The objective, regardless of the application of various systems, is to provide a relatively high capacity, highly reliable, and predictive safety assay.

Several areas of *in vitro* safety profiling underwent rapid development during the past couple of years. Dedicated chapters of the present book will discuss in detail organ- and system-specific toxicity/safety strategies, assays, and their implications. Here we will use two examples to demonstrate the development and application of early safety profiling capabilities.

Off-target or *in vitro* safety pharmacology panel[24]: Pharmacological targets for this assay panel are selected based on their association with known clinical adverse effects and then pooled into subpanels by their hit rate and the seriousness of the associated side effect(s). This assay set usually consists of approximately 70–80 targets (all associated with clinical ADRs). Potency at these frequently, but erroneously, called "antitargets"[25] gains relevance when compared to efficacious plasma concentrations in disease models. A large safety index measured between data generated in primary assays and off-targets might diminish or disappear entirely in cases where high plasma concentrations are required for therapy, or in cases of drug accumulation in an organ/tissue that carries the target, or competition with other molecules at metabolic enzymes. Thus, micromolar concentrations of drugs will appear in plasma and some tissues and could reach levels that might activate off-target proteins. Thus, high concentrations of drug candidates should be tested in the *in vitro* safety pharmacology assays to achieve this requirement. The BioPrint model gives a statistically correct predictive value between measured activities and clinical side effects, even at potencies over 10 μ*M*.[26] Also, some indications require the administration of potentially cytotoxic compounds at high doses close to the maximum tolerated dose (MTD) in oncology, transplantation, and indications of infectious diseases. Disease conditions might also alter the tolerated dose and exacerbate liabilities. Inhibition of the hERG channel, the most common off-target could be more serious, and triggers contraindication, in renal insufficiency or diabetes. On the other hand, even some serious side effects could be more tolerated in life-threatening diseases, particularly when acute treatment is required under hospitalized conditions. In rare cases, off-target liabilities could be balanced by an opposing effect at another target as in case of verapamil, which balances hERG channel inhibition by blocking the cardiac calcium channel.[27]

Testing for liabilities linked with largely hepatic functions is of a major interest, as hepatotoxicity is still the leading reason for late preclinical and more importantly clinical attrition. One can bundle early *in vitro* safety assays addressing liver function/toxicity into a suite comprising frontline tests for metabolism and drug–drug interactions, second-line tests for adduct formation, and more downstream assays for phospholipidosis, steatosis, and specific hepatocyte toxicity. The downstream assays can be used in an advanced format of high-content, multiparameter readouts for toxicology endpoints, for example the Cellumen approach using systems cell biology based on high-content screening.[28] Results are integrated, and the risk of hepatotoxicity is expressed as a score based on sophisticated algorithms.

10.3.2 Can *in vitro* discovery safety assays predict clinical performance?

Generation of a large volume of data in *in vitro* assays without correct interpretation does not speed up the selection of safe clinical candidates. The emphasis is on "the right data at the right time" in combination with right interpretation. Applying complex assays at an early stage without proper quality control (QC) and interpretation may produce misleading results, particularly when poor physicochemical properties compromise assay performance. For instance, safety/toxicology assays require high compound concentrations; consequently, poor solubility could be a major issue. (The same compounds will have problems in *in vivo* safety assays; bioavailability could be seriously compromised without time demanding and expensive formulation processes.) Thus, early assays are designed to be relatively simple and robust, and many have a built-in solubility control.

In general, two major aspects of *in vitro* safety profiling data generation should be considered.

Confidence in data

There are specific requirements of dynamic range and robustness of *in vitro* assays. In case the assay is designed only to signal an effect, a single-point determination in triplicate might be acceptable, with a defined follow-up format to test positives. However, for the support of SAR usually an IC_{50} or EC_{50} determination is preferred. The degree of occupancy required for therapeutic efficacy could be an issue; however, for uniformity and technical reasons, IC_{50} values are preferred for safety profiling. A good example is hERG inhibition, which is sufficient at an IC_{20} to cause prolongation of the QT interval in the electrocardiogram, but experimental data are represented as IC_{50}. The main reason is that the experimentally determined IC_{20} values would often fall into the "noise" range of the assay resulting in low confidence. The calculation for a safe TI with a value >30 was therefore adjusted to IC_{50} values.[7]

When *in vitro* safety assays are required to provide data for the calculation of a preclinical safety index, they use a broad range of concentrations. In case of complex cellular/electrophysiological assays, for example cardiac ion channels, this becomes a challenge because the extent of cell viability during the measurement could limit the success rate and render the assay expensive. However, time restriction might have serious effects on assay performance under circumstances when it limits the number of data points within a defined concentration range (see Figure 10.2), when the assay needs to accommodate slow equilibration or when extended duration of exposure is essential for the development of a complex effect (e.g., genetic toxicity or hepatotoxicity).

Poor solubility is one of the most significant limiting factors in early safety profiling. As all assays are performed up to high concentrations, compounds with poor solubility might precipitate or require high dimethyl sulfoxide (DMSO) concentration not tolerated by the assay. In addition, lipophilic compounds might stick to consumables. All of the above can contribute to generation of false negatives or "diminished" potency.

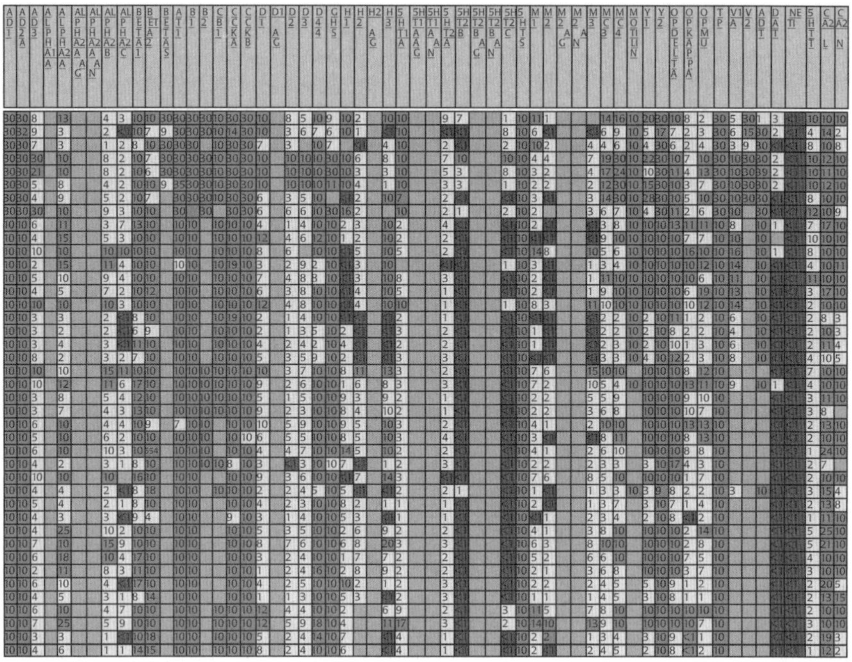

Figure 10-2: Heatmap of compounds submitted by a drug discovery project for off-target profiling. Each row represents a compound and columns are assigned to off-targets. This particular project has a serious problem with pharmacological promiscuity as compounds hit several targets at submicromolar potency. Red squares represent IC_{50} <1 μ*M*, yellow 1–10 μ*M*, and green >10 μ*M*. AG: agonist activity; AN: antagonist activity measured in functional assays. *See color plates.*

These assays also require a broad dynamic range to be able to differentiate between positive and baseline signals within a range from single-digit nanomolar to tens of micromolar concentrations.

At lead selection and optimization false negatives are more tolerated (high specificity): however, at clinical candidate selection – in an ideal situation – neither false positives nor false negatives are allowed (high sensitivity – high specificity).

It is of equal importance to determine the precision of the measurements. When in-house data on reference compounds are compared to those in the public domain, it is often found that published data might vary considerably between laboratories. However, these data are acceptable if the rank-order of potency was the same between different assay formats and clinical observations are in support of the findings.

Consistency/reproducibility of data is another major requirement for long-running drug discovery projects when scientists need to compare historical data to new results. This could become an issue if the assay format has been changed for various reasons. In these cases, consistency can be achieved by careful normalization. For the maintenance of high performance, most *in vitro* profiling assays use a set of compounds with diverse characteristics and potency at the target and apply them periodically. This is important as baselines might shift in automated systems, and cell line performance could vary between batches.

However, with careful QC of liquid handling and standardized cell line production parameters can be maintained at a steady level. Some cellular assays, which use harvested native cells, depend on large batches, often obtained from different donors or cadavers. It is important that these assays are recalibrated with new batches and the validation process repeated.

Even with the most attention to detail and quality, profiling assays encounter unexpected differences between data obtained from the same compound. These events need careful investigation. First, check whether data originated from the same batch: contamination or aggregation might be the reason behind differences in data. Importantly, different salt forms should be retested as they will have variable physicochemical properties with influence on solubility, permeability, and the like. Finally, equipment and human error have to be excluded.

Relevance of data

Lead optimization flowcharts include assay cascades for safety profiling. Such an example is the assay hierarchy for long QT testing, a major biomarker for arrhythmia. Statistical analysis shows that there is high correlation between hERG inhibition measured by manual patch clamp and clinical arrhythmogenesis associated with long QT[7]. However, even though manual patch clamp is the "gold standard" experiment, it is not feasible to use it for testing large number of compounds. Thus, one needs to find assays with qualities the same as or similar quality to those of manual patch clamp but with a much higher throughput at significantly lower cost. Ideally, a single assay with these later characteristics should replace manual patch clamp altogether. In reality, this rarely happens, and the most likely solution is that a combination of assays is introduced with various predictive levels and throughputs to filter compounds prior to using the manual patch clamp. This approach is built on assay cascades that are frequently if not always used in safety profiling. By the rule of thumb, the downstream prediction in the cascade should be incremental (starting at ~80 percent) with a very high level next to the gold standard assay. Most chapters in this book will describe such processes for various safety aspects.

In the long QT interval (LQT) testing cascade, the first component is an *in silico* QSAR-based tool that can "forecast" the hERG inhibition of molecules. Well-designed QSAR should be able to guide chemists to synthesize molecules with no or diminished hERG activity in the primary assay, which is most likely to be a binding assay. Compounds with potential efficacy in *in vivo* disease models will then proceed to the automated patch clamp assay to define their functional activity. This assay cascade is designed to deselect scaffolds/compounds with unacceptable hERG inhibition and to meet the compound requirement, turnaround time, capacity, and cost effectiveness during lead selection and optimization. It is also built on good correlation between the assays and above all on good predictive value for the *in vivo* nonrodent telemetry studies. Still, the question remains: How relevant are these assays to predict arrhythmogenesis in the clinic? The question is more than justified as a good correlation between *in vitro* (or even between *in vitro–in vivo*) data can be offset by many factors (e.g., the possible inhibition of other cardiac channels, receptors, and particular conditions such as a change in electrolyte equilibrium, pathological conditions, and formation of active metabolites). Some of these factors could be addressed in preclinical settings, but others could not. Under these conditions, a project with hERG liability has the choice to abolish hERG inhibition by SAR design or mitigate the effect to the extent that it offers an acceptable safety index. However, at this point one has to make sure that the compound is also tested for the other targets that could influence arrhythmogenesis.

Testing for hERG inhibition for the prediction of arrhythmogenesis is straightforward, but this is not the case for many other early safety-profiling assays, particularly for those that measure phenotypic changes as a common readout of effects at multiple targets. Therefore, *in vitro* profiling assays such as simple cellular assays to predict hepatotoxicity are less reliable. Cellular assays so far failed to provide high-quality hepatic phenotype maintained long enough to ensure prolonged compound exposure. Also, simple nonspecific readouts such as ATP depletion cannot differentiate between general cytotoxicity and specific liver toxicity. However, there is hope that novel, more complex assay arrangements and multiple high-content readouts of cellular functions will provide more predictive and higher throughput hepatotoxicity assays in the near future. Some recent developments to determine mitochondrial damage or phospholidosis have already shown improved predictive values.[29,30]

Certainly, most *in vitro* assays cannot predict (a) metabolite effects, (b) adverse effects associated by accumulation, and (c) drug actions at targets with mutations. Nevertheless, early safety-profiling assays have the power to detect trends toward certain adverse reactions and organ toxicity and to navigate drug discovery teams away from them. The major difficulty is estimating the impact of the data on the clinical performance determined by the human therapeutic index.

10.4 LEARNING FROM PAST MISTAKES

Clinical databases provide important information on toxicity and off-target related liabilities experienced in the clinic. Information on the so-called antitargets[25] is readily available and discussed in details. More importantly, at early phases of drug discovery, teams should avoid any side effect associated with undesirable off-targets so as not to co-optimize the potency at the primary target. *In vitro* safety pharmacology is an early profiling tool developed to address this issue by using a panel of off-targets, associated with clinical ADRs, designed to cover significant portion of both chemical and pharmacological space. This panel has been constantly evolving as new therapeutic target families are introduced bringing their bad-behaving members into scope and more functional assays enter the panels.[31] For example, with the advent of kinase inhibitor drugs, ever more off-target kinases are hit by these molecules. Therefore, high-throughput technologies for kinome profiling have been introduced at low cost [see Ambit[32,33]] which can address adverse effects linked with specific targets (e.g., Aurora[34]). Using these and other *in vitro* safety pharmacology panels (e.g., ion channels, GPCRs, proteases, enzymes, and nuclear receptors or their combinations) will provide information about off-target activity and could guide drug discovery teams to avoid or eliminate them.

Even though information is abundant, the relevance of the data should be determined. For example, how should a compound that inhibits PDE3 as an off-target with a nanomolar potency be positioned? It is known that PDE3 inhibition is associated with positive inotropy and could cause increased mortality in congestive heart failure (CHF) patients, but there is no evidence of similar effect in patients with no cardiac impairment.[35] A compound with off-target activity at PDE3 originally designed for the indication in cancer or for a patient population that rarely has concomitant CHF should not be lost for further development; however, if the indication is associated with serious cardiac conditions, the future of the molecule would be seriously questioned, particularly if the TI was very narrow. To put positive off-target findings in context, one needs to get information on drugs that have an effect on the same target.

Marketed drug databases are essential aids in this process as they give information about preclinical and clinical PK/PD, ADRs, black box labels, and drug withdrawals. Careful analysis of these data and their alignment with structural features is extremely important to learn from past mistakes. Careful monitoring of clinical ADRs is important to ensure the well-being of patients, but also to advance the learning process in drug discovery. Recent clinical studies highlighted side effects associated with defined pharmacological targets (e.g., the link between $5HT_{2b}$ agonism and cardiac valvulopathy[36] and the link between D_1 antagonism and Parkinsonism[24]). Databases such as Pharmapendium[37] and GVK[38] provide invaluable information for the prediction of ADRs for drug candidates.

As mentioned previously, major problems can arise if pharmacophores between primary therapeutic targets and off-targets (toxicophores) associated with ADRs are shared. In this case, teams should do a thorough SAR analysis and, based on the severity of overlap, either consider a different scaffold or switch to a different target for the same indication.

10.5 *IN SILICO* APPROACHES, DECISION SUPPORT TOOLS, AND MODELING

In silico tools make a significant contribution to the SAR-based early identification of potential toxicity. An increasing volume of published preclinical and clinical toxicity data are collected and used to build structure-related searchable databases. These expert knowledge databases can analyze chemical structures and match them with potential mechanisms of toxicity. DEREK for Windows (Lhasa Ltd.)[39] is one of such broadly used knowledge-based expert systems to provide toxicology alerts for new compounds. Although certainly not comprehensive, numerous efforts have been made to predict hepatotoxicity. Recently,

Cheng[40] reviewed *in silico* models of hepatotoxicity with the conclusion that no dose-prediction is in scope as today. However, continuing efforts, such as MCASE, based on postmarket adverse effect data[41] will continuously enhance and ultimately improve *in silico* prediction of liver toxicity.

One of the most advanced *in silico* predictions of any clinical liability is based on hERG QSAR and homology models[6]. Structural features of hERG inhibition have been discussed and published in detail, and major structural alerts are built into knowledge-based expert systems and broadly used by chemists[5]. Detailed information on available QSAR efforts to predict toxic effect is discussed in details elsewhere.[42,43,44]

10.5.1 Decision support tools: Data visualization

Various approaches have been developed to support risk assessment-based decision making. Because a large volume of data needs to be considered for this process, visualization tools are prominently featured. For example, a large volume of *in vitro* safety pharmacology data can be viewed together for the same project or for selected scaffolds and analyzed by their pattern of activity within a heatmap (Figure 10.3). It is easy to recognize from this heatmap that compounds within the same structural class hit several off-targets, which are part of the *in vitro* safety pharmacology panel and are associated with particular side effects. This heatmap prominently features strong nanomolar effect at 5HT2, H2, DAT, NET, and muscarinic receptor family. The tool directly links to the chemistry database with visualization of two-dimensional structures and to a "profiling WIKI" with information on adverse reactions, clinical data, and structures active at the same target. This type of tool can be powerful in the development of SAR for off-targets, but it also could be used for tracking project performance.

The heatmap is based on relatively simple processes: It uses data mining tools to provide quick access to comprehensive safety-related information. However, more sophisticated tools can introduce correlative assessment of various data and guide teams to the best utilization of the assays. At Novartis, we built a cardiac safety report that provides information on the correlation between QSAR bins and radioligand binding data for hERG inhibition and in parallel provides correlations between RLB, patch clamp data, and potency at the primary target (Figure 10.4). Modifiers of the RLB–patch clamp correlation are also highlighted by color-coding compounds with poor permeability/ solubility. An advanced form of the report can also perform similarity searches by chemical structures and biological characteristics.

10.5.2 How to drive lead optimization toward an acceptable therapeutic index

Comparison of SAR for the primary target and for a liability will determine the safety of compounds. Figure 10.5 demonstrates the performance of two projects that encountered potent activity at an antitarget and made attempts to

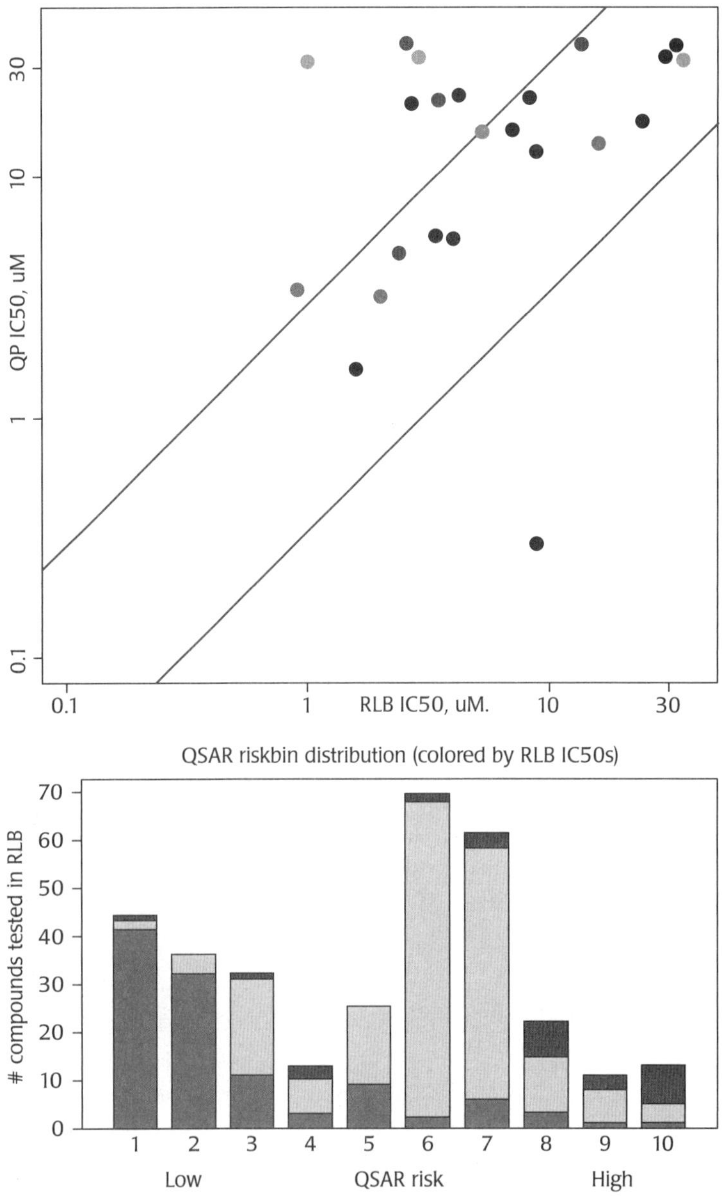

Figure 10-3: *In silico* tool for monitoring compound performance in three hERG inhibition assays. The lower panel shows correlation with the QSAR prediction (bin 1–10 forecasting hERG inhibition in an ascending order) and "matching" radioligand binding data (red: IC_{50} <1 μM, yellow: 1–30 μM; blue: >30 μM). Each dot represents a compound. The correlation suggests that the drug discovery team can use QSAR to predict hERG inhibition of molecules. The upper panel shows correlation of the radioligand binding and automated planar patch clamp (QPatch) IC_{50} data. The red lines mark the 3× difference in the IC_{50} that is acceptable for this correlation. The graph also highlights "alerts" such as low permeability (red dots), low solubility (green dots), or marginally positive effects in the radioligand binding and the QPatch assays (blue dots).

mitigate the liability. Both projects made an effort to preserve high activity at the primary target while reducing that to the off-target. *Project A* managed this successfully and provided couple of active compounds with much less activity

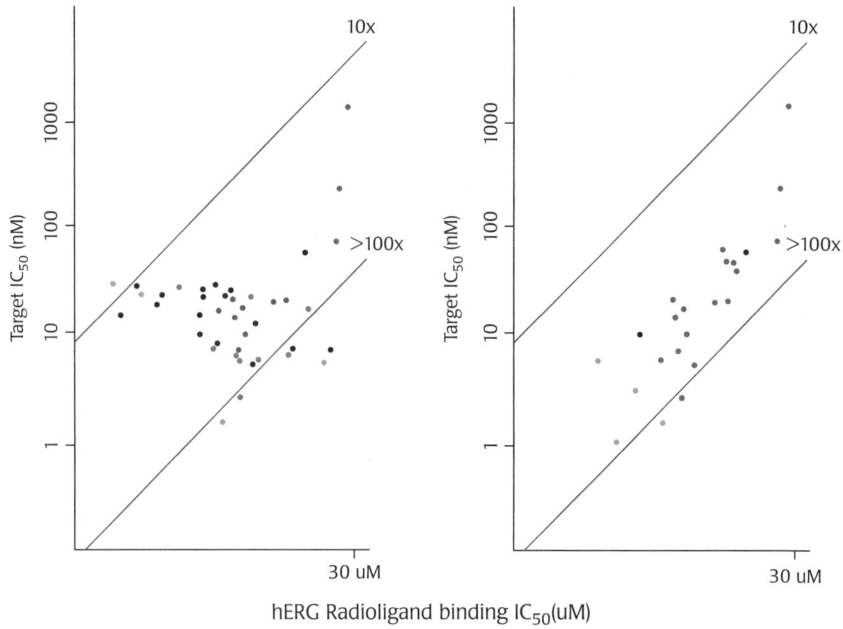

Figure 10-4: Correlation of hERG inhibition (RLB IC_{50}) with potency at the primary target (Target IC_{50}) for two different drug discovery projects. The left panel shows a loose correlation, which suggests there is little overlap between the two pharmacophores. This gives the project the opportunity to develop potent compounds for the primary target while mitigating hERG inhibition. The right panel demonstrates compound performance from a different project, where the primary and the hERG pharmacophore overlap to a great extent. Thus, there is a good correlation between primary and hERG inhibition. This is "poor prognosis" for hERG mitigation and predicts a difficult path forward. Projects with this kind of profile are advised to change scaffold to avoid lengthy mitigation process without guaranteed success. For the color codes, see explanation in Figure 10.3.

at the undesired target, but the efforts of *project B* failed, largely because of the tight overlap of the two pharmacophores, which prevented independent SAR modifications and eventually influenced activity at both targets in the same direction.

10.5.3 Moving away from *in vitro* affinity toward effective plasma and tissue concentrations

Most drug discovery projects identify one or two primary assays (biochemical or cellular) for routine use to monitor compound activity at the therapeutic target. The false security of "nanomolar" activity in these assays is still existent in the pharmaceutical industry, largely ignoring the fact that medicines behave in a complex way once in the organism, influenced by their PK/PD. Compensating or parallel processes can also diminish the effect of a potent drug candidate once applied *in vivo*. It should not be a surprise that often much higher plasma concentrations are needed for efficacy *in vivo* than concentration estimated based on *in vitro* experiments. Therefore, PD/PK data are required to predict possible

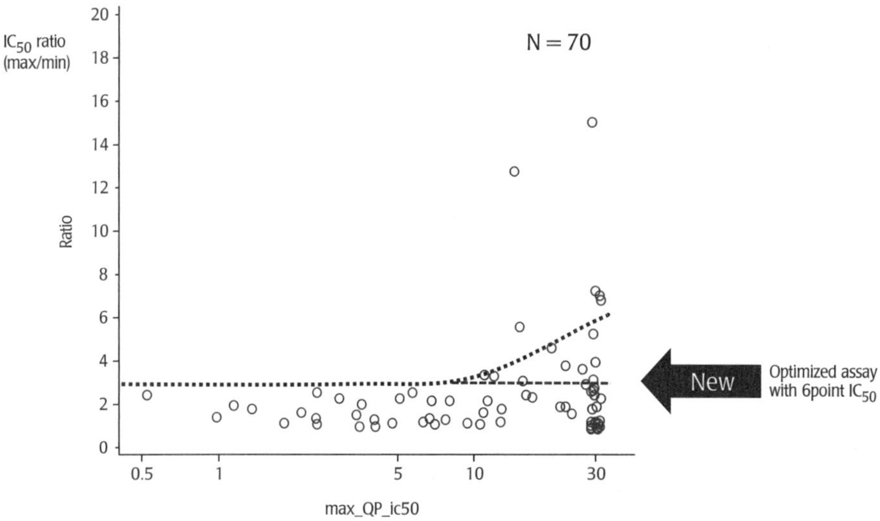

Figure 10-5: Critical analysis of assay performance: assessment of quality. The hERG QPatch assay was originally designed to provide an IC_{50} based on four concentrations due to time restraint. The requirement was to cover a dose range between 0.1 and 30 μ*M*. This was achieved by using 0.24, 1.2, 6.4, and 30 μ*M* concentrations of compounds. Results obtained from repeated experiments with the same compounds demonstrated that the quality of IC_{50} values between 10 and 30 μ*M* was poor, and in several cases the ratio in repeated experiments exceeded the 3× value. Consequently, an advanced version of the automated system allowed generating longer recordings with the application of six concentrations. Additional concentrations of 10 and 20 μ*M* filled the gap and increased the confidence in this range. In addition to this change, we also introduced a filter to avoid compounds with poor solubility and further increase assay quality.

adverse effects associated with organ-specific toxicities or with any recognized off-target activity. While at preclinical stages, no clinical data are available on a particular set of compounds. PK/PD studies in animal models could give some indication for clinical performance, particularly if it is performed in a relevant disease model. The broadly used cardiac safety evaluation for arrhythmogenesis prediction relies on hERG patch clamp IC_{50} values in comparison to free efficacious plasma concentration at C_{max}. This scheme was made possible by statistical analysis of human PD/PK data associated with arrhythmia and correlative hERG inhibition data. Unfortunately, translation of a large number of hits at off-targets into clinical ADRs is by far more difficult; therefore, most of the off-target safety pharmacology and *in vitro* toxicology assays rely on "flagging" adverse reactions. The BioPrint approach shows clearly that low micromolar activity at off-targets, regardless of the activity at the therapeutic target is likely to translate into ADRs at a significant level.[26,45] The underlying mechanisms can vary from high C_{max} accumulation in the heart or as an effect of a metabolite, just to mention a few.

It is most important to consider the indication. Some disease conditions, such as diabetes, congestive heart failure, and nephropathy predispose for arrhythmias. In a case when low level of hERG inhibition with an estimated 30 TI caused no prolongation of QT in healthy dogs and consequently in healthy volunteers, unexpected QT prolongation occurred when the drug was administered to patients with type 2 diabetes. This case clearly shows the necessity to test safety of compounds in relevant *in vivo* disease models whenever available.

10.6 CRITICAL EVALUATION AND CONCLUSIONS

Preclinical *in vitro* safety-profiling assays have to be used in an integrated environment, considering various elements of compound performance. There are few examples (e.g., the Ames test and broad-scale cytotoxicity assays) that, when applied appropriately, can support yes–no decision making during early phases of drug discovery. Most of the profiling assays, however, rely on results from other parallel-run assays and on the confirmation in downstream tests.

In some cases, on-target effects cannot be avoided, but depending on the indication, they could be tolerated. This issue is very important if a drug has been developed for a new target and no clinical data are available for ADRs. The case of Vioxx shows that on-target effects in the coagulation system can offset homeostasis and result in serious ADRs.[46] It is obvious that with further novel targets more unexpected side effects will emerge during careful clinical monitoring. Information obtained this way can be used to update preclinical testing panels and refine assays.

We have discussed specific considerations during safety assessment. Indication, patient population, disease conditions, and competition have a significant impact on the interpretation of safety/toxicology data. Recently, major efforts have been made to develop highly reliable and predictive biomarkers for both preclinical and clinical use. They can provide a significant bridge between clinical and *in vivo* performance. Early biomarkers have become an important component of safety evaluation. A good example of biomarker development is the advance in the detection of nephrotoxicity in both preclinical and clinical studies.[47] There are other areas, such as liver toxicity, where further development is essential to achieve better predictability. Genomic and proteomic approaches can provide fingerprints; however, interpretation of the data could be difficult, and specificity can be a serious issue.

Furthermore, possible conflicts between animal data and clinical performance could arise in case of species-specific targets, differences in metabolism, PK characteristics, pathway specificity, and different tissue distribution. For example, guinea pigs have a very high density of neurokinin-loaded neurons, and they are extremely sensitive to capsaicin, but humans are not. Therefore, blockade of neurokinin receptors might be much less effective in humans than in the guinea pig. Also, the majority of early profiling assays use human targets in transfected cells and recently native cells and tissues; however, preclinical *in vivo* toxicology is largely based on rat, dog, and monkey data. If compounds affect targets in a species-specific manner or are associated with diverse pathways, discrepancies may arise between in *vitro* and *in vivo* predictions. These discrepancies must be followed up on an individual basis.

Finally, we would like to address the term "idiosyncrasy" [(a) a peculiarity of constitution or temperament; an individualizing characteristic or quality; (b) individual hypersensitiveness (as to a drug or food)]. This term springs in place in case an unexpected severe side effect or toxicity appears in the clinic without any known mode of action. Most often it is referred to in the context of idiosyncratic drug-induced liver injury (DILI), which seems to appear sporadically without any dose-dependence and clear explanation. The term "idiosyncrasy" is temporary, in that it exists until the underlying mechanism is resolved. For example, drug-induced TdP was considered idiosyncratic until it became known to be associated with the inhibition of the hERG channel. DILI is different in many ways as a large number of various underlying mechanisms could be considered. Preclinical testing can take the possible elements of hepatotoxicity apart and then put them together in a multiple readout analysis.

In conclusion, recent advances in drug discovery chemistry and biomedical sciences have made it possible to generate valuable data in early preclinical setting to signal adverse clinical behavior of drug candidates. This progress enables pharmaceutical companies to guide projects toward safer molecules, by using SAR approaches. On the other hand, assays not associated with a particular target can use high-content multiple readouts and clinically validated biomarkers to enhance confidence in data, particularly when organ-specific toxicities are considered. The benefit of these efforts started to pay off; for example, LQT prediction by early testing has become routine during the past decade with the result that new medicines entering the clinic are devoid of drug-induced TdP.

At present, *in vivo* experiments are carrying the most weight in drug safety studies, regardless of early drug evaluation *in silico* or *in vitro*. The complexity of a living mammalian organism is not easy to model *in vitro* and will remain so for a long time. However, many adverse effects are overlooked in the classical *in vivo* toxicology evaluation. More clever approaches, discussed in the chapters of this book open new avenues in terms of increased precision and more relevant evaluation by introducing genetically altered animals to sensitize the system or by using disease models that make it possible to test drugs in the pathological environment equivalent to that of patients.

ACKNOWLEDGMENTS

Authors would like to acknowledge the many contributions of Steven Whitebread, Jacques Hamon, Dmitri Mikhailov, Gul Erdemli, Qiang Lu, and Mats Holmqvist to the content of this chapter. We also would like to extend a special thanks to Scott Biller for his advice and for the stimulating discussions and guidance.

REFERENCES

1. Lipinski CA. Drug-like properties and the causes of poor solubility and poor permeability. *J Pharm Toxicol Methods*. 2000;44:235–249.
2. Kola I, Landis J. Can the pharmaceutical industry reduce attrition rates? *Nat Rev Drug Discov*. 2004;3:711–716.
3. Cardiac Arrhythmia Suppression Trial II Investigators. Effect of the antiarrhythmic agent moricizine on survival after myocardial infarction. *New Engl J Med*. 1992;327:227–233.
4. Keating MT, Sanguinetti, MC . Molecular and cellular mechanisms of cardiac arrhythmias. *Cell*. 2001;104:569–580.
5. Jamieson C, Moir EM, Rankovic Z, et al. Medicinal chemistry of hERG optimizations: Highlights and hang-ups. *J Med Chem*. 2006;49:5029–5046.
6. Pearlstein R Vaz, R, Rampe D. Understanding the structure-activity relationship of the human ether-a-go-go-related gene cardiac K+ channel. A model for bad behavior. *J Med Chem*. 2003;46:2017–2022.
7. Redfern WS, Carlsson L, Davis AS, et al. Relationships between preclinical cardiac electrophysiology, clinical QT interval prolongation and torsade de pointes for a broad range of drugs: Evidence for a provisional safety margin in drug development. *Cardiovasc Res*. 2003;58:32–45.
8. Kramer JA, Sagartz JE, Morris DL. The application of discovery toxicology and pathology towards the design of safer pharmaceutical lead candidates. *Nat Rev Drug Discov*. 2007;6:636–649.
9. Leeson PD, Springthorpe B. The influence of drug-like concepts on decision-making in medicinal chemistry. *Nat Rev Drug Discov*. 2007;6:881–890.
10. Bender A, Jenkins JL, Glick M, et al. Analysis of pharmacology data and the prediction of adverse drug reactions and off-target effect from chemical structure. *Chem Med Chem*. 2007;2:1–14.
11. Wang J, Urban L, Bojanic D. Maximising use of in vitro ADMET tools to predict in vivo bioavailability and safety. *Expert Opin Drug Metab Toxicol*. 2007;3:641–665.
12. Wang J. Comprehensive assessment of ADMET risks in drug discovery. *Curr Pharm Design*, 2009;5(19):2195–2219.
13. Kerns EH, Di L. Physicochemical profiling: Overview of the screens. *Drug Discov Today Technol*. 2004;1:343–348.
14. Thomas VH, Bhattachar S, Hitchingham L, et al. The road map to oral bioavailability: An industrial perspective. *Expert Opin Drug Metab Toxicol*. 2006; 2:591–608.
15. Li AP. Building predictive ADMET models for early decisions in drug discovery. *Drug Discov Today*. 2001;6:357–366.
16. Ramot Y, Nyska A. Drug-induced thrombosis – Experimental, clinical, and mechanistic considerations. *Toxicol Pathol*. 2007;35:208–225.
17. Meyer CH, Schmidt JC, Rodrigues EB, et al. Risk of retinal vein occlusions in patients treated with rofecoxib (Vioxx). *Ophthalmologica*. 2005;219:243–247.
18. Zhu W, Zeng X, Zheng M, et al. The enigma of β2 adrenergic receptor Gi signaling in the heart. The good, the bad, and the ugly. *Circ Res*. 2005;97:507–509.
19. Shamovsky I, Connolly S, David L, et al. Overcoming undesirable HERG potency of chemokine receptor antagonists using baseline lipophilicity relationships. *J Med Chem*. 2008;51:1162–1178.
20. Obradovic T, Dobson G, Shingaki T, et al. Assessment of the first and second generation antihistamines brain penetration and role of P-glycoprotein. *Pharm Res*. 2007;24:318–327.
21. Faller B, Wang J, Zimmerlin A, et al. High-throughput in-vitro profiling assays: How useful for decision making? *Exp Opin Drug Metab Toxicol*. 2006;2:823–833.
22. Rubinstein AL. Zebrafish assays for drug toxicity screening. *Expert Opin Drug Metab Toxicol*. 2006;2:231–240.

23. Peterson RT, Nass R, Boyd WA, et al. Use of non-mammalian alternative models for neurotoxicological study. *Neurotoxicology*. 2008;29:546–555.
24. Whitebread S, Hamon J, Bojanic D, et al. In vitro safety pharmacology profiling: An essential tool for drug development. *Drug Discov Today*. 2005;10:1421–1433.
25. Vaz RJ, Klabunde T eds. *Antitargets: Prediction and Prevention of Drug Side Effects*. Wiley-VCH, Weinheim; 2008.
26. Krejsa CM, et al. Predicting ADME properties and side effects: The BioPrint approach. *Curr Opin Drug Discov Dev*. 2003;6:470–480.
27. Zhang S, Zhou Z, Gong Q, et al. Mechanism of block and identification of the verapamil binding domain to HERG potassium channels. *Circ Res*. 1999;84:989–998.
28. Giuliano KA, Johnston PA, Gough A, et al. Systems cell biology based on high-content screening. *Methods Enzymol*. 2006;414:601–619.
29. Cellumen. Cell Ciphr Toxicity Profiling. http://www.cellumen.com/solutions/cytotoxicity-csb.php., accessed date: 07. 05. 2010.
30. Morelli JK, Buehrle M, Pognan F, et al. Validation of an in vitro screen for phospholipidosis using a high-content biology platform. *Cell Biol Toxicol*. 2006;22(1):15–27.
31. Hamon J, Whitebread S, Techer-Etienne V, et al. *In vitro* safety pharmacology profiling: What else beyond hERG? 2009;1(4):645–665.
32. Ambit Biosciences. http://www.ambitbio.com. Accessed date: 07. 05. 2010.
33. Goldstein, DM, Gray GS, Zarrinkar PP . High-throughput kinase profiling as a platform for drug discovery. *Nat Rev Drug Discov*. 2008;7:391–397.
34. Lu LY, Wood JL, Ye L, et al. Aurora A is essential for early embryonic development and tumor suppression. *J Biol Chem*. 2008;283:31785–31790.
35. Robless P, Mikhailidis DP, Stansby GP. Cilostazol for peripheral arterial disease. Hoboken, NJ: John Wiley & Sons, 2008.
36. Elangbam CS, Job LE, Zadrozny LM, et al. 5-hydroxytryptamine (5HT)-induced valvulopathy: Compositional valvular alterations are associated with 5HT2B receptor and 5HT transporter transcript changes in Sprague-Dawley rats. *Exp Toxicol Pathol*. 2008;60(4–5):253–262.
37. Pharmapendium. https://www.pharmapendium.com.
38. GVK Biosciences. http://www.gvkbio.com. Accessed 08. 05. 2010.
39. Lhasa Ltd, DEREK. https://www.lhasalimited.org/index.php/derek/ Accessed 08. 05. 2010.
40. Cheng A. In silico prediction of hepatotoxicity. *Curr Computer-Aided Drug Design*. 2009;5:122–127.
41. Multicase Inc. Bioactive software. http://www.multicase.com. Accessed 09. 05. 2010.
42. Ekins S, ed. *Computational Toxicology*. Wiley-VCH, Hoboken NJ: 2007.
43. Ekins, S . Predicting undesirable drug interactions with promiscuous proteins *in silico*. *Drug Discov Today*. 2004;9:276–285.
44. Azzaoui K, Hamon J, Faller B, et al. Modeling promiscuity based on *in vitro* safety pharmacology profiling data *Chem Med Chem*. 2007; 2:874–880.
45. Whitebread S, Hamon J, Scheiber J, et al. Broad-scale in vitro pharmacology profiling to predict clinical adverse effects. *Am. Drug Discov*. 2008;1(7):1–5.
46. Mitchell JA, Warner TD. COX isoforms in the cardiovascular system: Understanding the activities of non-steroidal anti-inflammatory drugs. *Nat Rev Drug Discov*. 2006;5:75–86.
47. Dieterle F, Marrer E, Suzuki E, et al. Monitoring kidney safety in drug development: Emerging technologies and their implications. *Curr Opin Drug Discov Devel*. 2008;11:60–71.

11 Predictive toxicology approaches for small molecule oncology drugs

Timothy J. Maziasz, Vivek J. Kadambi, and Carl L. Alden

11.1 CANCER AS A WORLDWIDE DISEASE

Oncology therapeutic research and development represents the greatest opportunity today for pharmaceutical companies to significantly affect morbidity and mortality in the developed world. More than 12 million new cancer cases emerged worldwide in 2007. In 2009, approximately 560,000 people were projected to die from malignancies in the United States.[1] According to the World Cancer Center Report 2008, cancer is destined to become the leading cause of death on the planet by 2010.[2] The number of new cancer cases per year is predicted to triple by the year 2030, which represents 20 million to 26 million new cases and 13 million to 17 million additional deaths annually. Of equal significance is the number of new drugs undergoing testing for treatment of various forms of cancer. As of April 2009, 831 drugs and vaccines were in clinical development, which is a 32 percent increase over the number of oncologic agents in development in April 2008.[3]

This daunting unmet medical need, coupled with the rapid demise of the majority of cancer patients, requires that oncology drug development follow a much different paradigm than that used for the development of drugs for non-life-threatening diseases. The challenges of oncology drug development are underscored by the fact that phase 1 clinical trials commonly include patients with nonresponsive late-stage disease and a mean life expectancy of 3 to 5 months; patients treated with oncology drugs targeted against solid metastatic tumor disease (excluding a few cancers, such as hormone-dependent metastatic prostate cancer), typically have a mean life expectancy of only 1 to 2 years. Meanwhile, the 2009 Industry Profile report[3,4] shows the average length of time required to discover, develop, and register a new drug is 10 to 15 years. Novel, if not unconventional, thinking is clearly needed in all facets of pharmaceutical development to hasten the delivery of new drugs to the terminal cancer patient. It is not surprising then, that a recent report shows that the Food and Drug Administration (FDA) fast-track mechanisms, including accelerated approval with phase 2 data, priority review, and orphan drug status, are more commonly applied to submissions involving oncology drugs.[5]

With regard to toxicology/pathology strategies and testing paradigms that can help meet the challenges of developing therapeutic agents for the patient with late-stage cancer, this paper discusses the approaches successfully used to support research in identifying viable candidate molecules (early stage through the critical late lead optimization stage), as well as activities essential to filing successful investigational new drug (IND) requests and new drug applications (NDAs). Therapeutic strategies for the treatment of cancer involve a variety of modalities, including biologics (monoclonal antibodies), vaccines, and antisense (small interfering RNA) molecules. A discussion of the nuances of safety assessment for each of these modalities is beyond the scope of this chapter. Rather, the focus of this chapter is on the development of new small organic molecule entities directed at novel molecular targets. These small molecule drugs frequently are intended for adult patients with nonresponsive metastatic disease who are without medical options; however, the vision may be to expand their clinical use to front-line and pediatric indications.

11.2 ONCOLOGY THERAPY FOR THE LATE-STAGE CANCER PATIENT

Cancer is a complex disease, and it is unlikely that it can be managed with a single therapeutic modality. Consequently, a variety of mechanisms and targets are under active research to develop treatment for advanced-stage cancer. Although it is not the purpose of this chapter to provide a comprehensive review of anticancer therapy, it is important to define the types of therapeutic agents that are relevant to the toxicology/pathology strategies discussed here. The 10th edition of Goodman and Gilman's *The Pharmacological Basis of Therapeutics* lists the following classes of cancer chemotherapeutics: cytotoxic agents and antihormonal agents.[6] Cytotoxic agents include alkylating agents, antimetabolites, natural products (e.g., doxorubicin and bleomycin), and miscellaneous agents. Early generation cytotoxic agents, though a mainstay of cancer chemotherapy for many years, are well known for their marked clinical toxicity, which is due to their nonselective targeting of DNA and metabolic pathways common to both cancer and normal tissue with high replicative indices. The second-class, antihormonal agents are used for treatment of hormone-dependent cancers, including breast and prostate cancers. These drugs may typically follow the more traditional development pathway for drugs of chronic use since front-line therapy for these specific forms of cancer does not represent an area of unmet medical need.

Listed among the miscellaneous drugs in Goodman and Gilman's[6] is a tyrosine kinase inhibitor, imatinib. Now this agent is more representative of contemporary oncology therapy and is part of a third major class of cancer therapies known as molecular-targeted agents. These agents followed inroads into understanding the genomics of cancer cells,[7] and they represent the basis for the hope that breakthrough therapies for cancer patients are imminent. This therapeutic approach is hypothesized to limit tumor growth by reestablishing normal cell cycling and turnover.[8,9] Among the molecular mechanisms under consideration are kinase inhibitors, farnesyl transferase inhibitors, signal transduction inhibitors, cell cycle inhibitors, antiangiogenic agents, matrix metalloproteinase inhibitors, purinome inhibitors, proteasome inhibitors, and agents that inhibit DNA repair.[8,10–12] Specific agents have been reviewed by Rosa et al., 2008.[9,13]

Although agents acting through the aforementioned mechanisms were initially referred to as cytostatic, they are now frequently referred to as cytotoxic because they induce cell death.[9] Because it remains a difficult proposition to specifically target cancer cells, even these novel targets are associated with significant toxicity. Thus, remains the requirement for rigorous toxicology/pathology expertise in the discovery and development of these potential new anticancer drugs.

11.3 TOXICOLOGY/PATHOLOGY CHALLENGES IN THE DISCOVERY OF NEW ONCOLOGY DRUGS

The pursuit of newly identified targets in tumors and cancer cell lines holds great promise for oncology therapy; however, it also increases the risk for failure. It has been estimated that a molecule directed at a novel target has only about an 8 percent chance of success in achieving approval and marketing and that the probability for novel oncology drug success is even less.[14] Much of the risk lays with the fact that novel targets, by definition, lack validation through proof of efficacy in the clinic. Moreover, it is common for molecules active against novel targets to rapidly move through drug candidate selection and enter development well before the function of the target in normal tissues and physiology is fully understood.

Toxicology/pathology technologies can be applied to help define the physiological function of a target, as well as potential adverse effects resulting from inhibition of the target. Separating the beneficial effects of target inhibition in tumors from potential adverse effects that may occur with inhibition of the same target in normal tissues is challenging, especially when the target is widely expressed. This is often the case with oncology therapeutics that target mitosis because of the widespread physiological relevance of this process, these agents exhibit virtually no therapeutic index due to their concomitant efficacy and toxicity in fast turnover normal cells. This characteristic obscures the distinction between failures due to efficacy and toxicity and further complicates the development of oncology therapeutic agents. The failure rate of oncology drugs in development ranges from 74 percent to 95 percent with 30 percent of these failures attributed to either lack of efficacy or toxicity with lack of tolerability.[15,16] The inability to distinguish between these two factors in a clinical trial can be illustrated by the following: The standard practice for evaluating tolerability in phase 1 oncology clinical trials is to dose until a grade 3 (National Cancer Institute Toxicity Criteria) toxicity emerges (e.g., alanine aminotransferase (ALT) levels greater than 5 to 20 times the upper limit of normal). Even though grades 1 and 2 toxicities are common with most oncology agents, the appearance of grade 3 toxicity establishes the dose as greater than the maximum tolerated dose

Pre-LO

Assays:

- *In silico* mutagenicity
  - DEREK and PRISM
- *In silico* structural alerts
- Target expression in normal and tumor tissues
- Literature search

Deliverables:

- Assess mutagenic potential of scaffold
- Assess structural-based toxicity of scaffold
- Predict target-based effects

Early LO

Assays:

- hERG binding
- Genetic toxicity: modified Ames
- Sentinel toxicology studies in rats
- PK & ADME evaluations
- Kinase screen
- Broad pharmacology screen

Deliverables:

- Quality candidates for risk for QT disturbance and potential mutagenicity & ancillary pharmacology
- Early ID of potential structural- & mechanism-based toxicity
- Validation of drug-like properties

Late LO

Assays: (molecule with 95% purity):

- 1 cycle toxicology study in rats & dogs
- Preliminary safety pharmacology
  - Rats: mini-Irwin test
  - Dogs: surface ECG assessment
- Limited TK and PD assessment

Deliverables:

- Identify candidates with good probability of success in development
- Build case that toxicity profile is clinically acceptable
- Develop basis for dose-setting in GLP studies
- Define TK/PD/Toxicity inter-relationship

Figure 11-1: Recommended toxicology/pathology activities to support oncology drug discovery by stage.

(MTD) and terminates further dose escalation. Should, as is often the case, no patient benefit be observed at tolerated doses, it must be considered whether the dose-limiting toxicity prevents achievement of efficacious exposures or whether the target is truly viable as a therapeutic modality. This lack of clarity somewhat limits the usefulness of clinical experience in guiding drug discovery efforts to improve therapy. The convergence of toxicity with efficacy seen with many oncology agents presents a safety challenge that is not easily addressed, even by rational drug design. This makes it imperative for involvement of toxicology/pathology technologies and expertise in the process for selecting the most effective and best-tolerated oncology drug candidate.

11.4 CHALLENGES IN CANDIDATE SELECTION

The incorporation of toxicology/pathology technologies into drug discovery is now a well-established practice and is extensively reviewed in the literature.[17,18] A scheme for incorporating various toxicology/pathology activities into oncology drug discovery by stage is shown in Figure 11.1 and will be discussed in the subsequent sections of this chapter. One of the most significant challenges in evaluating molecules during the candidate selection process is to characterize the toxicity profile and to categorize the dose-limiting toxicity as pharmacology based or chemical structure based.

11.4.1 Classifications of adverse effects

The vast majority of drugs have molecular structures that are foreign to living organisms (xenobiotics) although many drugs are designed to mimic endogenous

Table 11-1. Categorization of toxicity

Adverse activity	Molecular basis	Structural component	Effect of structural optimization	Impact if dose limiting on candidate progression
Structural-based	Chemical reactivity of parent molecule or biotransformation to reactive metabolite	Toxicophore	Eliminate or reduce effect	Reject
Target-based	Activity against primary target	Primary pharmacophore	Potency can be changed	Accept
Off-target	Activity against unintended target(s)	Secondary pharmacophore or Nonselectivity against family of related targets by primary pharmacophore	Eliminate or reduce effect (may require changing structural template) Selectivity may be improved	Case-by-case

molecules. Drug molecules interact with cells, biochemical pathways and physiological systems by virtue of their structure; fundamentally then, the toxicities and adverse effects produced by any molecule ultimately reflect its structure (Table 11.1). Recognizing that some drug toxicities reflect the susceptibility of the individual (i.e., drug idiosyncrasy), the majority of adverse effects and toxicities can be placed into one of several major categories, including chemical-based, target-related, or off-target effects.[19] In the simplest case, the toxicity of a molecule can be due to the intrinsic reactivity of its structure or to its biotransformation to a reactive metabolite. Chemical-based reactivity initiates the molecular processes linked with cellular injury and death, including lipid peroxidation, covalent binding, mitochondrial dysfunction, and redox cycling.[19,20] Medicinal chemists are trained to recognize structural moieties that can increase the intrinsic toxicity of a molecule. These moieties are known as toxicophores and all good medicinal chemistry strategies for drug hunting will seek to avoid them.[21] Nonetheless, the identification of chemical-based toxicity remains incumbent on the toxicology/pathology group in supporting drug candidate selection.

The ability to identify chemical-based effects is essential because opportunities to improve the safety profile of oncology therapeutic agents, particularly cytotoxic agents, may often be limited to removal of chemical-based toxicity. To illustrate this, it is recognized that antimitotic agents produce some signal in liver function tests (LFTs) by virtue of the fact that they affect the relatively small population of cells in the liver undergoing mitosis. This effect is generally regarded to be clinically manageable based on experience with marketed agents.[22] In contrast, the clinical development of geldanamycin, which inhibits the activity of heat shock protein 90 (HSP 90), was discontinued after the appearance of dose-limiting liver toxicity that was shown to be related to its chemical structure and not the result of HSP 90 inhibition.[23] Subsequent efforts to identify a clinically useful HSP 90 inhibitor focused on structural modifications to remove the liver toxicophore.[24–26]

Pharmacological effects are related to a specific moiety on the molecular structure known as a pharmacophore. The pharmacophore is defined as "a set of structural features in a molecule that is recognized at the receptor site and is responsible for the molecule's biological activity."[27] The pharmacophore interacts with cellular macromolecules and receptors resulting in pharmacological activity and modulation of both disease and normal physiology. An important goal of the medicinal chemist working in drug discovery is to identify molecular structures exhibiting the desired pharmacological activity that can be further optimized to drug candidates. Ideally, the pharmacological activity of a molecule is only target-related (inhibition or activation of pharmacological systems related to the intended target), thus allowing optimization efforts by medicinal chemists to focus on increasing potency. This best-case scenario is not often realized and off-target pharmacological activity (also known as ancillary pharmacology) must also be addressed in optimization.[19,24,28] Off-target effects may result when there are unintended parallel structure–activity relationships for the primary target and some other unintended pharmacological target; or, as the result of loss of selectivity within a family of closely related macromolecules of which the target is a member (kinases and g-protein-coupled receptors are relevant examples). Even though adequate selectivity can usually be achieved with continued optimization, some off-target effects can be avoided only after changing to a different structural template.

These classifications of adverse effects are summarized in Table 11.1 and will be referred to again as they relate to the decision-making process for selection and advancement of drug candidates.

11.4.2 Target validation

Understanding the toxicological consequences of inhibiting a particular target or pathway can begin during drug discovery even before drug molecules are available for testing.[18,29] In fact, the first step in predicting the potential toxicity profile of a therapeutic agent is to understand the consequences of inhibition of its target. The distribution of the target in normal tissues and cells provides a useful, and perhaps underutilized, early readout for predicting the potential biological activity of new molecules. In fact, this should be considered essential information if the means are available to conduct these evaluations. Evaluation of target expression is possible through the same molecular technologies (immunohistochemistry, in situ hybridization, random polymerase chain reaction (rPCR), ribonucleic acid (RNA) and protein separation techniques) that are used in the initial characterization and cloning of the target. Arrays consisting of up to 40 tissues per species are typically evaluated from normal rodents, dogs, and humans as an adjunct to evaluation of tissue expression in tumor specimens. Unfortunately, many, if not most, targets of relevance for oncology are ubiquitous. Although the expression of the target in a tissue does not guarantee tissue-specific toxicity, this information becomes useful later, as an adjunct to the interpretation of *in vivo* toxicology results and the identification of potential target-based toxicity and potential species differences in toxicity response.

Mice in which the gene for a specific target has been deleted (i.e., knockout (KO) mice) have been utilized to help gain insight into the therapeutic viability of the target.[30] More recently, knockout mice have been utilized to address questions concerning toxicity and the potential adverse consequences of target inhibition. Even though knockout mice can be used to explore the role of a specific target or pathway in mechanisms of toxicity, the practice of equating a phenotype of a genetically ablated animal with a potential adverse drug effect carries with it many important caveats.[31,32] Moreover, many oncology targets involve pathways that are essential for normal embryo–fetal development, which significantly limits the utility of this approach. The use of provisional KO models as well as small interfering RNA (siRNA) technology may offer ways to avoid this limitation.

The literature provides a simple, but useful, adjunct for gaining early insight into the toxicological potential of a molecule. In many cases, modern pharmaceutical research suffers from the paucity of published information on the biological function of novel targets. Often, such information is gained only through the basic research that is initiated and supported by early efforts to discover drugs. And, in fact, the medicinal chemistry programs are a rich source of the probes necessary to study target function. Nonetheless, experienced toxicologists and pathologists conduct literature searches to ensure their awareness of anything known about a particular target.

Finally, validation of the target pathway by discovery biologists is an excellent opportunity to consider the viability of potential biomarkers of intended pharmacodynamic activity. Biomarkers can be applied in toxicology studies to refine the dosimetry of adverse effects and to help guide clinical dosing. The application of biomarkers as an adjunct to toxicology testing is also discussed later in this chapter.

11.4.3 Lead optimization

Although the terminology for the stages of candidate progression may vary across discovery organizations, the lead optimization stage is virtually universal. Lead optimization is the stage at which chemistry and biology screening becomes focused on a subset of the relevant chemical space with the ultimate goal of selecting clinical candidates. Nonclinical technologies are critical here to minimize the probability of candidate failure in early development.[33,34]

Early lead optimization – in vitro considerations

Initially, in early lead optimization, medicinal chemists are searching for the required level of potency and drug-like properties within one or more structural series. This is an appropriate juncture for the application of toxicology/pathology technologies to identify structures or structural moieties that may present chemical-based toxicity. However, it must be kept in mind that traditional cytotoxicity screening alone will not be enlightening with intrinsically cytotoxic molecules and that the kinds of *in vitro* assays that are typically used by toxicologists to screen large numbers of compounds for cytoxicity[17,35] are not likely to be useful with oncology therapeutics in their standard application. Instead, the discovery scientists will typically establish the cytotoxic consequences of target inhibition over a range of concentrations *in vitro*. A counterscreen will then be run, usually measuring inhibition of mitochondrial function, to define the concentration-response for nonspecific cytotoxicity. The separation of concentration–response curves for cell death and loss of mitochondrial function is evidence of pharmacological, or target-mediated, cytotoxicity.

The toxicologist can still use of *in silico* technology[36] to assess the chemical-based toxicity potential of various structural series and many molecular methodologies can still be applied, including covalent binding assays, mitochondrial assays and oxidative stress assays.[29,37]

There are some assays that are recommended for screening in early lead optimization because they are informative of potential problems that might manifest later in development as complications for patient tolerability. Besides, early awareness of these signals may help lead to improved molecules through further optimization. Some of these assays follow.

Ames assay. Bacterial reversion assays, like the Ames assay, offer reasonable cost and a higher throughput means of assessing the mutagenic potential of a compound and its metabolites. Clearly, some oncologic therapeutics target DNA as the basis for their efficacy (e.g., nitrogen mustards and nucleoside analogs), but with other contemporary targets, it would be prudent to avoid this structure-based liability whenever possible.

hERG assay. Interactions with rapid delayed rectifier potassium channel (e.g., that encoded by the human ether-a-go-go-related gene (hERG)) is ideally part of the early safety screening of candidate molecules because of the association of this activity with potentially deleterious cardiovascular (CV) outcomes.[38] Adverse cardiovascular effects are commonly seen with oncology therapeutic agents and can be structure based (e.g., adriamycin) as well as pharmacology based (e.g., Herceptin).[39] Since hERG interactions are often structurally based, appropriate high-throughput screening is useful to minimize the potential for adverse cardiovascular effects that may complicate development.

Receptor and enzyme screen. The potential for off-target activity is almost universally addressed in medicinal chemistry programs through a variety of broad receptor and enzyme screens that are available through commercial vendors.[29] These screens inform as to other pharmacological systems with which the molecule may interact thereby causing an adverse effect. Such screens augment the safety assessment in laboratory animals by providing corroborating data on human targets that mitigates potential interspecies differences in pharmacological action. Moreover, the screening data is useful in further guiding drug optimization and selection of molecules with improved human side-effect profiles, provided that the ancillary and desired target effects do not share a common structure–activity relationship. Common commercial screens can include >70 human receptors and enzymes and disclose whether a molecule is active on multiple pharmacological axes. The nature of this screen also facilitates evaluation of multiple compounds as a means of differentiation and determination of parallel structure–activity relationships.

Multiple kinase screens. These screens can provide an opportunity for differentiation and optimization of kinase inhibitors. Ancillary pharmacological activity is frequently seen with molecules that target kinases (e.g., tyrosine and serine/threonine kinases). This is a result of the common medicinal chemistry strategy of synthesizing adenosine triphosphate (ATP) analogs that competitively inhibit the binding of the nucleotide with the enzyme, and, subsequently, inhibit cellular signaling pathways.[40] Unfortunately, the analogy of ATP-binding sites among these kinases often leads to nonselective, even promiscuous, inhibition of multiple enzymes.[41] Accordingly, kinase inhibitors should be screened against multikinase panels (that are also available commercially) to gauge their selectivity for a target kinase.[40,42,43] However, there is debate concerning the utility of these results given the belief of some that increased selectivity may actually diminish efficacy against tumors. For example, Sutent (sunitinib malate) is a nonselective receptor tyrosine kinase (RTK) inhibitor whose efficacy is attributed to its broader kinase inhibition.[44] Because kinases are essential components of cellular signaling, it is not difficult to envision that the inhibition of kinase activity would have some consequence for normal tissue function. In reality, there is increasing evidence that discrete toxicities are associated with inhibition of specific kinases.[45–52] Therefore, it is equally plausible that the toxicity and side-effect profile of Sutent are, at least, partly explained by its nonselective kinase inhibition profile.[53] The relationship of kinase selectivity and optimal efficacy and safety remains poorly understood, and this no doubt continues to influence the interpretation of kinase screening results across the industry. It does seem certain that eventually sufficient information will be available to make kinase profiling a valuable tool for gaining insights into toxicity.

Although outside the scope of this chapter, the absorption, distribution, metabolism, and excretion (ADME) and pharmacokinetic (PK) properties of potential candidates should be screened at this stage to ensure that candidate molecule(s) will have favorable drug-like properties.[54,55] Because oncology agents are commonly administered intravenously, the need to characterize oral absorption characteristics should be determined by the intended clinical use or the commercial target. An increasing trend toward preference of oral routes presents significant additional challenges for candidate selection of agents. Achievement of favorable drug-like properties can be much more difficult for molecules with limited solubility in deriving satisfactory bioavailability values, for example.

In addition, the toxicologic hazard of cytotoxic molecules to liver and intestinal track may be significantly greater with oral routes of administration compared to parenteral routes.

Drug transporter screening is also encouraged at this point to gain insights into potential tumor resistance that could limit success of the molecule in the clinic. Enough metabolism studies should also be done to allow some prediction of potential drug–drug interactions, and some metabolite identification studies are necessary to characterize major metabolites and their potential pharmacological activity. Understanding the activity of a major metabolite is relevant for the PK/PD evaluations and also for the structure–activity analysis performed by the medicinal chemist. However, because of the significant toxicity produced by the parent molecule, the toxicity of metabolites is of lesser concern with oncology therapeutics.

Early lead optimization – in vivo considerations

Short-term *in vivo* studies are the mainstay for defining the toxicity profile of a molecule. These studies are often referred to as sentinel chemical toxicity tests and their impact during early lead optimization can be significant in guiding the direction of the medicinal chemistry program.[17] Beginning to build a database of *in vivo* toxicology results during the lead optimization stage pays dividends later in candidate selection because experience with a number of molecules will help clarify the patterns of effects that reflect the activity of the target class. Although there may not be sufficient compounds of interest available for *in vivo* toxicity testing early in lead optimization, it is prudent to consider conducting a preliminary toxicology study early with a sentinel molecule that, though not optimal for drug candidacy, may provide insights on adverse effects that are associated with either target modulation or the structural series. Testing other molecules of the class or series that are published in the literature can also be useful.

The design of a sentinel toxicity study is relatively straightforward and includes 3 to 5 days of dosing, small groups (three or four animals per dose), and three different doses. Endpoints to be evaluated include in-life observations (clinical signs, body weight, etc.), clinical pathology, gross pathology and microscopic evaluations, and evaluation of systemic exposure. Rats are typically the preferred species because of the massive historical database that exists for toxicology testing in this species. While it is common with non-oncology agents to assess lethality in preliminary studies to set the upper limit for doses in subsequent toxicity testing, this is not a useful practice with oncology agents, which tend to be potent molecules with high intrinsic and cumulative toxicity. Rather, the doses for a sentinel chemical study can be based on the tolerated doses from efficacy testing in the murine tumor models.

Although the limited value of mice for predicting human adverse responses is generally recognized in the toxicology/pathology community, and the National Cancer Institute (NCI) ceased using mice in toxicity testing in the early 1980s, the practice of assessing toxicity in the athymic (nude) mouse traditionally used in tumor models is still practiced in some organizations.[56] Much of the concern for the use of this mouse model derives from the fact that the animals are not intact: Nude mice have limited intestinal flora and are reared in barrier facilities because their T cell-mediated immunity is greatly impaired, as is their ability to mount a cytokine response.[57] This limits the relevance of this model for predicting toxicologic responses in humans, especially cancer patients who have marked systemic inflammation secondary to tumor necrosis and therapeutic intervention. The practice of using murine cancer models for toxicology assessment must then be considered a questionable practice for several reasons; its persistence in some organizations is more likely related to the fact that toxicity testing in mice requires smaller amounts of compound and, therefore, fewer chemistry resources to support these studies.

Though emphasis has been placed on structure-based effects thus far, shorter-term toxicology evaluations are also useful for early identification of pharmacology-based effects (i.e., target-related and ancillary effects). While target-related toxicity can definitely be dose limiting, it cannot necessarily be eliminated through structural modification, therefore, recognition of target-based toxicity is critical for understanding and predicting safety in the clinic. Strategically, stereochemical isomerism in the pharmacophore provides an excellent opportunity to differentiate target-related effects from chemical-based toxicity by assessing the difference in the toxicity profiles of the active and inactive enantiomers.

Late lead optimization

During the late lead optimization stage, the focus of toxicity testing shifts from screening and differentiation of a larger number of molecules to characterization of a single candidate or a small number of candidates. *In vivo* toxicology studies should be active by this stage. Successful profiling of potential candidates begins with the identification of the dose-limiting toxicity, including cause-of-death determinations. Elucidation of any noninvasive laboratory endpoints or premonitory changes that can be used to monitor the onset of toxicity will be invaluable in the design of subsequent GLP toxicity studies as well as to the clinical investigator. Finally, the interrelationship of toxicity, pharmacodynamic activity, and dose can be refined by the application of a biomarker of pharmacodynamic activity. This enables an understanding of how toxicity may develop in relation to the level and duration of target inhibition in the blood compartment as well as in tissues of interest.

11.4.4 Definitions of benchmark doses in oncology testing

The standard benchmarks typically used in toxicology studies including the no-observed-effect level (NOEL), no-observed-adverse-effect level (NOAEL), and lowest-observed-adverse-effect level (LOAEL) are usually not applicable with cytotoxic oncology molecules.[58,59] Rather, benchmarking in rat and dog studies with oncology therapeutics includes the dose that results in 10 percent mortality over the duration of the study (STD_{10}) in rats, and the highest nonseverely toxic dose (HNSTD), which is defined as a dose that does not produce death or moribundity during a study in rats or dogs. The application of these benchmarks to dose setting for clinical studies is defined later in this chapter. It should be mentioned that the common benchmark dose, the MTD, is often misused in oncology research in the manner in which this dose is defined. Some investigators refer to the dose that does not result in lethality within the duration of an efficacy study with a tumor model as an MTD. In clinical trials, the MTD is defined as the highest dose that does not result in grade three toxicities. Traditionally, the toxicology/pathology community defines MTD as the highest dose that does not result in alterations that would shorten the life span of the animal. In the development of drugs for treatment of late-stage cancer patients, there is no safety benefit to establishing this particular benchmark dose, nor does the MTD in an efficacy study carry significance for safety assessment. Therefore, in toxicology usage, it is preferable to use the HNSTD rather than MTD to ensure clarity in communication.

11.4.5 Building a candidate database

Results from limited toxicity studies of a relatively small number of analogs (1–3) with varying potency will support later candidate selection. The purposes are (a) to characterize dose-limiting toxicities, (b) to build a database that will enhance decision making, and (c) to build weight of evidence based on experience with multiple compounds that will enhance prediction of clinically relevant effects. Both purposes are facilitated by expanding the toxicity testing to include a nonrodent species. The choice of nonrodent species for safety assessments is traditionally based on similarity of metabolite profiles of the dog or nonhuman primate with the human profile based on any of several *in vitro* biotransformation systems. The rat is studied in tandem with the nonrodent species that provides the best coverage of human metabolite formation and exhibits pharmacological responsiveness. In oncology programs, a policy-based approach can be taken whereby the dog is used *de facto* as the nonrodent species. The reasons for this largely reflect the desire to minimize use of nonhuman primates and also because it is arguably unethical to use a nonhuman primate simply to confirm the severe toxicity of most oncology agents. The dog, on the other hand, is responsive to cytotoxic agents and is adequate to gauge most target-based toxicity.[56] Of interest though is the position held by some that a nonrodent species may not even be needed for preclinical safety evaluation of oncology therapeutic agents; this is based entirely on an analysis of a relatively small group of oncology agents in which it was showed that the rat reasonably predicts for human toxicity of anticancer drugs.[60] Although this is currently not a widely held practice within the pharmaceutical industry, nor is it recognized by the regulatory communities, it does illustrate the desire to streamline the process for moving new oncology medicines into patients.

As previously discussed, single high-dose lethality studies tend to not be illuminating with cytotoxic agents; therefore, concentrating efforts on understanding tolerability with repeated dosing is ultimately a more productive path for an oncology product. A useful starting point for late lead optimization toxicity testing is the rat toxicology study, which can involve either repeat-dosing for 7 days or a single therapeutic cycle as defined in a relevant efficacy model. The doses should bracket the optimally efficacious dose in the cancer model with allometric correction. Group sizes may again be modest (four or five per sex per dose suffices), and both genders should be included to account for the potential dimorphisms in the PK profile that can occur in rats, particularly with CYP3A4 substrates.[61] Once the STD_{10} and the HNSTD are defined in the rat, the dog study can be initiated using a starting dose allometrically scaled to the rat HNSTD. A single animal can be repeatedly dosed through 7 days, or for one cycle, with subsequent dosing of an additional dog or two to confirm tolerability. When the initial dose is not tolerated, a subsequent dose should be halved and given to a single animal more than 7 days, or one cycle, followed by confirmation with one or two additional dogs. Conversely, if no significant toxicity is observed with the initial dose, the subsequent dose can be doubled in a single dog more than 7 days, or a single cycle, with appropriate confirmation. Dosing two dogs at each of multiple dose levels can also be considered to more quickly define the HNSTD. Gender differences in metabolism are less common in dogs, so it is less critical to evaluate both sexes at this stage.[61]

Bridging from an efficacy model to a toxicology species is greatly facilitated through pharmacodynamic (PD) measurements. Extrapolation of toxicity conclusions across species and into humans is enhanced by understanding the PD–toxicity relationship through incorporation of appropriate biomarkers and PD endpoints into the toxicology studies. Many, if not most, pharmaceutical companies today expend significant resources to identify pharmacodynamic biomarkers as part of the translational medicine approach to clinical testing; ideally, the same biomarkers intended for clinical use should be applied in toxicology testing.[62,63] Such measurements can be extremely useful for confirming pharmacological activity of a drug candidate in tissues identified as target organs in toxicology studies to correlate toxicologic changes with pharmacodynamic changes.

Another reason to consider PD measurements as a platform for extrapolation is the fact that it is not uncommon for the PD half-life to be discordant with (greater than) the PK half-life. This means that a PD effect, including an adverse one, can be sustained even after the molecule has been cleared. It is important to recognize this possibility for drug candidates with dose-limiting toxicity related to target inhibition because the plasma/blood exposure may not fully predict the onset or reversal of toxicity. Finally, with highly potent oncology agents, it is common to see very narrow dose ranges in toxicology studies (i.e., on the order of tenths of a milligram between low and high doses). Although variability is expected with the PD readout, it does offer an alternative to characterizing the dose-dependence of toxicity in cases where interanimal variability may obscure or make it difficult to discern discrete exposures at each dose. Additionally the goal of the toxicology assessment is to characterize the full range of pharmacodynamic response, but not to explore pharmacologically inactive doses.

The guidance on the website of the International Conference on Harmonisation (ICH; *S9 Guidance for Nonclinical Evaluation for Anticancer Pharmaceuticals*) allows IND filings with quite limited ADME and PK studies with oncology therapeutics. This guidance enables many of the traditional PK/ADME characterizations to be conducted in parallel with clinical testing. Nonetheless, these evaluations are still highly important for refinement of the nonclinical safety assessment, and appropriate evaluations should be completed prior to IND filing. This includes sufficient testing to enable allometric scaling to project human PK properties, as well as to enable an initial assessment of the potential for drug–drug interactions.

11.5 CHALLENGES IN CANDIDATE DEVELOPMENT

11.5.1 Criteria for progression of a candidate

From a toxicology/pathology perspective, the decision to progress a drug candidate into development must include consideration of whether the toxicity profile can be tolerated and managed clinically, and what starting dose can be safely administered. The concept of a safety margin is irrelevant for most oncology agents because of the singularity of the dose relationships for efficacy and toxicity of cytotoxic agents, as shown in Table 11.2. Since potentially significant adverse effects are expected with clinical doses of a cytotoxic agent, the key question is whether patients can tolerate an optimally efficacious dose. A toxicity profile that is clinically manageable requires (a) a reasonable understanding of the nature of the dose-limiting toxicity, especially as related to the target; (b) a means of monitoring the onset of toxicity; and (c) the ability to reasonably gauge toxicity via PD readouts during dose escalation (Figure 11.2).

The nonclinical safety strategy should be designed to identify candidates with these attributes. Beyond that, case-by-case decision making is required for candidates that exhibit chemical-based or ancillary pharmacology-based (off-target) dose-limiting toxicity and the nature of the effect from the perspective of patient safety must be heavily weighted (Figure 11.3). A candidate exhibiting dose-limiting toxicity of a structural nature should be considered for rejection even for oncology use and regardless of the target tissue in favor of continued optimization.

Off-target effects, on the other hand, require case-by-case decision making. Clearly, a potentially useful drug should not be discarded based on a low-severity pharmacological side effect that can be monitored or is manageable (e.g., orthostatic hypotension). Conversely, a pharmacological effect posing a risk of serious critical organ dysfunction or injury to organ systems or tissues other than the gastrointestinal (GI) tract or hematopoietic tissues (i.e., CV system, CNS, or eye) would also form the basis for rejection, even in the oncology area, in favor of continued optimization.

Table 11-2. Examples of marketed oncology drugs showing absence of safety margins

		Highest tolerated dose (mg/m²)			Primary toxicities		
Drug	Human efficacious dose (mg/m²)	Rat	Nonrodent	Human	Rat	Nonrodent	Human
Bortezomid	1.3	0.6	0.6	1.8	GI tract Hematopoietic Lymphoid	GI tract Nerve hematopoietic	GI asthenia Neuropathy
Oxalplatin	85 (every 2 weeks)	114–138	35–45	85	Hematopoietic Kidney Liver	Heart GI tract Kidney Nerve Hematopoietic	Neuropathy GI tract Kidney Ototoxicity Hematopoietic
Doxataxel	75 (every 3 weeks)	1.2	7.5	75	Lymphopoietic Hematopoietic	Lymphoid Hematopoietic GI tract Skin	Neuropathy Hematopoietic
Irinotecan	124 (4 weeks on)	>120	32	124	Hemaotopoietic Lymphopoietic	Hemaotopoietic Lymphopoietic Cholinergic effects	Hematopoietic

Source: Summary Basis of Approval Documents and Product Labels. www.fda.gov/Drugs

- Are the toxicities consistent with the mechanism of target inhibition?
- Are the PK/PD/Toxicity inter-relationships defined?
- Can the toxicity be managed in the clinic?
- Can the toxicities be monitored?
- Are the toxicities reversible?
- Are any species differences understood?

Figure 11-2: Key nonclinical safety questions that need to be answered before moving a candidate into development.

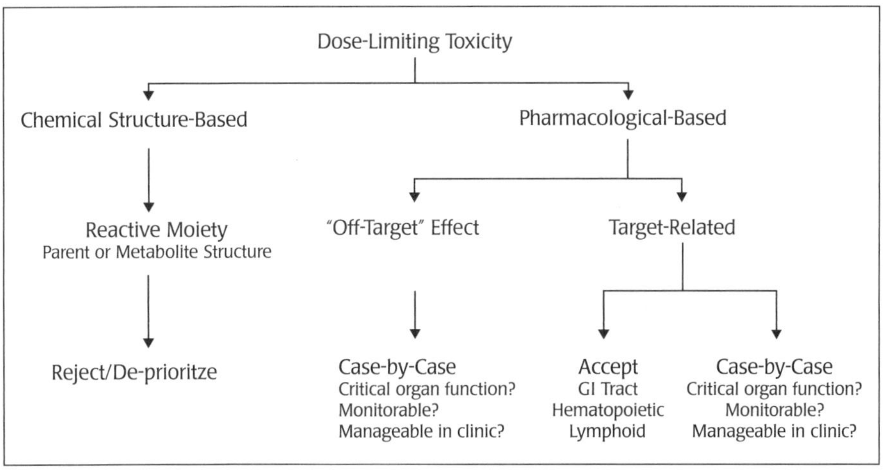

Figure 11-3: Decision tree for candidate advancement based on the toxicity profile.

11.5.2 IND-enabling (GLP-compliant) toxicology studies

The appropriate guidance for the conduct of toxicity testing to enable clinical trials with oncology therapeutics is the ICH S9 guidance document, Nonclinical Evaluation for Anticancer Pharmaceuticals. Good Laboratory Practice (GLP)-compliant toxicology studies of 28 days (total duration of in-life phase, not necessarily number of days of dosing) in rats and dogs are generally adequate to file an IND (Figure 11.4). Any additional testing indicated by specific liabilities of the molecule is determined on a case-by-case basis. The dosing cycles and route of administration must mimic or exceed the regimens planned in clinical testing, as discussed below.

Dose setting. The late discovery-stage toxicology studies need to provide an adequate basis for initiation of the GLP-compliant studies, including the selection of doses. A specific challenge in dose setting with molecules affecting cell turnover is their sharp dose-response curve. With molecules that target the cell cycle, the

IND Enabling

Activities:

- Ames assay (GLP)
- 28-day repeat-dose study (GLP) (rat and dog)

Deliverables:

- Toxicity benchmarks (HNSTD, STD10)
- Establish clinical safe starting dose
- Identify target organs & reversibility of toxicity
- Premonitory changes for toxicity
- Define the toxicity vs. TK vs. PD (target pharmaocology) relationship
- Understand any species differences
- Biomarkers

Phase 2

Activities:

- Subchronic 3-month repeat-dose toxicology study (rat and dog)

Deliverables:

- Define the progression of toxicity
- Clinical proof of concept

Phase 3

Activities:

- Segment II study
- Environmental impact assessment
- Workers safety studies

Deliverables:

- Registration package

Figure 11-4: Toxicology/pathology activities to support development of an oncology therapeutic agent for advanced disease requisite to a successful IND and **NDA** filing.

separation between doses (typically three dose levels) may be very limited, and there is often as little as a three- to fourfold difference between the doses causing minimal and maximal PD responses. The use of shorter-duration toxicology studies to set doses for longer-duration GLP-compliant studies will always involve some degree of uncertainty, even under the best of circumstances; however, it does not become advisable to conduct longer range-finding studies during the discovery stage to mitigate this risk if it costs wasted resources and animal use as well as delaying progression to the clinic. Rather, a better approach is to ensure that a mechanism is in place to execute timely decreases in dose (even on the weekends) in response to unanticipated deaths in the study. Finally, the typical precautions taken when transitioning from a test article prepared at the bench in medicinal chemistry laboratories to an active ingredient prepared by a process chemistry group should be observed. Potential changes in the exposure-dose profile that may result from changes in salt forms, solid state properties, and formulation should be explored with appropriate bridging PK studies.

Dosing regimens. The intended clinical route of administration should be used in the pivotal toxicology studies. However, there can often be uncertainty around the dosing schedule that will ultimately produce clinical efficacy at the time of transition into development. Therefore, the dosing schedule(s) used in the pivotal toxicology studies must take this uncertainty into consideration. One way to do this is to ensure that the toxicology studies include groups dosed with the regimen that produced maximal antitumor activity in the efficacy model. Inclusion of this dosing schedule in the pivotal toxicology studies will always be considered good practice. Daily dosing from a toxicology perspective represents the "worst case" scenario for most cytotoxic agents, and the disadvantage of defaulting to this dosing regimen is that only lower doses tend to be tolerated with this more rigorous schedule. This can result in a lower safe starting dose, which can slow the progress of clinical trials by increasing the number of dose

Table 11-3. Correspondence of dosing regimens in nonclinical toxicology studies and clinical trials

Clinical schedule	Nonclinical schedule
Once every 3 weeks	Single-dose study
Daily for 3 days every 3 weeks	Daily for 3 days
Daily for 5 days every 3 weeks	Daily for 5 days
Daily for 5–7 days on alternating weeks	Daily for 5–7 days on alternating weeks (2 dose cycles)
Once every 2 weeks	2 doses given 14 days apart
Once weekly for 3 weeks with 1 week off	Once weekly for 3 weeks
2 or 3 times per week	2 or 3 times per week
Continuous daily	Daily for 28 days
Weekly	Once weekly for 4 weeks

Source: S9 Nonclinical Evaluation For Anticancer Pharmaceuticals www.ich.org.

levels that are needed to reach evidence of an MTD. Moreover, this can provide another level of challenge to the team charged with manufacturing clinical supplies by increasing the number of strengths needed for clinical testing. In practice, cytotoxic agents are often dosed on cycles that include drug holidays to facilitate patient tolerability. In order to obviate this concern, an additional toxicology group(s) may be added to the pivotal studies to include the desired clinical regimen for safe starting dose determination. The inclusion of two different dosing regimens adds an order of complexity to the toxicology study, but may pay dividends in facilitating the clinical trials while conserving resources over the life of the project. The dosing regimens required in toxicology testing for various clinical plans as posted in ICH S9 are presented in Table 11.3.

Reversibility. The reversibility of any adverse effects should be addressed in the pivotal studies to demonstrate that patient recovery may be possible upon cessation of dosing should lack of patient tolerability necessitate this action.

Safe starting dose calculations. Initial doses for clinical testing are determined by establishing the STD_{10} in rats and the HNSTD in dogs. In the absence of knowledge of plasma exposures, it is generally recognized that the best method for normalizing exposures across species is represented by dosing based on body surface area as opposed to body weight (Table 11.4). The algorithm for calculating a safe starting dose based on toxicology benchmarks is shown in Figure 11.5. The STD_{10} on a mg/kg basis is allometrically scaled to a dose on a mg/body surface area (mg/m^2) basis. The safe starting dose then equals one-tenth of the rat STD_{10} in mg/m^2, if the dog can tolerate this dose. When this is not the case, the safe starting dose defaults to one-sixth of the dog HNSTD in mg/m^2. (ICH S9 Guidance Document) Achieving a precise STD_{10} obviously can be challenging. If significantly more than 10 percent of the rats die on test before scheduled necropsy, then the middle dose would be used for safe starting dose calculations, if there was not significant mortality in this lower dose.

Table 11-4. Interconversion of doses normalized to body weight and body surface area

Species	Conversion factor (S)	Body weight (mg/kg) (10 mg/kg used as example)	Body surface area (mg/m^2)
Human	37	10	370
Dog	20	10	200
Cynomolgus monkey	12	10	120
Rat	6	10	60
Mouse	3	10	30

Notes: Doses given as mg/m^2 divided by the conversion factor (S) = Dose given in mg/kg.
Doses given as mg/kg multiplied by the converstion factor (S) = Dose in mg/m^2.

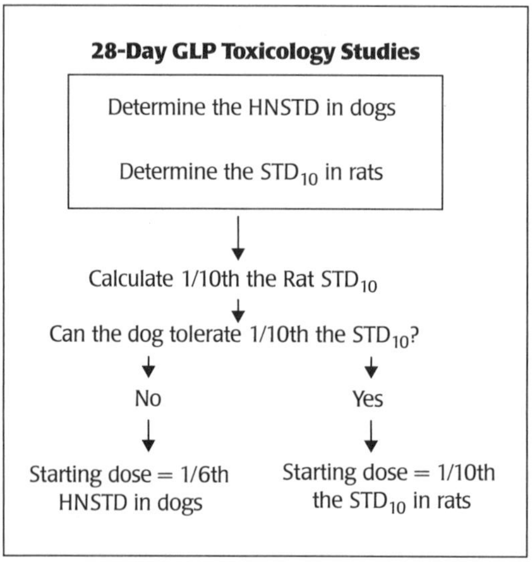

Figure 11-5: Algorithm for establishing the safe starting clinical dose for an oncology therapeutic agent.

The safe starting dose can be further decreased, if desired, with novel targets or other circumstances of potential toxicological concern. For example, if the dose-response curve is extremely sharp and if the PD effects are predicted to be more potent in humans, then a lower safe starting dose might be justified. However, the decision on the safe starting dose needs to include the consideration that many patients volunteer because of the belief that the drug candidate may provide benefit. Doses that are presumed to exert no PD effects certainly cannot be portrayed as potentially helpful.

11.5.3 Safety pharmacology

Safety pharmacology-related endpoints are typically evaluated directly in repeat-dose toxicology studies in rodents and nonrodents. These endpoints include (a) GI function – assessment of body weight gain/loss, stool consistency; (b) CNS function – behavioral effects such as stereotypy; (c) pulmonary function – cage-side observations including respiratory rate; (d) cardiovascular – oral mucosa color and capillary refill time, surface electrocardiograms, QTc assessment; and (e) renal function – urine and serum chemistry parameters, dehydration. This approach is consistent with ICH Guidance S9, which states that an "assessment of vital organ function should be available before the initiation of clinical studies; such parameters could be included in general toxicology studies. Standalone safety pharmacology studies need not be conducted to support studies in patients with late stage cancer or advanced disease."

In other cases, the necessity for safety pharmacology evaluation is based on known or predicted effects for the target class. For example, a comprehensive cardiovascular safety pharmacology evaluation on hemodynamics, mechanical, and electrical function might be considered necessary with small molecule inhibitors of tyrosine kinase because marketed products in this class (e.g., Sutent, Nexavar) exhibit adverse cardiovascular effects in animals and patients. The guidance on the ICH website (S7A *Safety Pharmacology Studies for Human Pharmaceuticals* and S7B *The Nonclinical Evaluation of the Potential for Delayed Ventricular Repolarization by Human Pharmaceuticals*) is applicable when there is specific cause for concern. The S7A guidance document addresses adverse drug effects on normal physiological function (including CNS, CV, respiratory, GI, and renal).

Adverse cardiovascular activity, in many therapeutic areas, tends to eliminate a candidate from further consideration. In contrast, cardiotoxicity is relatively common with treatment involving oncology therapeutic agents and includes a broad spectrum of adverse effects on cardiac structure, contractility, electrical conduction, and hemodynamics.[64–66] It has been estimated that, over time, oncology therapy may manifest as an up to eight-fold increase in mortality related to cardiac dysfunction.[67] Compared with the higher morbidity and mortality associated with progressive neoplastic disease, this relative risk for cardiovascular toxicity is typically viewed as acceptable by oncologists. Although the risk–benefit equation for oncology therapy is more tolerant of adverse cardiovascular effects, candidates possessing more benign cardiovascular profiles may be favorably differentiated from competitor oncology therapeutic agents.

11.5.4 Investigational new drug application

An investigational new drug application must be filed in order to initiate clinical testing. A successful IND for an oncology therapeutic must describe the toxicity profile of the agent and the rationale for safe testing in humans. This is greatly facilitated by ensuring that the regulatory summaries address the key pieces of information shown in Figure 11.6. Failure to do so could result in a clinical hold until any regulatory toxicology issues are resolved.

Preparation of the IND application is an appropriate time to ensure that the project clinicians are aware of and understand the toxicity profile of the clinical candidate. Clinical understanding of the interpretations and conclusions of the

- STD_{10} – the severely toxic dose with 10% mortality (rodent)
- HNSTD – the highest nonseverely toxic dose (dog)
- Dose-limiting toxicity and cause of death determination
- Target tissues for toxicity
- Biomarkers for key adverse effects
- Reversibility of effects
- PD/TK/Toxicity relationships

Figure 11-6: Key information to be included in the nonclinical toxicology summary for an IND application to support the first in human clinical plan.

toxicologist/pathologist is critical for initiation of clinical testing. It goes without saying that a good partnership between nonclinical safety scientists and their clinical counterparts is essential.

Finally, prior to submission of the IND, it is worth taking steps to ensure that the strengths of the clinical formulation prepared by the pharmaceutics group will support the safe starting dose and the dose escalation plan for the clinic. This becomes very important should regulatory authorities disagree with the safe starting dose and ask for a dose reduction; therefore, any decisions regarding the strengths of clinical formulation to be manufactured should anticipate this possibility and provide an appropriate contingency.

11.5.5 Longer-term toxicity studies for cancer chemotherapeutics

The ICH S9 guidance document states that 13-week studies should be completed before initiating phase 3 clinical trials and that, in most cases, these studies are sufficient to support registration. Genetic toxicity testing must be conducted prior to registration. Formerly, Segment II (teratology) reproductive toxicology testing in both rat and rabbit were also required for registration. However, under current ICH S9 Guidance, Segment II evaluations are no longer required for genotoxic agents that affect the cell cycle.

It may be possible to delay the initiation of 13-week studies until proof-of-concept is achieved, during phase 2. Although this would reduce the initiation of futile toxicology studies in an area with an inherently high rate of failure, this is also not yet a standard practice. In the end, toxicology testing is not expected to be limiting for progression of clinical testing or registration of molecules that provide benefit for the late-stage cancer patient.

Another unique feature of clinical testing of oncology medicines is that it is unethical to stop treating a cancer patient volunteer should they wish to continue on the trial. The implication of this is that the duration of the initial

Table 11-5. Leading cancer types causing death of children by chronological age group

Age (years)	Cancer type (top 4 cancer types by age group)			
0–4	Brain and CNS	Leukemia	Endocrine	Soft tissue
5–9	Leukemia	Brain and nervous system	Endocrine	Hodgkin's lymphoma
10–14	Leukemia	Brain and nervous system	Bones/joints	Hodgkin's lymphoma
15–19	Brain and nervous system	Leukemia	Bones/joints	Soft tissue/ non- Hodgkin's lymphoma

Source: National Cancer Institute SEER Pediatric Monograph, "Cancer Incidence and Survival Among Children and Adolescents: United States SEER Program 1975–1995" (1999). www.cancer.gov

phase 1 patient exposure can be prolonged at the patient's discretion. Under this scenario, the risks defined by existing animal toxicity data and outlined in the informed consent document are potentially undefined. The implication is that the duration of exposure of patients can exceed the duration of exposure in animals, and potential new toxicities might be discovered in patients.

11.5.6 Other considerations

Progression from late-stage to front-line therapy

The typical testing paradigm used in non-oncology therapeutic areas has limitations when applied to the development of novel oncology therapeutics, and may actually confer substantial competitive disadvantage for the sponsor that chooses the more traditional approach. However, it must also be recognized that a traditional testing paradigm might be more appropriate when the ultimate therapeutic goal is front-line therapy. This will especially be the case for treatment of tumor types where patient longevity is significant (life expectancy >3–4years, e.g., prostate or mammary cancers), or for which viable therapeutic options are already available. Under these circumstances, the guidance document on the ICH website (M3 *Nonclinical Safety Studies for the Conduct of Human Clinical Trials and Marketing Authorization for Pharmaceuticals*) should be followed.

Pediatric testing and combination therapy considerations

Traditionally, the clinical testing of drugs in pediatric populations has been supported primarily by toxicology studies with adult animals coupled with safety data from clinical studies in adult populations. The rationale for toxicology studies in neonatal and juvenile animals is to assess drug-related effects on the postnatal development of organ systems that are not functionally mature (e.g., brain, kidney, lung, reproductive tissues, immune, hematopoietic, and skeletal systems). The major cancers found in pediatric and adolescent patients typically occur in developing tissues (see Table 11.5), which makes it likely that most oncology therapeutic agents will target developing tissues.[68]

Although the risk–benefit analysis typically supports clinical transition into pediatric patients, there may be considerations that require the attention of the nonclinical safety professional. Differences between adult and child tumors can complicate the extrapolation of efficacy from adult to pediatric patients.[69] This, in turn, may alter the MTD of the agent and the corresponding tolerability in children. Moreover, pediatric populations may require different clinical formulation that should be assessed for suitability for use in children.

Clinical trials often will include testing of the therapeutic candidate in combination with other marketed therapeutics or even with other molecules in clinical development. Pharmacology testing may explore combination therapy largely to differentiate simple additivity from true opportunities for synergistic efficacy. In these cases, the toxicologist/pathologist must be vigilant for a substantive shift in toxicity that may occur with altered pharmacodynamic activity.

11.6 CONCLUSIONS

Because of the magnitude and complexity of neoplastic disease, modified paradigms are used for advancing new treatments for cancer through nonclinical testing and into clinical trials. Because of the complexity of drug development in general, it is essential that the toxicologist/pathologist supporting oncology projects engage as early as possible to ensure selection of quality candidates and a reasonable understanding of the consequences of target inhibition.

Drugs used in the treatment of advanced-stage cancers, by their nature, typically produce significant toxicity at ordinary clinical doses. The role of the toxicologist/pathologist is to provide the oncologist with an assessment of whether the toxicity profile of a candidate drug is tolerable and can be managed in the clinic.

The era of targeted therapy hopefully will deliver a breakthrough in therapy for the late-stage cancer patient. Perhaps novel targets whose activities are limited to cancer cells will be identified. These agents may improve the toxicity profile of oncology therapeutics; however, until that occurs, it will be incumbent on toxicologists and pathologists to identify and manage the toxicology challenges associated with anticancer therapy.

ACKNOWLEDGMENTS

The authors thank Mr. Vilmos Csizmadia, Ms. Elaine Zhang, Ms. Alexis Khalil, and Dr. Craig D. Fisher for critical review and assistance in preparation of the manuscript.

The authors also wish to thank Sage Publications for granting copyright permission to use the following work for preparation of this book chapter: T. Maziasz, V. J. Kadambi, L. Silverman, E. Fedyk, and C. L. Alden, "Predictive Toxicology Approaches for Small Molecule Oncology Drugs," *Journal of Toxicologic Pathology,* 2010; 38(1): 148–164.

REFERENCES

1. Jemal A, Siegel R, Ward E, et al. Cancer statistics, 2009. *CA Cancer J Clin.* 2009;59(4):225–249.
2. Boyle P, Levin, B., ed. 2008. *World Cancer Report 2008.* Lyon Cedex: World Health Organization. www.who.int. Accessed February 2009.
3. Christel MD. From pipeline to market: Pipelines bulk up as industry shakes up R&D, a surge in clinical projects spurs hope. *R&D Directions.* 2009;15:12–89.
4. PhRMA. (2009). *Pharmaceutical Industry report: industry profile 2009.* www.phrma.org. Accessed February 2009.
5. DiMasi JA, Grabowski HG. Economics of new oncology drug development. *J Clin Oncol.* 2007;25(2):209–216.
6. Griffith J, Hardman LEL, Gilman AG. *Goodman & Gilman's The Pharmacological Basis of Therapeutics.* (Section IX, Table IX-1) 10th ed. McGraw-Hill Professional United States of America,;2001.
7. Gibbs JB. Mechanism-based target identification and drug discovery in cancer research. *Science.* 2000;287(5460):1969–1973.
8. Saijo N, Tamura T, Nishio K. Problems in the development of target-based drugs. *Cancer Chemother Pharmacol.* 2000;46(Suppl):S43–45.
9. Saijo N. What are the reasons for negative phase III trials of molecular-target-based drugs? *Cancer Sci.* 2004;95(10):772–776.
10. Haystead TA. The purinome, a complex mix of drug and toxicity targets. *Curr Top Med Chem.* 2006;6(11):1117–1127.
11. Knapp M, Bellamacina C, Murray JM, et al. Targeting cancer: The challenges and successes of structure-based drug design against the human purinome. *Curr Top Med Chem.* 2006;6(11):1129–1159.
12. Iglehart JD, Silver DP. Synthetic lethality – A new direction in cancer-drug development. *N Engl J Med.* 2009;361(2):189–191.
13. Rosa DD, Ismael G, Lago LD, et al. Molecular-targeted therapies: Lessons from years of clinical development. *Cancer Treat Rev.* 2008;34(1):61–80.
14. Marchetti S, Schellens JH. The impact of FDA and EMEA guidelines on drug development in relation to Phase 0 trials. *Br J Cancer.* 2007;97(5):577–581.
15. Kola I, Landis J. Can the pharmaceutical industry reduce attrition rates? *Nat Rev Drug Discov.* 2004;3(8):711–715.
16. Walker I, Newell H. Do molecularly targeted agents in oncology have reduced attrition rates? *Nat Rev Drug Discov.* 2009;8(1):15–16.
17. Sasseville VG, Lane JH, Kadambi VJ, et al. Testing paradigm for prediction of development-limiting barriers and human drug toxicity. *Chem Biol Interact.* 2004;150(1):9–25.
18. Kramer JA, Sagartz JE, Morris DL. The application of discovery toxicology and pathology towards the design of safer pharmaceutical lead candidates. *Nat Rev Drug Discov.* 2007;6(8):636–649.
19. Smith DA, Schmid EF. Drug withdrawals and the lessons within. *Curr Opin Drug Discov Devel.* 2006;9(1):38–46.
20. Liebler DC, Guengerich FP. Elucidating mechanisms of drug-induced toxicity. *Nat Rev Drug Discov.* 2005;4(5):410–420.
21. Hughes JD, Blagg J, Price DA, et al. Physiochemical drug properties associated with in vivo toxicological outcomes. *Bioorg Med Chem Lett.* 2008;18(17):4872–4875.
22. Shanholtz C. Acute life-threatening toxicity of cancer treatment. *Crit Care Clin.* 2001;17(3):483–502.
23. Supko JG, Hickman RL, Grever MR, et al. Preclinical pharmacologic evaluation of geldanamycin as an antitumor agent. *Cancer Chemother Pharmacol.* 1995;36(4):305–315.
24. Campillos M, Kuhn M, Gavin AC, et al. Drug target identification using side-effect similarity. *Science.* 2008;321(5886):263–266.

25. Lang W, Caldwell GW, Li J, et al. Biotransformation of geldanamycin and 17-allylamino-17-demethoxygeldanamycin by human liver microsomes: Reductive versus oxidative metabolism and implications. *Drug Metab Dispos.* 2007;35(1):21–29.
26. Nowakowski GS, McCollum AK, Ames MM, et al. A phase I trial of twice-weekly 17-allylamino-demethoxy-geldanamycin in patients with advanced cancer. *Clin Cancer Res.* 2006;12(20 Pt 1):6087–6093.
27. Guner OF. *Pharmacophore Perception, Development, and Use in Drug Design (Iul Biotechnology Series 2).* (See Preface). International University Line; La Jolla, CA, 2000.
28. Smith DA, Johnson DE, Park BK. Editorial overview: Safety of drugs can never be absolute. *Curr Opin Drug Discov Devel.* 2006;9(1):26–28.
29. Houck KA, Kavlock RJ. Understanding mechanisms of toxicity: Insights from drug discovery research. *Toxicol Appl Pharmacol.* 2008;227(2):163–178.
30. Zambrowicz BP, Sands AT. Knockouts model the 100 best-selling drugs – Will they model the next 100? *Nat Rev Drug Discov.* 2003;2(1):38–51.
31. Ryffel B. Impact of knockout mice in toxicology. *Crit Rev Toxicol.* Mar 1997;27(2):135–154.
32. Bolon B. Genetically engineered animals in drug discovery and development: a maturing resource for toxicologic research. *Basic Clin Pharmacol Toxicol.* 2004;95(4):154–161.
33. Lesko LJ, Rowland M, Peck CC, et al. Optimizing the science of drug development: Opportunities for better candidate selection and accelerated evaluation in humans. *Pharm Res.* 2000;17(11):1335–1344.
34. Caldwell GW, Ritchie DM, Masucci JA, et al. The new pre-preclinical paradigm: Compound optimization in early and late phase drug discovery. *Curr Top Med Chem.* 2001;1(5):353–366.
35. Atterwill CK, Wing MG. In vitro preclinical lead optimisation technologies (PLOTs) in pharmaceutical development. *Toxicol Lett.* 2002;127(1–3):143–151.
36. Merlot C. In silico methods for early toxicity assessment. *Curr Opin Drug Discov Devel.* 2008;11(1):80–85.
37. Wallace KB. Mitochondrial off targets of drug therapy. *Trends Pharmacol Sci.* 2008;29(7):361–366.
38. Aronov AM. Tuning out of hERG. *Curr Opin Drug Discov Devel.* 2008;11(1):128–140.
39. Ng R, Better N, Green MD. Anticancer agents and cardiotoxicity. *Semin Oncol.* 2006;33(1):2–14.
40. Davies SP, Reddy H, Caivano M, et al. Specificity and mechanism of action of some commonly used protein kinase inhibitors. *Biochem J.* 2000;351(Pt 1):95–105.
41. Fedorov O, Marsden B, Pogacic V, et al. A systematic interaction map of validated kinase inhibitors with Ser/Thr kinases. *Proc Natl Acad Sci USA.* 2007;104(51):20523–20528.
42. Goldstein DM, Gray NS, Zarrinkar PP. High-throughput kinase profiling as a platform for drug discovery. *Nat Rev Drug Discov.* 2008;7(5):391–397.
43. Karaman MW, Herrgard S, Treiber DK, et al. A quantitative analysis of kinase inhibitor selectivity. *Nat Biotechnol.* 2008;26(1):127–132.
44. Overington JP, Al-Lazikani B, Hopkins AL. How many drug targets are there? *Nat Rev Drug Discov.* 2006;5(12):993–996.
45. Castoldi RE, Pennella G, Saturno GS, et al. Assessing and managing toxicities induced by kinase inhibitors. *Curr Opin Drug Discov Devel.* 2007;10(1):53–57.
46. Marshall J. Clinical implications of the mechanism of epidermal growth factor receptor inhibitors. *Cancer.* 2006;107(6):1207–1218.
47. Lacouture ME. Mechanisms of cutaneous toxicities to EGFR inhibitors. *Nat Rev Cancer.* 2006;6(10):803–812.
48. Larkin JM, Eisen T. Kinase inhibitors in the treatment of renal cell carcinoma. *Crit Rev Oncol Hematol.* 2006;60(3):216–226.
49. Illanes O, Anderson S, Niesman M, et al. Retinal and peripheral nerve toxicity induced by the administration of a pan-cyclin dependent kinase (cdk) inhibitor in mice. *Toxicol Pathol.* 2006;34(3):243–248.

50. Kerkela R, Grazette L, Yacobi R, et al. Cardiotoxicity of the cancer therapeutic agent imatinib mesylate. *Nat Med.* 2006;12(8):908–916.
51. Clark JW, Eder JP, Ryan D, et al. Safety and pharmacokinetics of the dual action Raf kinase and vascular endothelial growth factor receptor inhibitor, BAY 43-9006, in patients with advanced, refractory solid tumors. *Clin Cancer Res.* 2005;11(15):5472–5480.
52. Ramiro-Ibanez F, Trajkovic D, Jessen B. Gastric and pancreatic lesions in rats treated with a pan-CDK inhibitor. *Toxicol Pathol.* 2005;33(7):784–791.
53. Patyna S, Arrigoni C, Terron A, et al. Nonclinical safety evaluation of sunitinib: A potent inhibitor of VEGF, PDGF, KIT, FLT3, and RET receptors. *Toxicol Pathol.* 2008;36(7):905–916.
54. Balani SK, Miwa GT, Gan LS, et al. Strategy of utilizing in vitro and in vivo ADME tools for lead optimization and drug candidate selection. *Curr Top Med Chem.* 2005;5(11):1033–1038.
55. Leeson PD, Springthorpe B. The influence of drug-like concepts on decision-making in medicinal chemistry. *Nat Rev Drug Discov.* 2007;6(11):881–890.
56. Tomaszewski JE. Multi-species toxicology approaches for oncology drugs: the US perspective. *Eur J Cancer.* 2004;40(6):907–913.
57. Jackson Lab (2009). The Jackson Lab Mice Database. jaxmice.jax.org/strain. Accessed February 2009
58. Dorato MA, Engelhardt JA. The no-observed-adverse-effect-level in drug safety evaluations: use, issues, and definition(s). *Regul Toxicol Pharmacol.* 2005;42(3):265–274.
59. Lewis RW, Billington R, Debryune E, et al. Recognition of adverse and nonadverse effects in toxicity studies. *Toxicol Pathol.* 2002;30(1):66–74.
60. Newell DR, Silvester J, McDowell C, et al. The Cancer Research UK experience of preclinical toxicology studies to support early clinical trials with novel cancer therapies. *Eur J Cancer.* 2004;40(6):899–906.
61. Paulson SK, Maziasz TJ . *Role of metabolism and pharmacokinetics in the development of celecoxib.* In: Krishna, R, ed. *Applications of Pharmacokinetics Principles in Drug Delivery* Kluwer Academic/Plenum, New York, NY: 2003.
62. Hsieh FY, Tengstrand E, Lee JW, et al. Drug safety evaluation through biomarker analysis – A toxicity study in the cynomolgus monkey using an antibody-cytotoxic conjugate against ovarian cancer. *Toxicol Appl Pharmacol.* 2007;224(1):12–18.
63. O'Connell D, Roblin D. Translational research in the pharmaceutical industry: From bench to bedside. *Drug Discov Today.* 2006;11(17–18):833–838.
64. Yamamoto DS, Viale PH. Cyclooxygenase-2: From arthritis treatment to new indications for the prevention and treatment of cancer. *Clin J Oncol Nurs.* 2003;7(1):21–29.
65. Loerzel VW, Dow KH. Cardiac toxicity related to cancer treatment. *Clin J Oncol Nurs.* 2003;7(5):557–562.
66. Force T, Krause DS, Van Etten RA. Molecular mechanisms of cardiotoxicity of tyrosine kinase inhibition. *Nat Rev Cancer.* 2007;7(5):332–344.
67. Simbre VC, Duffy SA, Dadlani GH, et al. Cardiotoxicity of cancer chemotherapy: implications for children. *Paediatr Drugs.* 2005;7(3):187–202.
68. Young JL, Jr., Ries LG, Silverberg E, et al. Cancer incidence, survival, and mortality for children younger than age 15 years. *Cancer.* 1986;58(Suppl 2):598–602.
69. U.S. Department of Health and Human Services, Food & Drug Administration, Center for Drug Evaluation and Research and Center for Biologics Evaluation and Research. *Guidance for industry: Pediatric Oncology Studies in Response to a Written Request.* Rockville, MD; 2000.

12 **Mechanism-based toxicity studies for drug development**

Monicah A. Otieno and Lois D. Lehman-McKeeman

12.1 INTRODUCTION

Drug attrition during discovery and development continues to be a major hurdle for drug approval. Even as the number of investigational new drug (IND) filings increased between 1986 and 2006, new drug applications (NDA) remained flat during the same time period due to attrition.[1] The major reason for drug attrition in the clinic is preclinical toxicity, accounting for 35 percent of terminated drugs, followed closely by clinical efficacy and clinical safety.[1–3] Attrition due to preclinical toxicity is even higher (~70 percent) when compounds that fail prior to candidate drug nomination are considered.[4] Toxicologists need to learn from the success of approaches employed in drug metabolism and pharmacokinetics (DMPK) where attrition due to unfavorable PK has been reduced from a high of 40 percent in 1991 to only 6 percent in 2001.[2] This success was achieved by applying a variety of *in vivo* and *in vitro* approaches including predictive *in silico* and *in vitro* assays prior to preclinical and clinical administration.[5,6]

The traditional toxicologist manages nominated candidate drugs through the rigors of clinical development; however, in the rising need to reduce drug attrition, there is a paradigm shift in training toxicologists to evaluate the safety of pharmacological targets or new chemical entities (NCEs) through all phases of drug discovery and development. However, toxicologists are faced with a tougher hurdle in reducing attrition than groups in drug metabolism and pharmacokinetics. The clinical success of predicting PK is based on well-defined endpoints – clearance, absorption, and metabolic stability – that can be evaluated to obtain good oral bioavailability. In contrast, toxicity can occur in multiple organs with complex mechanisms involving those directly related to the intended pharmacology or resulting from exaggerated pharmacology, off-target pharmacology or direct organ toxicity. An evaluation of 88 candidate drugs at Bristol-Myers Squibb found that both target and chemistry-related toxicities contributed significantly to compound failure and the major toxicities were cardiovascular, hepatotoxicity, and teratogenicity.[7] Toxicity testing for cardiac safety and hepatic toxicity are discussed in detail in Chapters 3 and 4, respectively. Because of the high attrition attributed to teratogenicity, a proactive approach that combines literature assessment and *in vitro* screening assays has been implemented at Bristol-Myers Squibb to evaluate NCEs for their teratogenic potential early in the drug discovery process.[8] The high concordance of malformations detected with *in vitro* teratogenicity assays compared to *in vivo* findings[8] provides confidence in the predictive value of these assays.

The purpose of this chapter is to discuss approaches that can be taken to differentiate mechanisms of toxicities due to the pharmacological target (target-related effects) or chemotype (chemistry-related effects). This distinction is fundamentally important for assessing the potential risk for toxicity in humans, and such insight can also help to direct efforts in compound synthesis and identification of off-target liabilities. The examples outlined provide examples of approaches that can be applied either prospectively to influence decisions in discovery on the safety of a target or chemical series or retrospectively to investigate mechanisms of toxicity for clinical candidates.

12.2 MECHANISTIC APPROACHES TO EVALUATE TOXICITY DUE TO THE PHARMACOLOGICAL TARGET

Toxicities due to primary pharmacology, referred to as a target-related toxicity in this chapter, can be undesirable, depending on the phenotype and the intended patient population. The risk associated with this type of toxicity is lack of a therapeutic index between the efficacious and toxic dose in both preclinical and clinical studies. Knowing the mechanisms for a target-related toxicity can guide the development of a clinical safety biomarker or influence a decision to abandon the target altogether. Toxicologists working in drug discovery can identify potential hazards as soon as pharmacological targets are identified. Initial investigations are literature-based with a focus on the target tissue distribution, similarities to other targets, cross-species similarities, and knockout or transgenic phenotypes. Potential for toxicity from such evaluations can be tested by *in vitro* or *in vivo* methods. Small interfering RNA (siRNA) knockdown of a target gene and use of inactive enantiomers are other approaches that can be used to investigate target-related toxicities.

12.2.1 Use of tissue distribution to evaluate target-related toxicity

An approach taken to investigate target-related toxicity for a novel or existing target is to profile its tissue distribution; if a target is highly expressed in organs other than those intended for therapeutic modulation, then an *in vivo* study with a tool molecule can ascertain whether there are potential target-related liabilities in the organs with highest expression. An example of this approach was taken to evaluate potential liabilities in testes of acetyl-coenzyme A carboxylase (ACC) inhibitors.

ACC is the rate-limiting enzyme in fatty acid synthesis and fatty acid oxidation, and its inhibition is attractive for treatment of metabolic diseases.[9,10] Indeed, ACC2 knockout mice are resistant to diet-induced obesity and type 2

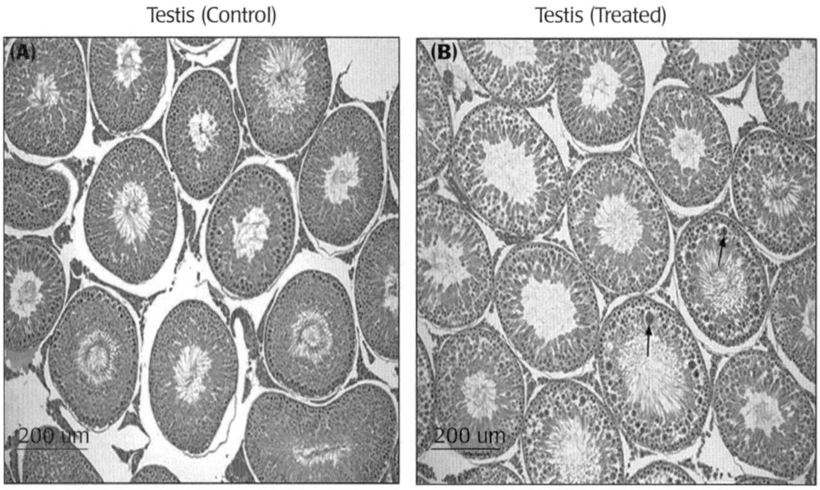

Figure 12-1: Testicular toxicity in rats given a small molecule non-specific ACC inhibitor for 14 days. (A) Testis from control (B) Testis from treatment group. Note necrotic and degenerative round spermatids, including synctia (arrows), and reduced cellularity of seminiferous epithelium in several tubes.

diabetes,[11] and small molecule inhibitors of ACC ameliorate signs of metabolic syndrome in rats.[9,12] ACC exists as two isozymes: ACC1 is present in the lipogenic tissues adipose, liver, testis, and mammary glands, whereas ACC2 is present in the oxidative tissues liver, skeletal muscle, and heart.[9,10,13,14] Testicular germ cells undergoing meiosis have increased ACC activity and fatty acid synthesis,[15,16] and depletion of acetyl-coenzyme A, a substrate required for ACC activity, causes testicular toxicity in Zucker obese rats.[17] Di(2-ethylhexyl) phthalate, an established testicular toxicant,[18] significantly decreases ACC1 expression in the testes,[19] suggesting a possible, although unproven causal relationship. Based on this information, it was deemed prudent to evaluate the effect of small molecule ACC inhibitors on testicular toxicity. As such, both obese and lean rats given an efficacious dose of a non-isotype-specific ACC inhibitor developed testicular toxicity after 2 weeks of dosing (Figure 12.1) (personal communication). Necrotic and degenerative round spermatids with reduced cellularity of seminiferous epithelium of the testis were noted. Thus, published information on tissue distribution and target organ toxicity directed an assessment for potential liabilities and guided decisions on how to proceed with the target.

12.2.2 Use of knockout animals to confirm target-related toxicity

The phenotypes observed in genetically manipulated animals can be extremely valuable in identifying potential issues associated with a pharmacologic target. Depending on the severity of the phenotype and the anticipated risk–benefit associated with the therapeutic indication, characterization of the model phenotype or studies with tool molecules can confirm the hazard and possible human risk.

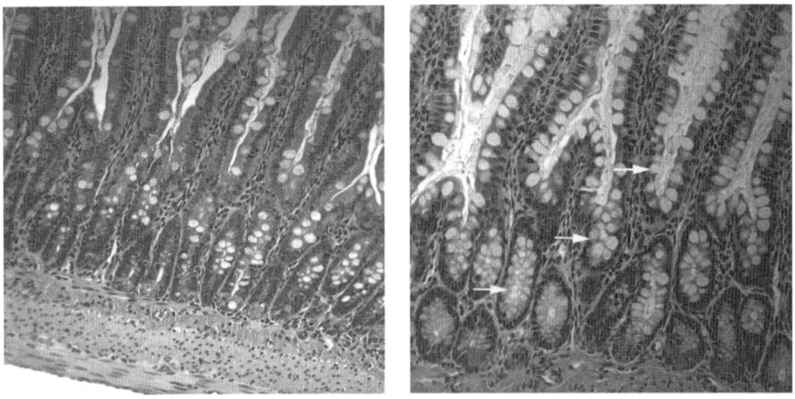

Figure 12-2: γ-Secretase inhibitors that modulate Notch processing cause intestinal goblet cell metaplasia. (A) Duodenum from vehicle control and (B) goblet cell metaplasia (arrows) in duodenum after 3 days of 30 μmol/kg benzodiazepine. Adapted by permission from Oxford University Press: *Toxicol. Sci.*, 82, 341–358, copyright (2004).

An example where a putative target-related toxicity can be supported with the knockout phenotype is illustrated with γ-secretase inhibitors. The therapeutic target for γ-secretase inhibitors is amyloid precursor protein in brain; however, this prevents processing of another γ-secretase substrate Notch, whose cleavage induces transcription of genes that are important in cellular differentiation of the immune and gastrointestinal systems. (For reviews see References 20, 21.) Dosing of rodents for 5 to 15 days with γ-secretase inhibitors has been associated with gastrointestinal toxicity (Figure 12.2), specifically goblet cell metaplasia, increased enteroendocrine cells, and reduced absorptive cells.[22–24] Deletion of Notch is embryonic lethal;[25] however, animals lacking Hes-1, a downstream effector gene of the Notch signaling pathway, show abnormalities in intestinal cell differentiation.[26] This provides an example where information from knockout animals can be used to confirm a target-related effect. Discovering molecules that selectively inhibit amyloid precursor protein without affecting Notch has been challenging; however, a safety biomarker for the undesirable side effect would be useful in clinical development of γ-secretase inhibitors. Increases in the gene products for Rath-1 and adipsin, regulated by Hes-1, have been detected in feces of rats treated with γ-secretase inhibitors[22,23] that presented with intestinal toxicity, which identifies the proteins as potential biomarkers for the gut lesions.

Genetically manipulated models can also help to determine whether toxicities observed during preclinical safety evaluation are directly related to the pharmacologic target. For example, corticotropin releasing factor (CRF) receptor antagonists cause marked hepatic changes including hypertrophy and hyperplasia and alteration of thyroid hormone homeostasis in rats.[27] However similar hepatic effects are also observed in CRF receptor null mice given CRF antagonists, thereby confirming that the effects are not related to the intended target pharmacology, but rather are due to off-target effects.

12.2.3 Use of siRNA approaches to evaluate target-related toxicity

RNA interference is another tool that can be used to investigate toxicities due to primary pharmacology by essentially silencing the target in a specific organ. The basic tenet for siRNA technology is formation of a double-stranded RNA against a target sequence triggering its mRNA degradation thus silencing the gene.[28,29] Inhibition of gene expression with siRNA can be used to study the contribution of a target to a toxicological outcome or study the mechanisms of toxicity mediated by a pharmacologic target. siRNA has been used to elucidate the mechanisms for PPARα activation-induced liver hypertrophy and tumorigenecity in rodents.[30] In these studies two siRNAs for PPARα were administered to mice and by a subtractive analysis with genes from a PPARα inducer, a set of sixteen transcripts in the liver was identified as essential for liver hypertrophy. With the premise that the mechanism for liver hypertrophy should be the same regardless of the pharmacological target or chemical insult, the gene signature obtained from the siRNA studies against PPARα was interrogated against a training set of genes from 211 rats treated with 30 non-PPARα compounds that induce liver hypertrophy to build a predictive model. The training set was further validated with an independent set of genes from 107 rats treated with 17 non-PPARα compounds and a nine-gene model was produced that was highly predictive of liver hypertrophy. These genes revealed that the potential mechanisms for liver hypertrophy mediated by PPARα included pathways that increased cell proliferation, altered lipid metabolism, or affected the Golgi apparatus. This provides an example where using siRNAs was useful in revealing the potential mechanisms for a toxicological outcome.

siRNAs can also be used to confirm the role of a target on a toxicological outcome; this was used to confirm that A1 adenosine receptors are responsible for hypoxia-induced cardiac malfunction in chick embryos.[31] Hypoxia-induced abnormalities including cardia bifida and looping defects, believed to be caused by binding of adenosine to its receptors, were significantly reduced in the presence of SiRNA targeting the A1 adenosine receptors.

12.2.4 Use of inactive enantiomers to evaluate pharmacologic target-related toxicity

A powerful approach to evaluating target-related toxicity is the use of biological inactive enantiomers. Since the inactive structure is a mirror image of the active isomer, the potential for chemistry-related toxicity is essentially equivalent, but target-related toxicities will differ. An inactive enantiomer has been used to elucidate the mechanism for thrombocytopenia by ABT-737, a potent small molecule inhibitor of the antiapoptotic proteins BCl-X_L, BCl-2, and BCl-w.[32] These proteins are overexpressed in several tumors[33] and contribute to cancer cell progression by preventing cell death.

Intravenous infusion of 15 mg/kg ABT-737 in dogs resulted in a concentration-dependent reduction in circulating platelets with a decrease of 100 percent at

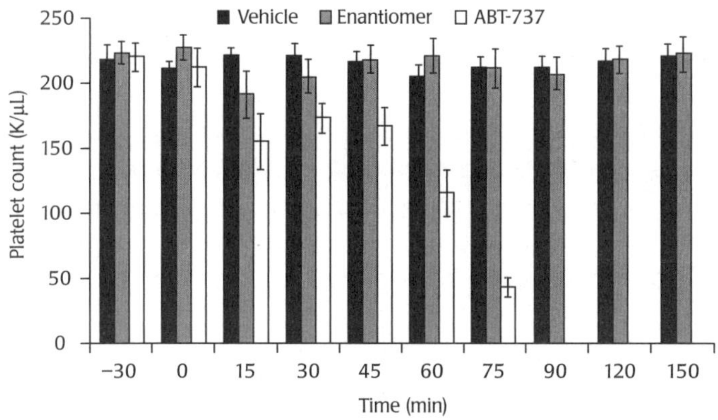

Compound	[30-min], μM	[60-min], μM	[90-min], μM	[150-min], μM
ABT-737	7.6±0.8	38.4±6.3	159.7±14.2	29.4±4.2
Enantiomer	9.4±0.8	36.3±3.0	130.0±12.6	20.7±2.6

Figure 12-3: Thrombocytopenia in dogs given ABT-263, but not its inactive enantiomer, at equivalent exposures. Adapted by permission from Macmillan Publishers Ltd: *Cell Death and Differentiation*, 14, 943–51, copyright (2007).

maximal plasma concentrations of ABT-737.[34] In contrast, thrombocytopenia was not detected with the inactive enantiomer of ABT-737 (Figure 12.3) at equivalent exposures implicating inhibition of BCl proteins as the cause for decreased platelet counts. Although ABT-737 is potent against BCl-2, BCl-X_L, and BCl-w, inhibition of BCl-X_L is the likely cause for reduction of platelets. BCl-X_L is highly expressed in platelets compared to the other antiapoptotic proteins[34]; moreover, BCl-X_L knockout or heterozygote mice develop thromboytopenia from increased platelet clearance by apoptosis.

12.3 MECHANISTIC APPROACHES TO EVALUATE CHEMISTRY-RELATED TOXICITIES

12.3.1 Background

As new chemical entities are identified and optimized during the drug discovery process, it is important that chemical moieties with potential liabilities be avoided during the chemical design process, and if not, then tested to confirm lack for toxicity. The best example is risk assessment for NCEs containing aromatic amine, amide, or sulfonamide groups that can potentially cause genotoxicity;[35] these functional groups continue to be designed into molecules during the lead identification stages, however, they are often removed before candidate drug selection or tested early for genotoxicity with established *in silico* and *in vitro* approaches.[36]

Compounds with reactive functional groups are avoided, whenever possible, during the drug design process. Formation of reactive metabolites has been linked to idiosyncratic toxicities in the clinic;[37,38] therefore, judicious drug design coupled with covalent binding assays are used to guide decisions regarding potential safety risks from reactive metabolites[39–41] in order to avoid costly late-stage drug withdrawal.

Hemolytic anemia has been described for drugs containing sulfonamides, quinones, anilines, and carboxylic acids resulting from oxidative damage or covalent binding to red blood cells.[42–49] NCEs with these functional groups should be carefully evaluated for reactive metabolite formation early in drug discovery.

Cationic and ampiphilic molecules with high LogP are known to cause phospholipidosis,[50,51] a disorder of lysosomal phospholipid accumulation commonly found in the lung and liver. *In vitro* assays[52,53] can be used to test compounds fulfilling these physicochemical properties, and if positive, the compounds can either be redesigned early in the drug discovery process or undergo a risk assessment provided for compound progression.

12.3.2 Compound metabolism as the determinant of toxicity

Biotransformation and generation of reactive intermediate metabolites are associated with a variety of toxicities and idiosyncratic reactions.[37] Toxicologists should always consider how drug disposition and fate contribute to toxicity, as target organ dosimetry, biotransformation, and detoxification reactions can be important determinants of toxicity. In all cases, understanding how biotransformation may differ across species, with emphasis on human metabolism, is an important component in determining whether preclinical effects are predictive of and relevant for human safety evaluation.

As an example, the nonnucleoside reverse transcriptase inhibitor, efavirenz (Sustiva), produces marked acute renal tubular epithelial cell necrosis in rats, with no similar renal changes noted in monkeys. Based on these findings, the metabolic fate of efavirenz was evaluated in rats, monkeys, and humans using both *in vitro* (liver and kidney S9, microsomal, and cytosolic fractions) and *in vivo* (analysis of urinary metabolites) approaches. Evidence for species differences in metabolism was derived from a comprehensive evaluation of the urinary metabolites of the drug, which revealed a rat-specific glutathione (GSH) conjugate in urine.[54,55] Although GSH conjugation is typically a detoxification reaction, there are numerous examples of compounds for which the intrarenal processing of the conjugate leads to a nephrotoxic intermediate.[56] Rats treated with acivicin to inhibit λ-glutamyltranspeptidase (GGT) and thereby block the renal hydrolysis of the efavirenz-GSH conjugate decreased the severity and incidence of proximal tubule necrosis,[57] establishing that metabolism of the GSH conjugate, which was formed only in rats, was directly involved in toxicity. In this example, efavirenz-induced renal toxicity was determined to be specific to rats and not predictive for humans and supported the further development of the compound.

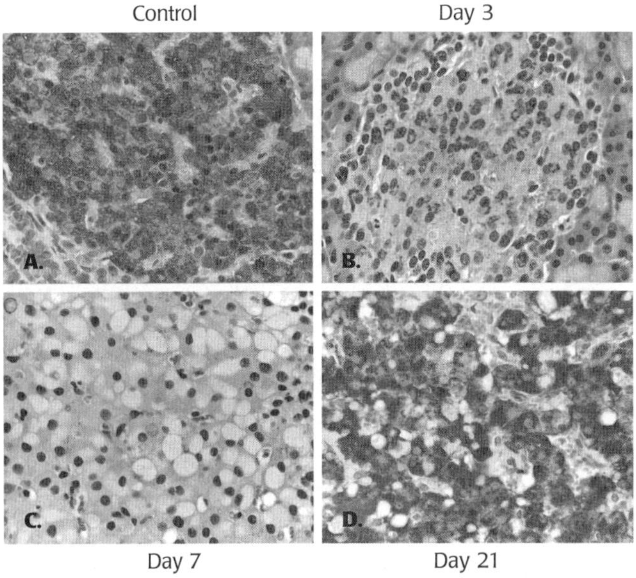

Figure 12-4: Treatment with AR-M10090 resulted in decreased insulin staining and vacuolation of the pancreas (B, C) compared to controls (A). Insulin staining was restored after removal of drug (C). Adapted by permission from Oxford University Press: *Toxicol. Sci.*, 105, 221–29, copyright (2008).

12.3.3 *In vivo* and/or *in vitro* studies investigating chemistry-related toxicities.

In cases where a chemistry-related toxicity is encountered during drug discovery, mechanistic studies can sometimes launch an *in vitro* assay that predicts *in vivo* findings; such assays are useful tools for evaluating structure-activity relationships (SAR) against the toxicity. For example, rats given the delta-opioid agonist AR-M100390 developed vacuoles in the β-cells of the pancreas associated with complete depletion of insulin (Figure 12.4).[58] Intracellular insulin levels were also depleted in pancreatic cells treated with AR-M100390 and other structurally related molecules that cause the same lesion *in vivo* (Figure 12.5). Mechanistic studies revealed that the compounds inhibited insulin2, but not insulin1 mRNA, which was important for human risk assessment because rats have two insulin genes, whereas higher species, including man, have a single insulin gene that is similar to the rodent insulin2 gene.[59] The *in vitro* assay was subsequently used to establish SAR against insulin depletion and to select molecules without this liability.

Another example where the chemotype was responsible for the toxicological outcome was teratogenicity in rats given SB-236057, a 5HT1B receptor inverse agonist.[60] SB-236057 is structurally similar to cyclopamine, a known teratogen,[61] which suggested that teratogenicity by SB-236057 was likely chemistry related. *In vitro* studies with rat embryos found that SB-236057 was teratogenic and produced axial and posterior somite formations similar to the skeletal defects

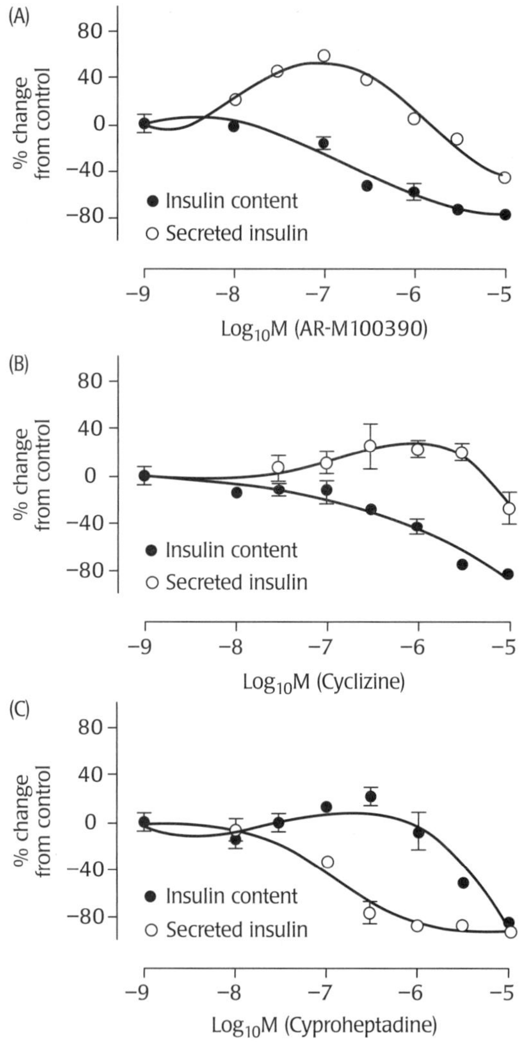

Figure 12-5: Intracellular (closed circles) and secreted insulin (open circles) in RINm5F cells treated with (A) AR-M10090, (B) cyclizine, and (C) cyproheptadine. Adapted by permission from Oxford University Press: *Toxicol. Sci.*, 105, 221–29, copyright (2008).

observed *in vivo* (Figure 12.6).[62] *In vitro* mechanistic studies revealed that teratogenicity by SB-236057 was due to alteration of the Notch1 pathway. These examples highlight the value of *in vitro* assays that predict *in vivo* toxicity because they are facile in studying mechanisms of toxicity and understanding SARs against specific toxicities.

12.4 IMPACT OF MECHANISTIC STUDIES ON INTEGRATED RISK ASSESSMENT FOR A DEVELOPMENT MOLECULE

Mechanistic studies attempt to put preclinical findings into context for human risk assessment. The critical issue is whether the mechanism of toxicity is common across species and if it will occur in man. As described previously, in the case of efavirenz, toxicity noted in rats was not predictive of similar adverse

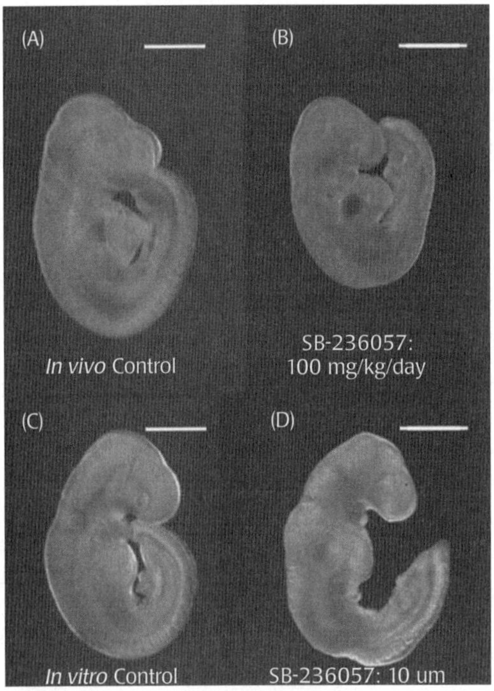

Figure 12-6: Comparison of malformations in embryos harvested from dams given 100 mg/kg/day of SB-236057 (B) or cultured for 48 h with 10uM SB-236057 (D). A,C: The respective control vehicle-treated embryos were normal. Embryos from *in vivo* or *in vitro* treatment groups exhibited abnormal patterned, missing somites, and/or shortened caudal extension. Adapted by permission from Wiley-Liss Inc.: Birth Defects Research (Part A), 70, 789–807, copyright (2004).

effects in humans, and this potent nonnucleoside reverse transcriptase inhibitor is widely used as part of highly active antiretroviral therapy for the treatment of human immunodeficiency virus.

Another example where an integrated risk assessment may inform on human risk is provided by neurokinin (NK) receptor antagonists, which cause testicular toxicity in dogs, but not rats.[63,64] The NK3 antagonist Talnetant produces testicular lesions preceded by decreases in testosterone in dogs from doses of 0.3 to 1 g/kg, but rats and mice tested up to 1 g/kg do not develop testicular toxicity.[64] Other chemically diverse NKR antagonists, such as Osanetant and SCH 206272, also cause the same lesion in dogs, and like Talnetant, SCH 206272 also does not produce testicular lesions in rats.[63,64] Testicular toxicity with such structurally diverse molecules suggests that the effect is related to NKR pharmacology. Receptor binding and functional assays find that the rat and human NK receptors differ in their response to antagonists by up to two orders of magnitude compared to the human receptors,[65–67] but there is no available data on dog receptors. Gerbil and guinea pigs NKR are functionally similar to human receptors,[68] raising the possibility that the species-specific testicular toxicity in the dog could be due to functional differences between the rat and dog receptor. The integrated risk assessment to man in this case could involve the following: comparing receptor response toward antagonists between the dog and human NK receptors, determining whether common mechanisms for toxicity are shared between dog and man by *in vitro* methods, and/or including testosterone as a biomarker in the clinical plan.

12.5 CONCLUSION

Mechanistic studies performed during drug discovery and development are critical for establishing the potential for adverse effects in humans. Mechanistic studies conducted early during the target identification phase can provide important information on potential liabilities that may influence whether a target represents a viable option for additional research. Mechanistic studies directed toward assessing chemistry-related toxicities can provide important information that may help to direct lead identification and optimization stage, and mechanistic studies carried out late in clinical development often help to answer regulatory questions regarding clinical safety. Ultimately, mechanistic studies provide critical information that allows for an informed human risk assessment, contributes to minimizing the likelihood of identifying untoward and unpredicted adverse effects in the clinic, and ultimately aids in successfully advancing new compounds through drug development.

ACKNOWLEDGMENTS

The authors acknowledge their colleagues Evan Janovitz, Frederic Moulin, and Karen Augustine-Rauch for their contributions and critical evaluation of the manuscript.

REFERENCES

1. Federsel HJ. Handing over the baton: Connecting medicinal chemistry with process R&D. *Drug News Perspect.* 2008;21(4):193–199.
2. Kola I, Landis J. Can the pharmaceutical industry reduce attrition rates? *Nat Rev Drug Discov.* 2004;3(8):711–715.
3. Kola I. The state of innovation in drug development. *Clin Pharmacol Ther.* 2008;83(2):227–230.
4. Kramer JA, Sagartz JE, Morris DL. The application of discovery toxicology and pathology towards the design of safer pharmaceutical lead candidates. *Nat Rev Drug Discov.* 2007;6(8):636–649.
5. Chaturvedi PR, Decker CJ, Odinecs A. Prediction of pharmacokinetic properties using experimental approaches during early drug discovery. *Curr Opin Chem Biol.* 2001;5(4):452–463.
6. Wishart DS. Improving early drug discovery through ADME modelling: An overview. *Drugs R D.* 2007;8(6):349–362.
7. Car BD. Enabling technologies in reducing drug attrition due to safety failures. *American Drug Discov.* 2006;1:53–56.
8. Augustine-Rauch KA. Predictive teratology: Teratogenic risk-hazard identification partnered in the discovery process. *Curr Drug Metab.* 2008;9(9):971–977.

9. Harwood HJ, Jr. Acetyl-CoA carboxylase inhibition for the treatment of metabolic syndrome. *Curr Opin Investig Drugs*. 2004;5(3):283–289.
10. Kim KH. Regulation of mammalian acetyl-coenzyme A carboxylase. *Annu Rev Nutr.* 1997;17:77–99.
11. Abu-Elheiga L, Oh W, Kordari P, Wakil SJ. Acetyl-CoA carboxylase 2 mutant mice are protected against obesity and diabetes induced by high-fat/high-carbohydrate diets. *Proc Natl Acad Sci USA*. 2003;100(18):10207–10212.
12. Harwood HJ, Jr., Petras SF, Shelly LD, et al. Isozyme-nonselective *N*-substituted bipiperidylcarboxamide acetyl-CoA carboxylase inhibitors reduce tissue malonyl-CoA concentrations, inhibit fatty acid synthesis, and increase fatty acid oxidation in cultured cells and in experimental animals. *J Biol Chem*. 2003;278(39):37099–37111.
13. Conde E, Suarez-Gauthier A, Garcia-Garcia E, et al. Specific pattern of LKB1 and phospho-acetyl-CoA carboxylase protein immunostaining in human normal tissues and lung carcinomas. *Hum Pathol*. 2007;38(9):1351–1360.
14. Widmer J, Fassihi KS, Schlichter SC, et al. Identification of a second human acetyl-CoA carboxylase gene. *Biochem J*. 1996;316 (Pt 3):915–922.
15. Bajpai M, Gupta G, Jain SK, et al. Lipid metabolising enzymes in isolated rat testicular germ cells and changes associated with meiosis. *Andrologia*. 1998;30(6):311–315.
16. Whorton AR, Coniglio JG. Fatty acid synthesis in testes of fat-deficient and fat-supplemented rats. *J Nutr.* 1977;107(1):79–86.
17. Saito M, Ueno M, Ogino S, et al. High dose of *Garcinia cambogia* is effective in suppressing fat accumulation in developing male Zucker obese rats, but highly toxic to the testis. *Food Chem Toxicol*. 2005;43(3):411–419.
18. Park JD, Habeebu SS, Klaassen CD. Testicular toxicity of di-(2-ethylhexyl)phthalate in young Sprague-Dawley rats. *Toxicology.* 2002;171(2–3):105–115.
19. Itsuki-Yoneda A, Kimoto M, Tsuji H, et al. Effect of a hypolipidemic drug, Di (2-ethylhexyl) phthalate, on mRNA-expression associated fatty acid and acetate metabolism in rat tissues. *Biosci Biotechnol Biochem*. 2007;71(2):414–420.
20. Imbimbo BP. Therapeutic potential of gamma-secretase inhibitors and modulators. *Curr Top Med Chem*. 2008;8(1):54–61.
21. Wolfe MS. Selective amyloid-beta lowering agents. *BMC Neurosci*. 2008;9(Suppl 2):S4.
22. Milano J, McKay J, Dagenais C, et al. Modulation of notch processing by gamma-secretase inhibitors causes intestinal goblet cell metaplasia and induction of genes known to specify gut secretory lineage differentiation. *Toxicol Sci*. 2004;82(1):341–358.
23. Searfoss GH, Jordan WH, Calligaro DO, et al. Adipsin, a biomarker of gastrointestinal toxicity mediated by a functional gamma-secretase inhibitor. *J Biol Chem*. 2003;278(46):46107–46116.
24. Wong GT, Manfra D, Poulet FM, et al. Chronic treatment with the gamma-secretase inhibitor LY-411,575 inhibits beta-amyloid peptide production and alters lymphopoiesis and intestinal cell differentiation. *J Biol Chem*. 2004;279(13):12876–12882.
25. Huppert SS, Le A, Schroeter EH, et al. Embryonic lethality in mice homozygous for a processing-deficient allele of Notch1. *Nature*. 2000;405(6789):966–970.
26. Suzuki K, Fukui H, Kayahara T, et al. Hes1-deficient mice show precocious differentiation of Paneth cells in the small intestine. *Biochem Biophys Res Commun*. 2005;328(1):348–352.
27. Wong H, Lehman-McKeeman LD, Grubb MF, et al. Increased hepatobiliary clearance of unconjugated thyroxine determines DMP 904-induced alterations in thyroid hormone homeostasis in rats. *Toxicol Sci*. 2005;84(2):232–242.
28. Elbashir SM, Harborth J, Lendeckel W, et al. Duplexes of 21-nucleotide RNAs mediate RNA interference in cultured mammalian cells. *Nature*. 2001;411(6836):494–498.
29. Elbashir SM, Lendeckel W, Tuschl T. RNA interference is mediated by 21- and 22-nucleotide RNAs. *Genes Dev*. 2001;15(2):188–200.

30. Dai X, De Souza AT, Dai H, et al. PPARalpha siRNA-treated expression profiles uncover the causal sufficiency network for compound-induced liver hypertrophy. *PLoS Comput Biol.* 2007;3(3):e30.
31. Ghatpande SK, Billington CJ, Jr., Rivkees SA, et al. Hypoxia induces cardiac malformations via A1 adenosine receptor activation in chicken embryos. *Birth Defects Res A Clin Mol Teratol.* 2008;82(3):121–130.
32. Chauhan D, Velankar M, Brahmandam M, et al. A novel Bcl-2/Bcl-X(L)/Bcl-w inhibitor ABT-737 as therapy in multiple myeloma. *Oncogene.* 2007;26(16):2374–2380.
33. Buolamwini JK. Novel anticancer drug discovery. *Curr Opin Chem Biol.* 1999;3(4):500–509.
34. Zhang H, Nimmer PM, Tahir SK, et al. Bcl-2 family proteins are essential for platelet survival. *Cell Death Differ.* 2007;14(5):943–951.
35. Nesnow S, Bergman H. An analysis of the Gene-Tox Carcinogen Data Base. *Mutat Res.* 1988;205(1–4):237–253.
36. Contrera JF, Matthews EJ, Kruhlak NL, Benz RD. In silico screening of chemicals for genetic toxicity using MDL-QSAR, nonparametric discriminant analysis, E-state, connectivity, and molecular property descriptors. *Toxicol Mech Methods.* 2008;18(2–3):207–216.
37. Walgren JL, Mitchell MD, Thompson DC. Role of metabolism in drug-induced idiosyncratic hepatotoxicity. *Crit Rev Toxicol.* 2005;35(4):325–361.
38. Kalgutkar AS, Gardner I, Obach RS, et al. A comprehensive listing of bioactivation pathways of organic functional groups. *Curr Drug Metab.* 2005;6(3):161–225.
39. Shu YZ, Johnson BM, Yang TJ. Role of biotransformation studies in minimizing metabolism-related liabilities in drug discovery. *Aaps J.* 2008;10(1):178–192.
40. Baillie TA, Cayen MN, Fouda H, et al. Drug metabolites in safety testing. *Toxicol Appl Pharmacol.* 2002;182(3):188–196.
41. Baillie TA. Metabolism and toxicity of drugs. Two decades of progress in industrial drug metabolism. *Chem Res Toxicol.* 2008;21(1):129–137.
42. Trepanier LA. Idiosyncratic toxicity associated with potentiated sulfonamides in the dog. *J Vet Pharmacol Ther.* 2004;27(3):129–138.
43. Adams JG, Heller P, Abramson RK, et al. Sulfonamide-induced hemolytic anemia and hemoglobin Hasharon. *Arch Intern Med.* 1977;137(10):1449–1451.
44. Itano HA, Hollister DW, Fogarty WM, Jr, et al. Effect of ring substitution on the hemolytic action of arylhydrazines. *Proc Soc Exp Biol Med.* 1974;147(3):656–658.
45. Stonier PD, Edwards JG. Nomifensine and haemolytic anemia. *Pharmacovigilance.* 2002:155–166.
46. Sanford-Driscoll M, Knodel LC. Induction of hemolytic anemia by nonsteroidal anti-inflammatory drugs. *Drug Intell Clin Pharm.* 1986;20(12):925–934.
47. Munday R, Smith BL, Munday CM. Structure-activity relationships in the haemolytic activity and nephrotoxicity of derivatives of 1,2- and 1,4-naphthoquinone. *J Appl Toxicol.* 2007;27(3):262–269.
48. Singh H, Purnell ET. Hemolytic potential of structurally related aniline halogenated hydroxylamines. *J Environ Pathol Toxicol Oncol.* 2005;24(1):67–76.
49. Arndt PA, Garratty G. The changing spectrum of drug-induced immune hemolytic anemia. *Semin Hematol.* 2005;42(3):137–144.
50. Nonoyama T, Fakuda R. Drug-induced phospholipidosis – Pathological aspects and prediction. *J. Toxicol. Pathol.* 2008;21:9–24.
51. Reasor MJ, Kacew S. Drug-induced phospholipidosis: Are there functional consequences? *Exp Biol Med (Maywood).* 2001;226(9):825–830.
52. Morelli JK, Buehrle M, Pognan F, et al. Validation of an in vitro screen for phospholipidosis using a high-content biology platform. *Cell Biol Toxicol.* 2006;22(1):15–27.
53. Nioi P, Perry BK, Wang EJ, et al. In vitro detection of drug-induced phospholipidosis using gene expression and fluorescent phospholipid based methodologies. *Toxicol Sci.* 2007;99(1):162–173.

54. Mutlib AE, Chen H, Nemeth G, et al. Liquid chromatography/mass spectrometry and high-field nuclear magnetic resonance characterization of novel mixed diconjugates of the non-nucleoside human immunodeficiency virus-1 reverse transcriptase inhibitor, efavirenz. *Drug Metab Dispos.* 1999;27(9):1045–1056.
55. Mutlib AE, Chen H, Nemeth GA, et al. Identification and characterization of efavirenz metabolites by liquid chromatography/mass spectrometry and high field NMR: Species differences in the metabolism of efavirenz. *Drug Metab Dispos.* 1999;27(11):1319–1333.
56. Dekant W. Chemical-induced nephrotoxicity mediated by glutathione S-conjugate formation. *Toxicol Lett.* 2001;124(1–3):21–36.
57. Mutlib AE, Gerson RJ, Meunier PC, et al. The species-dependent metabolism of efavirenz produces a nephrotoxic glutathione conjugate in rats. *Toxicol Appl Pharmacol.* 2000;169(1):102–113.
58. Otieno MA, Bavuso N, Milano J, et al. Mechanistic investigation of *N,N*-diethyl-4-(phenyl-piperidin-4-ylidenemethyl)-benzamide-induced insulin depletion in the rat and RINm5F cells. *Toxicol Sci.* 2008;105(1):221–229.
59. Melloul D, Marshak S, Cerasi E. Regulation of insulin gene transcription. *Diabetologia.* 2002;45(3):309–326.
60. Solomon HM, Posobiec LM, Augustine KA. SB-236057 with potent teratogenicity in rats, rabbits and mice. *Birth Defects Res. Part A: Clin. Mol. Teratol.* 2003;67:357.
61. Keeler RF, Binns W. Teratogenic compounds of *Veratrum californicum* (Durand). V. Comparison of cyclopian effects of steroidal alkaloids from the plant and structurally related compounds from other sources. *Teratology.* 1968;1(1):5–10.
62. Augustine-Rauch KA, Zhang QJ, Leonard JL, et al. Evidence for a molecular mechanism of teratogenicity of SB-236057, a 5-HT1B receptor inverse agonist that alters axial formation. *Birth Defects Res. Part A: Clin. Mol. Teratol.* 2004;70:789–807.
63. Losco PE, Leach MW, Sinha D, et al. Administration of an antagonist of neurokinin receptors 1, 2, and 3 results in reproductive tract changes in beagle dogs, but not rats. *Toxicol Pathol.* 2007;35(2):310–322.
64. Dennis M, Wier PJ, Giardina GA. Anti-androgens and methods for treating disease. *PCT Int. Appl.* 2000, WO00043008(A1):1–16.
65. Sarau HM, Griswold DE, Potts W, et al. Nonpeptide tachykinin receptor antagonists: I. Pharmacological and pharmacokinetic characterization of SB 223412, a novel, potent and selective neurokinin-3 receptor antagonist. *J Pharmacol Exp Ther.* 1997;281(3):1303–1311.
66. Petitet F, Beaujouan JC, Saffroy M, et al. NK-1 tachykinin receptor in rat and guinea pig brains: Pharmacological and autoradiographical evidence for a species difference. *Peptides.* 1993;14(3):551–559.
67. Emonds-Alt X, Bichon D, Ducoux JP, et al. SR 142801, the first potent non-peptide antagonist of the tachykinin NK3 receptor. *Life Sci.* 1995;56(1):PL27–32.
68. Beaujouan JC, Torrens Y, Saffroy M, et al. A 25 year adventure in the field of tachykinins. *Peptides.* 2004;25(3):339–357.

13 **Fish embryos as alternative models for drug safety evaluation**

Stefan Scholz, Anita Büttner, Nils Klüver, and Joaquin Guinea

13.1 INTRODUCTION

Approval of new medicinal products requires demonstration of their efficacy and safety. Therefore, development of new drugs is processed in distinct phases including basic research, lead discovery/development, preclinical testing, and final clinical trials. Drug safety is initially evaluated preclinically in laboratory animals (rodents and other mammals). Preclinical safety data are then submitted to appropriate authorities such as the U.S. Food and Drug Administration (FDA) or the European Medicines Agency (EMEA) for the approval of subsequent clinical trials in human subjects.[1] Clinical trials are performed in three phases in human patients with increasing number of volunteers starting with 20 to 80 healthy volunteers in phase I and ending with about 200 to 2,000 people in phase III to demonstrate that the drug offers significant clinical benefit. In these studies only part of the patients receive the new drug, the remainder are treated with a placebo or comparator.[2]

Due to the thorough preclinical and clinical trial phases development of new drugs has become a lengthy (10–15 years) and expensive process. From the early identification of lead compounds to preclinical and clinical trials expenditures of $0.5 to 2 billion are estimated (see References 3, 4, 5, and references therein). Although the actual cost estimates for new drugs may be inflated in some calculations and only valid for compounds with new molecular entities, all estimates demonstrate the enormous investments associated with the development of a new drug.[4,6,7] The costs are primarily caused by the preclinical and clinical testing phase and failure of the majority of candidate drugs to survive until the market application stage. On average, only 8 percent of compounds from the phase 1 clinical trial reach the market,[5] and toxicity is a leading cause of attrition at all stages of the drug development process.[8] In clinical phases I–III, toxicity caused one-third of the drug development projects to be closed. Despite the extensive testing for approval, 2.9 percent of the drugs are withdrawn from the market after approval.[1] More than 90 percent of these withdrawals were caused by hepatotoxicity and cardiovascular toxicity.[9]

The submission of new drugs for approval is negatively correlated with the increasing budget spent on the development of new medicines. Hence, concern has been raised that the increasing costs are limiting the development of new drugs.[5] The high costs may particularly interfere with the development of medicines against untested therapeutic areas and explain the preference for areas of known clinical values.[10]

The current status of drug development has not only been criticized for its costs but for the high demand of experimental animals as well. For instance, in 2005 about 12.1 million nonhuman vertebrates have been used for experimentation and other scientific purpose in the European community.[11] More than 50 percent of these animals have been used for research, production, and quality control of human and veterinary medicines or for toxicological and other safety evaluation. Thirty percent have been used due to requirements of European community (EC) legislation including the approval of new drugs. Thus, a large proportion of the animal experiments can be attributed to the safety evaluation for the development of new medicinal products. There is a strong societal demand for replacing and reducing these experiments by alternative methods.[12,13] Also current legislation supports the use of alternative methods such as *in vitro* or other nonanimal methods (e.g., the EU *Directive 86/609/EEC*). Since preclinical studies involving animal experimentations are responsible for more than one-third of the costs of drug development,[3,4] reduction of animal experiments would also contribute to the development of a more cost-effective drug approval process.

There is an urgent need to reduce costs and the number of animals associated with the development of new drugs. One of the primary goals is to prioritize for compounds entering the preclinical and clinical testing phases (i.e., shifting the potential attrition of drugs foreseen for market approval to a very early stage of development).[14] Various measures have been proposed for reducing the number of compounds entering the preclinical and clinical phase. (a) Limited pathophysiological and mechanistic understanding has been identified as one criterion for failure in clinical trials.[5] The inclusion of toxicogenomics in the early drug development would increase our understanding of drug toxicity and the corresponding risk factors, result in the development of biomarkers for chronic effects and, hence, improve the accuracy of the prediction of drug toxicity in the human population from experimental findings.[1,15] (b) Development of new compounds should consider adverse drug responses when searching for more potent compounds and include toxicity estimation in the early screening of candidate drugs.[15] (c) Small animal models such as lower vertebrates and/or their embryos or invertebrates may be implemented in an efficient preclinical screening system and reduce the number of compounds subjected to later time-consuming and expensive trials.[5,12,15]

In the present chapter we suggest the use of fish embryos as a powerful screening system that could be used to prioritize compounds for later testing using rodent or other mammalian models and clinical trials. We describe the peculiarities of the model, provide examples that show promising applications, and discuss potential limitations and future research perspectives.

13.2 THE FISH EMBRYO MODEL

An efficient screening system in preclinical development and safety evaluation of drugs would ideally be characterized by (a) the capability to represent ADME (absorption, distribution, metabolism, and excretion) properties of a complex organism, (b) the detection of specific toxic effects in different cell types and organs, (c) the demonstration of effects of chemicals on functionality (e.g., movement, photosensitivity, blood circulation), (d) the assessment of the vulnerability of highly sensitive, critical developmental stages (e.g., gastrulation, neurulation), (e) an extensive background in developmental genetics, (f) easy experimental handling and dosing, and (g) the possibility to analyze at a small scale with potential high throughput capacity. With respect to this features, cellular *in vitro* models are of limited capacity since they do not represent the complex interaction between tissues of an organism, and toxicity may greatly depend on the model (type of primary cell or cell line) and its capabilities (e.g., for metabolism).

In contrast, these features are provided by lower vertebrate embryos and invertebrates. Due to the striking homologies between vertebrates, the use of invertebrates is of limited relevance for the screening of drug safety and efficacy. For instance, Gunnarson et al.[16] compared the sequence similarities of selected human drug orthologues in various species (Table 13.1). With respect to the selected drug targets, mouse shows a similarity of 89–99 percent based on sequence homology. *Xenopus* and zebrafish exhibited a 16 to 93 percent and 47 to 90 percent similarity, respectively. For invertebrates homologies were significantly lower, and some of the drug targets could not even be identified.

Among the lower vertebrates, fish embryos of some species, such as zebrafish (*Danio rerio*) and medaka (*Oryzias latipes*), are of particular interest, since they produce a large number of transparent embryos that can be easily manipulated and observed in microtiter well plates (Table 13.2). Their genomes are sequenced and are accessible via the ensembl Web site (http://www.ensembl.org/index.html). Standard biomolecular tools such as transgenesis, mutations screening, systems biology techniques, and functional genomics are available for both species. The zebrafish model has been extensively reviewed.[17–20] The medaka, a model fish that has been traditionally used in Japan, has emerged as a second teleost model providing some complementary features.[21–23] Both species require similar husbandry conditions with respect to light cycle, temperature, and water quality.[23,24] Their evolutionary distance is about 115–200 Myr. However, their embryonic development shares the characteristics of egg-laying teleost and vertebrates in general (Figure 13.1). Early development is fast in zebrafish and medaka, with about 5 and 10 days of development, respectively, to free swimming feeding larvae.

In the zebrafish (Figure 13.1, upper panel), the newly fertilized egg shows cytoplasmatic movements generating a non-yolky blastodisc. After the first cleavage the cells divide at about 15-minute intervals. At around 24 hours, the heart is

Table 13-1. Examples of predicted orthologs with specific drug interactions in distantly related species supported in the literature[a]

Human target	Drug or class of drugs	*M. musculus*	*G. gallus*	*X. tropicalis*	*X. laevis*	*G. aculeatus*	*D. rerio*	*D. melanogaster*	*D. pulex*	*C. elegans*	*A. thaliana*	*C. reinhardtii*	*D. discoideum*	*S. cerevisiae*	*T. thermophila*	*E. coli*	*S. elongatus*
IMDH2: Inosine-5′-monophosphate dehydrogenase 2	Mycophenolate mofetil	99	95	93	93	89	90	66	74	52	46	52	60	61	29	37	18
ALDH2: Aldehydede hydrogenase	Disulfiram	94	85	80	79	78	77	69	74	66	59	57	50	49	47	39	–
HMDH: HMG-CoA reductase	Statins	93	86	74	93	75	77	44	41	25	30	–	29	32	10	–	–
SC6A4: 5HTtransporter	SSRIs	93	76	57	–	69	66	49	49	42	–	–	–	–	–	–	–
SCN5A: Sodium channel protein type 5 subunit alpha	Neuroactive drugs blocking voltage-gated sodium channels	94	76	56	16	61	62	41	40	–	–	19	–	–	14	–	–
ESR1: Estrogen receptor	Estrogens	89	77	69	69	46	46	–	–	–	–	–	–	–	–	–	–
AGTR1:Type-1 angiotensin II receptor	Certain antihypertensive agents	94	76	61	62	38	47	–	–	–	–	–	–	–	–	–	–

Source: Reprinted from *Environmental Science & Technology*, vol. 42, issue 15, Lina Gunnarsson et al., "Evolutionary Conservation of Human Drug Targets in Organisms used for Environmental Risk Assessments" Aug 1, 2008, with permission from Elsevier.

[a] Sequence similarities to the human drug target are given as percentages. Note that the ortholog prediction in *X. laevis* is based on comprehensive EST data and not on a fully sequenced genome. Abbreviations: SSRI, selective serotonin reuptake inhibitor; HMG-CoA, 3-hydroxy-3-methylglutaryl-coenzyme A reductase; –, ortholog absent.

Table 13-2. Zebrafish and medaka, two popular teleost models in developmental biology, genetics, drug research, and (eco)toxicity

The **zebrafish** (*Danio rerio*) is one of the most popular model organisms in drug development, developmental genetics and (eco)toxicology (see, for instance, reviews of [17–20,25,26,33]). The zebrafish is a small tropical teleost native to the rivers of India and South Asia.[27] Its rapid development, easy maintenance in the laboratory, and large number of offspring provides advantages for experimental studies. The extensive genetic characterization, corresponding functional data, disease models, and availability of a large number of transgenic lines with reporter genes are in particular useful for studying drug interactions (photo: Andre Künzelmann, UFZ).	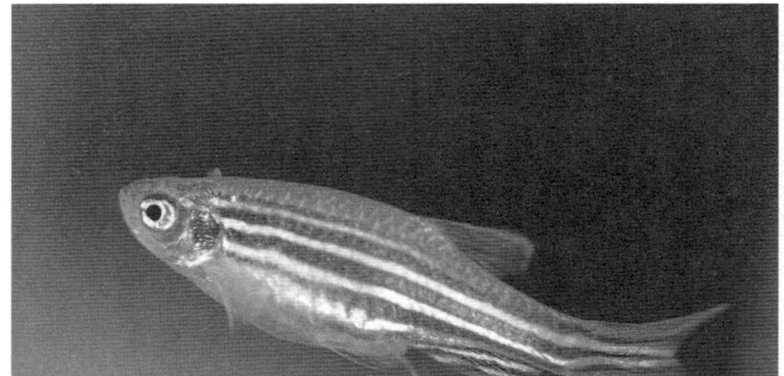
The **medaka** (*Oryzias latipes*) is a teleost native to Japan, Korea, China, and Taiwan[23]. Similar to the zebrafish, it produces transparent embryos that allow easy observation and manipulation. Medaka is a popular model organism in Japan and the first fish species in which stable transgenesis was established. It provides some complimentary features to the zebrafish such as adaptation to a wide range of temperatures.[22] The identification of sex specific markers, secondary sex characters and a sex determination gene have lead to increasing attraction of the medaka as a model for research on sex determination and differentiation[23,28] (photo: Andre Künzelmann, UFZ).	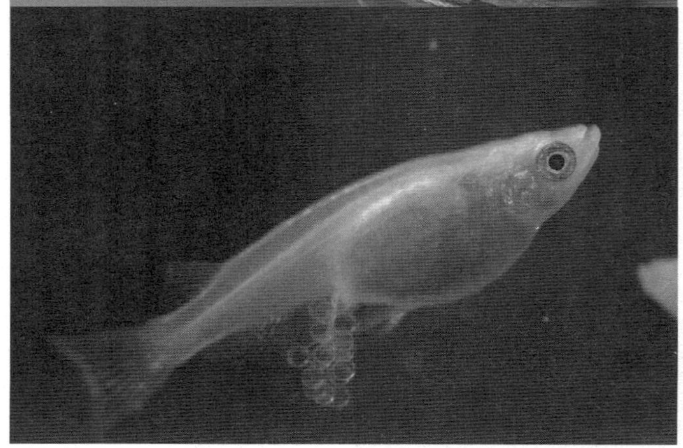

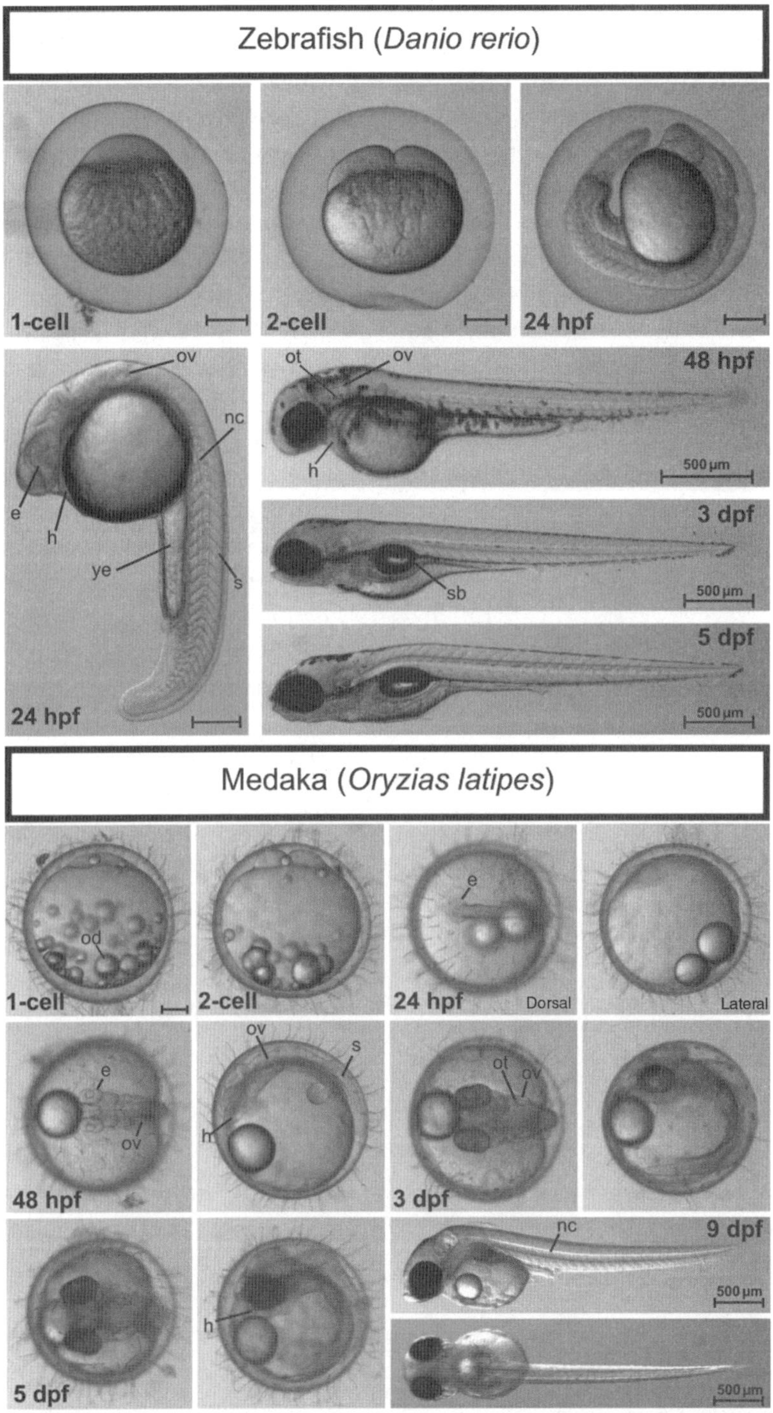

Figure 13-1: Selected developmental stages of zebrafish and medaka embryos and larvae. Embryos were raised in glass Petri dishes at 26°C. The chorion of 24-hpf-old zebrafish was manually removed with forceps. The chorion of Medaka embryos is tough and has not been removed due to the fragility of the yolk sac. Abbreviations: dpf, days postfertilization; e, eye; h, heart; hpf, hours postfertilization; nc, notochord; od, oil droplet; ot, otolith; ov, otic vesicle; s, somite; sb, swim bladder; ye, yolk extension. Scale bars = 200 µm if not otherwise indicated.

visible as a cone-shaped tube, and the heart beat can be observed. Furthermore, spontaneous contractions of the tail and trunk can be detected. Formation of pigmentation begins in the retinal epithelium, and after 48 hpf pigmentation is clearly visible in all parts of the body. After 48 hpf the liver primordia and swim bladder are developed, and a nearly complete circulation system is established. Hatching occurs at around 3 days, but independent feeding cannot be observed before 5 dpf when morphogenesis is completed, the swimbladder is inflated, and all major organs are developed.

In the medaka (Figure 13.1, lower panel), eggs are characterized by oil droplets. Upon fertilization and formation of the blastodisc, oil droplets are displaced toward the vegetal pole and begin to fuse. The chorion is covered with attachment filaments, which usually keep the eggs attached to the female's body. The first cleavages last approximately 35 min at 26°C. Compared to the zebrafish embryo, development is slower. After 24 hpf, the embryonic body develops as a solid rod of cells. At this time, eye morphogenesis is just initiated, and no somites are yet formed. The heart *anlagen* is formed around 30 hpf and melanophores appear on the yolk sphere in the same time. The onset of blood circulation can be detected after about 2 days. The anterior allocation of the heart is completed after 6 days of development, and the blood flow in the embryo is clearly visible. The *anlagen* of the liver and pancreas can be detected around 2 dpf. Hatching and feeding of fish can be observed at 9–10 dpf, when all major organs are developed.

Fish embryos are considered as alternatives to the testing of adult animals and are thus not regulated by current legislation.[29] The stage of development at which this risk is considered to be sufficient for protection is that at which the normal locomotion and sensory functioning of an individual independent of the egg or mother can occur. There is no clear demarcation for this stage, and it has, for instance, been controversially discussed for fish embryos.[30] However, current legislation considers the last third of development within the egg or mother as the appropriate stage of manifestation of sentience in vertebrates. For a fish, amphibian, cephalopod, or decapod, stages prior to the capability of feeding independently are considered as nonprotected stages.[31,32]

It is clear, that cross reading from simple animal models to humans or higher vertebrates is limited. Therefore, it is unlikely that models such as the fish embryo test will ever serve as surrogate to preclinical testing using mammalian species. However, screening and prioritizing of compounds using fish embryo could substantially reduce costs associated with preclinical and clinical studies. Since fish embryos could also be useful for lead development and screening for the identification of compounds with certain mode of actions, they could be used to calculate an initial therapeutic index (i.e., the ratio of the toxic dose to the dose required for the therapeutic effects). With increasing information on the action and toxicity of drugs in the fish embryo, the predictivity may also improve, for instance, by identification of interspecies biomarkers of toxicity that can be used for the comparison of toxic responses between species.

13.3 ACUTE AND CHRONIC TOXICITY

Information on the acute toxicity represents the base set of information required for the approval of drugs as well as for the registration of new industrial chemicals, pesticides, and biocides. For the environmental risk assessment of industrial chemicals, fish embryos have been suggested as surrogate for testing of adult fish.[33–35] Indeed, when data for 173 chemicals were compared, toxicity in zebrafish embryos showed a correlation of $r^2 = 0.89$ with the geometric mean of acute toxicities of various fish species.[35] The correlation line is close to the line of unity. For approval of drugs, acute toxicity is most frequently tested in mouse or rat, by oral, intraperitoneal, or intravenal application of the candidate compound. Whether fish embryos can be used as a surrogate for predicting rodent (and human) acute toxicity remains, however, questionable. As shown by Parng et al.[36] for 11 out of 18 randomly selected drugs, the LC_{50} of zebrafish closely matched the LD_{50} of mice (less than tenfold deviation from a perfect match). For the remaining compounds, zebrafish embryos showed a higher sensitivity of up to 3 orders of magnitude. Since this result might be biased by the selection of compounds and their physicochemical properties and mode of action, we performed another comparison using LC_{50} of fathead minnow (a teleost often used for acute fish toxicity estimation) with LD_{50} in rat or mouse with a selection of 57 chemicals (Figure 13.2). The compounds included in the comparison were covering a broad range of toxicities, physicochemical characteristics (Henry's low coefficient, octanol–water partition coefficient), and various mode of actions.[37] Although the correlation of acute toxicities seemed to be weak, the observation of Parng et al.[36] that fish or fish embryos exhibit a higher sensitivity could be confirmed. The deviating acute toxicities may partially result from the comparison of doses and water-borne concentrations. Fish are continuously exposed via the water, and equilibrium between the water and the fish body is established during the experiment. In rodents single doses via feeding or injection are applied. Some compounds may be rapidly excreted via the kidney or – in case of high volatility – the lungs. Differences in systemic distribution and metabolism may also account for the differences. Further research will be necessary to identify the major constraints for the weak correlation and/or to identify methods (experimental or computational) to establish a significant correlation between the acute fish (embryo) and rodent toxicity. Despite the weak correlation of acute toxicity between fish and rodents, an area of particular value for fish embryo assays would be, however, the comparison of acute toxicity and therapeutic doses. This would be particularly feasible if the drug target or the effect on the drug target, respectively, can be assessed in the embryo simultaneously.[38]

An example for the use of fish embryo assays for the development of efficient nanosized PAMAM (polyamidoamine) dendrimers drug delivery tools is reported in Reference 39. PAMAM dendrimers with amino functional groups were toxic and attenuated growth and development of zebrafish embryos at

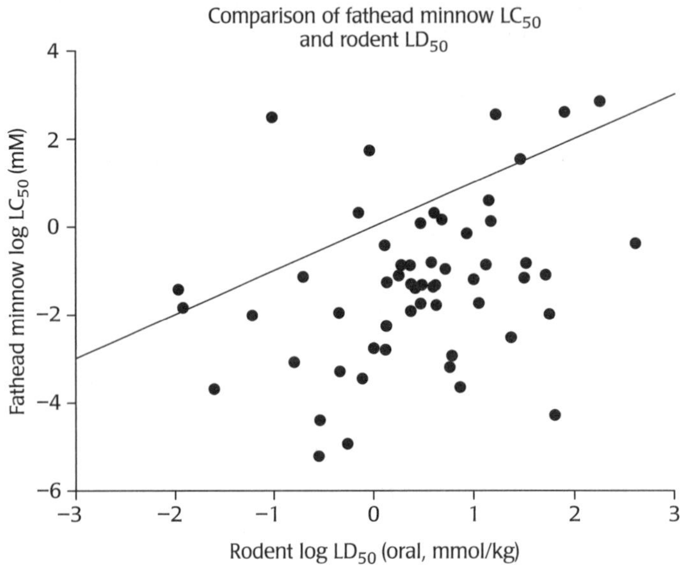

Figure 13-2: Relationship of acute toxicities in the teleost fathead minnow and rodents (mice and rats). Data for fathead minnow LC_{50} concentrations originated from the U.S. EPA ECOTOX database and comprised a list of reference chemicals with a wide distribution of physico-chemical properties and different toxicities (extracted from[37]). Corresponding rodent LD_{50} were extracted from the Halle Registry of Cytotoxicity (kindly provided by K. Tanneberger, Swiss Federal Institute of Aquatic Science and Technology, CH) and/or the ChemIDplus Lite database (http://chem.sis.nlm.nih.gov/chemidplus/chemidlite.jsp). Generally LD_{50} of mice and rats were close together. In case data of both organisms were available, the geometric mean was used. The line represents the line of unity (i.e., where LC_{50} of rodent would perfectly match the LD_{50} of rodents).

sublethal concentrations. Dendrimers with carboxylic acid terminal functional groups, however, were not toxic to zebrafish embryo. The authors concluded that zebrafish embryos were an ideal system for assessing the initial toxicity of novel nanotherapeutic agents and prioritizing further research.

The relevance of acute toxicity test for the safety validation of drugs has been questioned, since acute toxicity data are generally not used to decide whether a drug is submitted for a clinical trial.[39] In contrast, the estimation of potential chronic effects is of high relevance for human therapy. Drugs are applied in subacute doses and side effects can particularly arise during long-term treatment. Therefore, in preclinical studies chronic toxicity is evaluated in 6–12 months treatment of rodents.[40] A prescreening model would need to extrapolate from short- to long-term effects. Changes in gene expression, protein, or metabolomic patterns could be indicators of a potential chronic toxicity, since it can be assumed that any toxic effect starts from an initial molecular interaction. Fish embryos could be used to identify these early interactions and to correlate them with potential chronic toxicity. While this has been principally shown for gene expression patterns and chronic toxicity in fish,[41,42] further research is needed to establish meaningful markers for chronic toxicity and with cross-validity among different species.

13.4 GENOTOXICITY

Genotoxic compounds have the potential to be human carcinogens and/or mutagens and, hence, may induce cancer and/or heritable defects. Therefore, the assessment of genotoxicity is included in the preclinical safety evaluation of drugs.[43,44] Assays for the evaluation of genotoxicity are also available for fish embryos, but have yet not been applied for the testing of human drugs or drug candidates. For instance, single-strand breaks have been detected by the comet assay in zebrafish embryos exposed to river sediments.[45,46] Furthermore, transgenic lines of zebrafish and medaka have been constructed that allow quantification as well as the specific analysis of the mutational spectra by DNA sequencing.[47,48] The transgenic zebrafish strain harbors an *Escherichia coli* plasmid containing the rpsL gene. When the plasmid is extracted from the zebrafish embryo genomic DNA and used for transformation of an appropriate *E. coli* host strain, mutations of the rpsL gene result in the appearance of colonies. The medaka transgene harbors multiple copies of a bacteriophage lambda vector with the cII gene as a mutational target. The recovery of cII mutants from fish genomic DNA by lambda *in vitro* packaging is used to measure the mutagenic effects.[49] The advantage of an embryo-based assay is – as mentioned earlier – the complex interaction between the tissues of an intact organism and a better representation of ADME. However, whether these fish embryo assays correlate with rodent *in vivo* assays and offer any advantages over existing *in vitro* alternatives remains to be elucidated.

13.5 DEVELOPMENTAL TOXICITY

Developmental disorders can occur as severe side effects of drug treatment. Historically, one of the most tragic cases has been the induction of limb abnormalities in humans by the sedative thalidomide. The thalidomide case of 1961 can be seen as a turning point for the awareness of teratogenic effects caused by drugs.[50] As a consequence, extensive testing of drug candidates is required for drug approval. Developmental toxicity testing is currently assessed following the OECD guidelines 414[51] or 421[52] (Annex VI of the European Directive 92/32/EEC) with two animal species (preferred species are rat and rabbit). However, correlation of developmental toxicities from historical data within mammalians is far from being ideal and barely reaches a predictivity of above 50 percent for humans.[53]

Many possible alternative models have been explored during the last decades (e.g., whole rate embryo culture and primary or permanent embryonic stem cells[54]). Furthermore, different attempts have been made to develop QSAR approaches for the prediction of teratogenic effects.[55–57] Fish embryos also appear to be a promising alternative test system for the reliable and cost-effective identification of potential human teratogenic compounds.[58] An experimental advantage is their extracorporal development and the transparency of the eggs of some species that facilitates observation of teratogenic effects. They have already been used in the assessment of developmental toxicity. Particularly the studies of Bachmann and Nagel[59,60] that tested forty-one teratogens can be highlighted. Correlations with mammalian toxicity were found in thirty-six compounds (88 percent), with one false positive (2 percent) and four false negatives (10 percent) in the zebrafish embryo test. Although the selection of compounds in this study may have been biased and the study did not have a focus on potential difficult compounds, it can be considered as a proof-of-concept that the use of zebrafish for predicting human developmental toxicity is principally possible. Interestingly, thalidomide – which failed to demonstrate teratogenic effects in some mammalian strains – has recently been shown to provoke teratogenic effects in zebrafish embryos. Using transient gene knock-down the protein cereblon was confirmed to be the primary target of thalidomide.[61]

However, as can be expected from species differences within mammalians, the fish embryo developmental tests based on morphological and functional endpoints may not be able to sufficiently predict human developmental toxicity as required by regulatory agencies. However, improved species read-across could be achieved by including toxicogenomic profiles into the analysis (e.g., the analysis of patterns of genes wherein an altered regulation is involved in developmental disorders). Stigson et al.[62] have recently demonstrated the use of differential transcription as potential marker for teratogenic compounds. Species-specific teratogenic effects might also be attributed to different metabolic capacities (i.e., ability to metabolically activate or deactivate certain compounds). Therefore, the use of a mammalian metabolic activation system has been suggested for testing of teratogenic effects in fish embryos. Busquet et al.[63] demonstrated that only by addition of male rat liver microsomes during the first 2 hours of exposure in zebrafish embryos could induce developmental effects of cyclophosphamide and ethanol.

Provided that an endpoint related to the therapeutic effect can be measured in the fish embryo as well, the parallel measurement of this endpoint and teratogenic effects can be used as first information on the efficacy of the compound and for prioritization of compounds with a high therapeutic index. An example is given in Table 13.3[64] and Figure 13.3 for compounds potentially inhibiting the sonic hedgehog (shh) signaling pathway. Some type of cancers (medullablastomas) are caused by deregulation of the shh signaling pathway. Compounds inhibiting this pathway by binding the membrane proteins PATCHED or SMO are potential anticancer agents and have already been shown to reduce the growth of medulla blastomes.[65] It is possible to identify shh-inhibiting candidate compounds using a cellular reporter gene assay for the expression of *Gli1*, a target gene of the shh pathway.[66] In medaka, similar to birds and mammals, shh inhibitors such as cyclopamine cause cyclopia or holoprosencephaly, respectively, a disorder that is characterized by failure of the embryo's forebrain to divide and form a bilateral hemisphere during development.[67,68] The cyclopia phenotype can be used to analyze the potential shh-inhibiting capacity of candidate compounds. Various compounds that have been identified to inhibit the expression

Table 13-3. Induction of the cyclopia phenotype in 4 dpf medaka embryos exposed to various concentrations of cyclopamine and SANT-2

Compound	Concentration (μ*M*)	Eye field distance	Developmental delay (%)	Hemorrhage (%)	Lethality (%)
Control	–	113 ± 22	–	–	–
Cyclopamine	6.25	87 ± 11*	–	–	–
	25	66 ± 23*	70–80	–	–
	50	n.a.	80	–	5–10
	100	n.a.	80	–	5–10
SANT-2	5	118 ± 33	–	–	–
	25	126 ± 6	80	20	–
	50	n.a.	80	50	10
	100	n.a.	80	50	10

Notes: The cyclopia phenotype was quantified by measuring the distances of the eye field (see also Figure 13.3). Medaka embryos were exposed from 2 h postfertilization. Ethanol was used as a vehicle. Final concentration of ethanol was 1% including controls. Percentages refer to the proportion of embryos showing the appropriate effect. Experiments were replicated three times with 20–30 animals per compound and concentration. Hemorrhage represented the most common noncyclopia teratogenic effects. Developmental delays refers to percentage of embryos showing an up to 10-h delay according to the stage map of Iwamatsu.[64] * Statistically significant different if compared to controls ($p > .05$). n.a. = not analyzed.

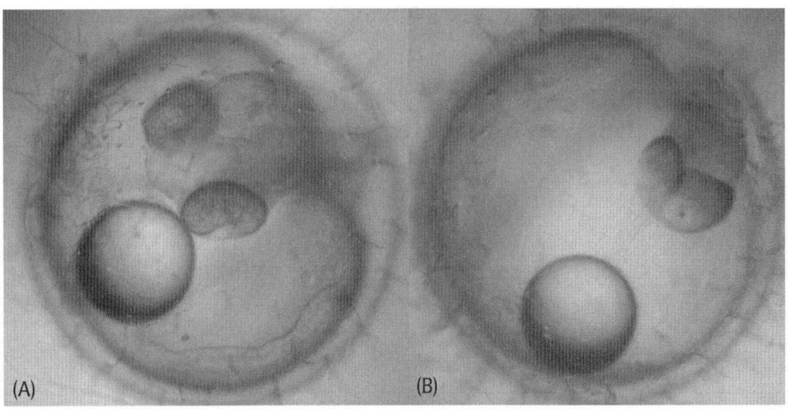

Figure 13-3: Induction of the cyclopia phenotype in 4-dpf medaka embryos exposed to 50 μ*M* cyclopamine. Note the reduced distance between the eye fields in embryos treated with cyclopamine (B) in contrast to controls (A). Medaka embryos were exposed from 2 h postfertilization. Ethanol was used as a vehicle. Final concentration of ethanol was 1 percent including controls.

of the shh-target gene *Gli1* were analyzed in 4-dpf-old medaka embryos for their ability to induce the cyclopia phenotype.[69] The cyclopia phenotype was quantified by measuring the distances of the eyes which is reduced in embryos exposed to cyclopamine. Although some of the compounds such as SANT-2 were potent inhibitors (>tenfold more efficient than cyclopamine) they did not induce the cyclopia phenotype in medaka embryos (Figure 13.3). Furthermore, both cyclopamine and SANT-2 induced developmental delay, other teratogenic effects such as hemorrhages, and reduced survival at higher concentrations. Thus, potential side effects of these compounds may interfere with any specific effect that could be of therapeutic interest. Thus, compounds with lowest toxicity with respect to specific phenotypes may be used for further development of drug candidate compounds.

13.6 ORGAN TOXICITY

13.6.1 Cardiotoxicity

For many noncardiac drugs interference with the physiology and function of the heart, such as the prolongation of ventricular repolarization (QT prolongation) and cardiac arrhythmia has been reported.[70] These effects can be associated with life-threatening diseases such as torsades de pointes. Therefore, international guidelines for the evaluation of drug safety require the evaluation of QT prolongation.[71]

One of the main mechanisms involved in drug-induced cardiac disfunction is the inhibition of the KCNH2 potassium channel. The ionic mechanisms controlling repolarization of the zebrafish heart are highly similar to higher vertebrates, particularly with respect to the KCNH2 channel.[20] The zebrafish heart can be easily observed in embryos from 24 hpf (at 28°C) when the rhythmic activity is established. From 42 hpf, heart chambers can be identified.[72] Thus, a number of studies have used zebrafish embryos to assess the effect of drugs, drug candidates, or libraries of small molecules on cardiac function (Table 13.4). It was found that, for at least 77 percent of the drugs known to interfere with cardiac function, these effects were also observed in the zebrafish embryo. The assays were generally conducted by visual observation and counting of the heart rate over a period of 15 seconds in the transparent embryos. Automatic analysis is possible using power spectral analysis, which has shown to reveal the same result as manual counting of the heart beat rate.[73]

13.6.2 Hepatotoxicity

Severe liver injury caused by drugs is an important factor in failure of drug approval. Drug-induced liver injury is the leading cause for acute liver failure in the United States.[74] Therefore, the liver is a primary target organ in the repeated dose rodent studies performed as part of the nonclinical studies.[75] Zebrafish embryos have also been suggested for the screening of liver toxicity.[76] During embryonic development of the zebrafish, the liver is differentiated within 96 hpf. At 72 hpf, liver cells and bile are visible. At 96 hpf, liver extends from the left side of the embryo across the midline to the esophagus, and hepatic blood flow is present. Many typical liver biochemical characteristics (e.g., lipid metabolizing enzymes, HMG-CoA lyase, peroxisome proliferators-activated receptors, carboxylases, biotin, and cytochrome P450 enzymes) have been reported to be present in zebrafish.[76] Screens for hepatotoxicity of drugs using early life stages of zebrafish have thus far only been reported for 6-dpf larvae[76,77] using phenotypic and protein biomarkers for assessment of toxicity. The study by Vanparys et al.[77] analyzed twenty-one drugs or reference compounds. Two false positives (out of seven known nonhepatotoxic compounds) and two false negatives (out of fourteen known hepatotoxic compounds) were observed. Further research and inclusion of additional markers may lead to the optimization of the zebrafish hepatotoxicity screen and allow the use of earlier embryonic stages as well. Furthermore, inclusion of metabolic activation systems such as described for teratogenicity assays could improve correlation to humans (see earlier discussion). However, it must be noted that the use of simple screening systems such as fish embryos is probably restricted to liver hepatotoxicity that is not associated with low-frequency idiosyncratic effects, metabolic variability in man, or unidentified interactions with other agents or factors.[75] These idiosyncratic rare side effects are probably difficult to be detected in any kind of animal model.

13.6.3 Neurotoxicity

Neurotoxicity is responsible for the withdrawal of many drugs and is therefore considered as important target in the safety evaluation of drug candidates. According to a study of the pharmaceutical company Bristol-Myers Squibb, about 8 percent of historical drug attritions could be attributed to adverse effects on the central or peripheral nervous system.[78] Neurotoxic drugs can act on a wide variety of different neuronal target cells, such as, for instance, motoneurons and cells of the otic, the visual system, or the brain. Analysis of neurotoxicity in preclinical studies is labor intensive and/or technically difficult and involves the study of morphological, behavioral, and functional endpoints in rodents or dogs.[79,80] Zebrafish embryos or early larval stages have already been used to screen for neurotoxic effects of drugs, and recent reviews have analyzed drugs with known effects in humans in zebrafish early life stages.[20,76] For instance, drugs known to affect vision in humans were assessed by an optokinetic or optomotor response assay in larvae[80,81] (Table 13.4). Ototoxic effects were analyzed using the lateral line cells in zebrafish larvae. These cells are structurally closely related to mammalian inner ear cells[82,83] (Table 13.4). Furthermore, locomotor assays have been used to assess the seizure liability and movement disorders caused by drugs[84,85] (Table 13.4). If the different assays for neurotoxic effects in zebrafish are compared with known effects in humans, 68–100 percent of the neurotoxic compounds would have been identified in the zebrafish assay.[20]

13.6.4 Gastrointestinal toxicity

Gastrointestinal toxicity evaluated with zebrafish early life stages has been described in one study.[81] The potential impact of drugs on gut function was analyzed in 7-dpf zebrafish larvae by recording the frequency of gut contraction.

Table 13-4. Examples of studies using zebrafish embryos for the evaluation of drug organ toxicity

Organ	Reference	Description
Heart (cardiotoxicity)	[86]	Hundred compounds were screened for the effect on the heart rate by 15-s video recordings in 2 dpf zebrafish embryos. Of 23 drugs that were known to cause repolarization abnormalities in human, 22 were also positive in zebrafish embryos.
	[87]	Of 13 tested drugs 12 provoked a reduced heart beating rate in 3 dpf zebrafish embryos.
	[81]	The QT-prolongation effect of 9 drugs were tested in 3 dpf old zebrafish embryo. Five of the tested compounds were known human hERG blocking compounds, 2 drugs were associated with trachycardia. Four compounds also showed a mild to strong tachycardial or bradycardial effect in zebrafish. Atrial and ventricular contraction rates were recorded over a period of 15 s.
	[88]	Nine compounds known to provoke QT prolongation and nine compounds with no know effects in humans were analyzed in 3 dpf zebrafish embryos by counting the heart rate over a period of 15 s. Seven and 8 of the positive control compounds induced bradycardy or atriventricular dissociation, respectively. Propranolol was identified as a false positive albeit effects were observed at concentration 1,000-fold above the clinical concentrations.
Liver (hepatotoxicity)	[77]	Twenty-one drugs or reference compounds with known hepatoxicity have been screened in 6-dpf zebrafish larvae.
Neurotoxicity	[80]	Effects on the visual system were tested by the optokinetic and optomotor response assay in 8-dpf zebrafish larvae using 27 drugs including 19 compounds known to cause effects on human vision. Thirteen of the positive compounds provoked effects in zebrafish as well. Two false positives could be attributed to having direct effects on movement not related to disturbance on the visual system.
	[81]	The optomotor response assay using 8-dpf zebrafish was used to test 9 different drugs with know effects on human vision. Seven of the tested compounds were positive in zebrafish larvae as well.
	[82]	Neuromast hair cells in the zebrafish lateral line of 6 dpf larvae exposed to 5 known ototoxic drugs were stained with DASPEI. Morphometric analysis of neuromast cells revealed ototoxic effects for all of the tested compounds.

Organ	Reference	Description
	[83]	Ototoxic effects of 1040 FDA approved drugs were screened in 5-dpf embryos by fluorescence staining of lateral line hair cells. Seven known included ototoxic drugs were positively identified. Fourteen compounds were additionally classified as ototoxic. Validation of two of these compounds in an *in vitro* preparation of mouse utricles confirmed the loss of hair cells.
	[84]	Seizure liability was analyzed in 7-dpf larvae exposed to 25 drugs (17 known positive and 8 known negative compounds). Larvae were videotracked and increased swimming speed and activity, circular movements – as indicators of seizure-like locomotor activity – were quantified. Four false negative and 3 false positive compounds were detected.
	[85]	Three antipsychotic drugs were tested in 10- to 19-dpf zebrafish larvae. Locomotor activity was recorded by 5-min video tracking, and the frequency of erratic movements (rapid bouts, vertical or sideway swimming) was determined. Two of the drugs had a strong neurotoxic effects in larvae. A third compound, olanzapine, exhibited – similar to known effects in human – only mild effects on locomotion.
Gastrointestinal toxicity	[81]	The potential impact of drugs on gut function was analyzed for 10 drugs in 7-dpf zebrafish larvae by recording the frequency of gut contraction after 1 h of exposure. Compounds that were found to reduce the number of gut contractions have been also reported to inhibit gastrointestinal motility in humans.

Note: Only examples that investigated a minimum of three compounds have been listed.

Compounds that were found to reduce the number of gut contractions have been also reported to inhibit gastrointestinal motility (see Table 13.4).

13.6.5 Toxicity to other organs

There are many other organs and organ systems that principally could be targets of drug side effects. For some of these organs such as the lung, the appropriate structure in fish (embryos) is missing, and fish embryos would not be useful as a screening model. However, for many other organs, such as pancreas, kidney, or the immune system, fish embryos or early life stages could principally be used to analyze organ toxicity (Table 13.4). Already promising examples are reported, but no systematic study evaluating a larger group of drugs has been published. For instance, Hentschel et al.[89] demonstrated that the nephrotoxic drug gentamycin caused acute renal failure-like effects in embryonic zebrafish. Gentamycin was injected at 50–55 hpf, and renal failure was quantified by determining the percentage of fish with edema, the decrease in clearance of injected fluorescing dyes, and histopathological investigation in 72- and 96-hpf embryos.

Early life stages of zebrafish have also been proposed as models to study the immune response. The innate immune response or components of the underpinning signaling pathways are already established in zebrafish embryos, and proinflammatory responses provoked by pathogens have been observed.[90–93] However, immune modulation by drugs has yet not been addressed in fish embryos.

13.7 ENVIRONMENTAL RISK ASSESSMENT OF MEDICINAL PRODUCTS

Traditionally, safety evaluation of new drugs has been exclusively focused on potential adverse effects on human health. However, in the last decades, human pharmaceuticals have been found in surface and ground waters. Albeit they have been detected in low concentrations ranging from ng/L to μg/L levels,[94,95] concerns have been raised that exposure may harm aquatic organisms.[96,97] Environmental concentrations of human pharmaceuticals are related to their prescription rates and their persistence.[98,99] Due to their continuous use and high prescription rates, human drugs are – primarily via sewage effluents – released into the aquatic environment leading to a chronic low-level exposure of aquatic organisms. Therefore, appropriate regulations that request data on the potential toxicity to aquatic organisms have been established by the FDA and the EMEA.[100,101] These regulations do not have any effect on the approval of a drug, but may lead to constraints for risk minimization measures, such as instructions for safe disposal of nonused products.

The environmental risk assessment for the registration of human pharmaceuticals follows the principles that have been established for the regulation of pesticides, biocides, and chemicals.[102] Data on the (chronic) toxicity of algae, invertebrates, and fish are required. To identify potential chronic effects on fish, the EMEA guideline for the ERA of human pharmaceuticals requests data obtained by the fish early life stage test.[103] These effects may also be predicted from alternative short-term experimental setups, such as exposure to fish embryos. Therefore, various research groups have recently aimed at the identification of subacute biomarkers in the fish embryo, particularly genes or proteins of which the expression was changed by the exposure to chemicals.[42] For changes in transcription levels, it has already been shown that analysis of gene expression as an additional endpoint increases the sensitivity of the zebrafish embryo test and is observed for many compounds in the same range of concentration that provoked effects in the fish early life stage test.[41]

13.8 LIMITATIONS AND RESEARCH PERSPECTIVES

It must be noted that in some of the studies cited in this chapter, particularly those that found a 100 percent agreement of fish early life stages and human effects, only a very small number of drugs has been investigated. To demonstrate the suitability of embryo/larval assays, an extended research with an increased number of compounds will be necessary. Furthermore, the level of effective concentrations and doses, for both therapeutic and adverse effects, has not been compared systematically between fish embryos/larvae and mammalians. The relationship of effect levels, should, however, be considered when a decision is made for the use of fish embryos as a screening system.

The advantage to screening for drug toxicity at a very small scale may be partially compensated by the difficulty to observe effects on an organ or cell-specific level. Therefore, transgenic strains that harbor a reporter gene such as GFP expressed in a specific organ could be of particular interest for the development of new fish embryo assays. This could, for instance, allow an easier monitoring of inflammation and its modulation by drugs in zebrafish with GFP fluorescence in neutrophilic cells,[104] or analysis of heart arrhythmic effects in zebrafish with green fluorescing myocardium.[105] Furthermore, the analysis of the expression of organ-specific biomarker genes is greatly facilitated.[106]

In many of the described assays, particular those for neurotoxicity, postembryonic stages older than 5 dpf were used. According to the current legislation and practice[33,34] and the 3Rs concept,[107] these assays would have rather been accepted as refinement than as replacement of animal experiments. Further optimization of the tests may lead to the possibility to explore earlier embryonic life stages. For instances, ototoxicity was already observed in 5-dpf eluteroembryos.[83] Furthermore, it has been observed that zebrafish embryos exposed to organophosphate pesticides exhibit a reduced locomotion response to tactile sensitization already in 3-dpf embryos (N. Klüver, unpublished data). This type of response may also be useful to study the potential neurotoxicity of drug candidates in embryonic stages.

A further limitation in the fish embryo assays is the potential poor absorption of drugs, their different metabolic capacity, and species differences, which could result in the failure to detect a compound exhibiting adverse health effects in humans. Poor absorption via the skin has been made responsible for failure to induce toxic effects of some drugs in zebrafish embryos. In these examples microinjection of the compound instead of water-borne exposure has partially improved the agreement with known human data.[20] To reduce false negatives caused by poor absorption, chemical analytics should routinely be included in fish embryo assays in order to monitor the uptake of the drug candidate into embryonic tissues. However, chemical analytics of embryonic concentrations have only been considered in some of the studies (e.g., Reference 81). Reduced metabolic capacity of fish embryos – as mentioned earlier – might be compensated by supplementation of exposure media with mammalian metabolic activation systems.[63] Furthermore, species differences might be partially compensated by establishing robust molecular biomarkers with species cross validity. Toxicogenomic profiles in zebrafish embryos show distinct characteristics related to the type and concentration of the compound to which embryos have been exposed.[108] These changes in expression profiles could be used to establish biomarkers for potential adverse effects with improved species cross-validity.[15]

13.9 CONCLUSION

Reduction of animal experiments and costs associated with drug development is a key to improving the identification of new and safe medicines and making these drugs affordable for citizens of less-developed countries. Strategies that allow the early identification of potentially adverse side effects appear particularly effective in reducing the budget that is spent for drug development. Fish embryos would represent a powerful system that could be used as a prescreening model in order to limit the number of compounds entering preclinical and clinical trials. They address economic (fast, small-scale analysis, high-throughput capacity) as well as ethical societal demands (replacement of mammalian experiments). Zebrafish has been the preferred model, and systematic studies for drug safety evaluation have to date not been reported for the medaka, albeit this species exhibited similar features. Due to its evolutionary differences, medaka may serve as a complimentary model that could overcome species pecularities or provide advantages for specific endpoints. Exploitation of both models may provide better correlation to mammalian method. Therefore, research using medaka embryos as a drug toxicity model needs to be intensified and compared to the zebrafish.

Especially in combination with alternative approaches such as toxicogenomics or a phase 0 clinical trial based on microdosing, fish embryo assays have a strong potential for reducing drug developmental costs in the near future.[15,109] This is also demonstrated by a growing number of enterprises in which lead development and initial preclinical safety evaluation is performed with embryos of one of the most popular teleost model, the zebrafish (e.g., Zygogen, Phylonix Pharmaceuticals, ZF-Biolabs, ZF-Screen, Summit, Biotecont). As has been highlighted in this chapter, recent investigations have demonstrated a high predictive power of the zebrafish embryo model. However, in some cases, the reports on the efficacy of the fish embryo model for drug safety evaluation is rather anecdotal. Hence, further systematic research is needed to improve the correlation between the fish embryo, rodent modes, and/or humans and to define the domain of applicability.

REFERENCES

1. Li AP. Accurate prediction of human drug toxicity: A major challenge in drug development. *Chem Biol Interact.* 2004;150(1):3–7.
2. Greener M. Drug safety on trial – Last year's withdrawal of the anti-arthritis drug Vioxx triggered a debate about how to better monitor drug safety even after approval. *Embo Rep.* 2005;6(3):202–204.
3. DiMasi J, Hansen R, Grabowski H. The price of innovation: New estimates of drug development costs. *J Health Econ.* 2003;22(2).
4. Adams CP, Brantner VV. Estimating the cost of new drug development: Is it really $802 million? *Health Affairs.* 2006;25(2):420–428.
5. FDA. Challenge and opportunity on the critical path to new medicinal products. Retrieved from http://www.fda.gov. 2004.
6. Light DW, Warburton RN. Setting the record straight in the reply by DiMasi, Hansen and Grabowski. *J Health Econ.* 2005;24(5):1045–1048.
7. Riggs TL. Research and development costs for drugs. *Lancet.* 2004;363(9404): 184–184.
8. Kramer JA. Designing safe drugs: what to consider? *Expert Opin Drug Discov.* 2008;3(7):707–713.
9. Schuster D, Laggner C, Langer T. Why drugs fail – A study on side effects in new chemical entities. *Curr Pharma Design.* 2005;11(27):3545–3559.
10. Woosley RL, Rice G. A new system for moving drugs to market. *Issues Sci Technol.* 2005;21(2):63–68.
11. Commission of the European Communities. Fifth Report on the Statistics on the Number of Animals used for Experimental and other Scientific Purposes in the Member States of the European Union {SEC(2007)1455}. 2007.
12. Knight A. Non-animal methodologies within biomedical research and toxicity testing. *ALTEX Alternat Tierexp.* 2008;25(3):213–231.
13. Taylor K, Gordon N, Langley G, et al. Estimates for worldwide laboratory animal use in 2005. *Altern Lab Anim.* 2008;36(3):327–342.
14. Fieldent MR, Kolaja KL. The role of early in vivo toxicity testing in drug discovery toxicology. *Expert Opin Drug Saf.* 2008;7(2):107–110.
15. Amir-Aslani A. Toxicogenomic predictive modeling: Emerging opportunities for more efficient drug discovery and development. *Technol Forecast Social Change.* 2008;75(7):905–932.
16. Gunnarsson L, Jauhiainen A, Kristiansson E, et al. Evolutionary conservation of human drug targets in organisms used for environmental risk assessments. *Environ Sci Technol.* 2008;42(15):5807–5813.
17. Chakraborty C, Hsu CH, Wen ZH, et al. Zebrafish: A complete animal model for in vivo drug discovery and development. *Curr Drug Metab.* 2009;10(2): 116–124.
18. Redfern WS, Waldron G, Winter MJ, et al. Zebrafish assays as early safety pharmacology screens: Paradigm shift or red herring? *J Pharmacol Toxicol Method.* 2008;58(2):110–117.

19. Zon LI, Peterson RT. In vivo drug discovery in the zebrafish. *Nat Rev Drug Discov.* 2005;4(1):35–44.
20. Eimon PM, Rubinstein AL. The use of in vivo zebrafish assays in drug toxicity screening. *Expert Opin Drug Metabol Toxicol.* 2009;5(4):393–401.
21. Wittbrodt J, Shima A, Schartl M. Medaka – A model organism from the far East. *Nat Rev Genet.* 2002;3(1):53–64.
22. Shima A, Mitani H. Medaka as a research organism: Past, present and future. *Mech Dev.* 2004;121(7–8):599–604.
23. Yamamoto T-O. *Medaka (Killifish): Biology and Strains.* Tokyo: Keigaku Publishing Company; 1975.
24. Westerfield M. *The Zebrafish Book. A Guide for the Laboratory Use of Zebrafish (Danio rerio).* 4 ed. Eugene: University of Oregon Press; 2000.
25. Coverdale LE, Lean D, Martin CC. Not just a fishing trip – Environmental genomics using zebrafish. *Curr Genom.* 2004;5(5):395–407.
26. Hill AJ, Teraoka H, Heideman W, et al. Zebrafish as a model vertebrate for investigating chemical toxicity. *Toxicol Sci.* 2005;86(1):6–19.
27. Eaton RC, Farley RD. Spawning cycle and egg production of zebrafish, *Brachydanio rerio*, in the laboratory. *Copeia.* 1974;1(1):195–209.
28. Nanda I, Kondo M, Hornung U, et al. A duplicated copy of DMRT1 in the sex-determining region of the Y chromosome of the medaka, *Oryzias latipes. Proc Natl Acad Sci USA.* 2002;22(18):11778–11783.
29. Fleming A. Zebrafish as an alternative model organism for disease modelling and drug discovery: Implications for the 3Rs. NC3Rs, Iss. 10, National Centre for the Replacement, Refinement and Reduction of Animals in research. Retrieved from www.nc3rs.org.uk. 2007:1–7.
30. Urho L. Characters of larvae – what are they. *Folia Zool.* 2002;51(3):161–186.
31. EFSA. Opinion on the "Aspects of the biology and welfare of animals used for experimental and other scientific purposes". *EFSA J.* 2005;292:1–46.
32. Anonymous. *Animals (Scientific Procedures) Act 1986.* London: HMSO; 1986.
33. Nagel R. DarT: The embryotest with the zebrafish *Danio rerio* – A general model in ecotoxicology and toxicology. *ALTEX Alternat Tierexp.* 2002;19(Suppl 1/02): 38–48.
34. Braunbeck T, Boettcher M, Hollert H, et al. Towards an alternative for the acute fish LC(50) test in chemical assessment: The fish embryo toxicity test goes multi-species – An update. *ALTEX.* 2005;22(2):87–102.
35. Lammer E, Carr GJ, Wendler K, et al. Is the fish embryo toxicity test (FET) with the zebrafish (*Danio rerio*) a potential alternative for the fish acute toxicity test? *Comp Biochem Physiol Part C: Toxicol Pharmacol.* 2009;149(2):196–209.
36. Parng C, Seng WL, Semino C, et al. Zebrafish: A preclinical model for drug screening. *Assay Drug Devel Technol.* 2002;1(1):41–48.
37. Schirmer K, Tanneberger K, Kramer N, et al. Developing a list of reference chemicals for testing alternatives to whole fish toxicity tests. *Aquat Toxicol.* 2008;90(2):128–137.
38. Heiden TCK, Dengler E, Kao WJ, et al. Developmental toxicity of low generation PAMAM dendrimers in zebrafish. *Toxicol Appl Pharmacol.* 2007;225(1):70–79.
39. Robinson S, Delongeas J-L, Donald E, et al. A European pharmaceutical company initiative challenging the regulatory requirement for acute toxicity studies in pharmaceutical drug development. *Regul Toxicol Pharmacol.* 2008;50(3):345–352.
40. FDA. International Conference on Harmonisation; Guidance on the Duration of Chronic Toxicity Testing in Animals (Rodent and Nonrodent Toxicity Testing). Notice. *Fed Reg.* 1999;64:34259–34260.
41. Weil M, Sacher F, Scholz S, et al. Gene expression analysis in zebrafish embryos: A potential approach to predict effect concentrations in the fish early life stage test. *Environ Toxicol Chem.* 2009;28(9):1970–1978.

42. Scholz S, Fischer S, Gündel U, et al. The zebrafish embryo model in environmental risk assessment – Applications beyond acute toxicity testing. *Environ Sci Pollut Res.* 2008;15:394–404.
43. ICH. International Conference on Harmonisation of Technical Requirements for Registration of Pharmaceuticals for Human Use: Guidance for Industry S2B Genotoxicity: A Standard Battery for Genotoxicity Testing of Pharmaceuticals. Retrieved from http://www.fda.gov. 1997.
44. Lorge E, Gervais V, Becourt-Lhote N, et al. Genetic toxicity assessment: Employing the best science for human safety evaluation. Part IV: A strategy in genotoxicity testing in drug development: Some examples. *Toxicol Sci.* 2007;98(1):39–42.
45. Kosmehl T, Krebs F, Manz W, et al. Differentiation between bioavailable and total hazard potential of sediment-induced DNA fragmentation as measured by the comet assay with zebrafish embryos. *Journal of Soils and Sediments.* 2007;7(6): 377–387.
46. Kosmehl T, Hallare AV, Reifferscheid G, et al. A novel contact assay for testing genotoxicity of chemicals and whole sediments in zebrafish embryos. *Environ Toxicol Chem.* 2006;25(8):2097–2106.
47. Amanuma K, Takeda H, Amanuma H, et al. Transgenic zebrafish for detecting mutations caused by compounds in aquatic environments. *Nat Biotechnol.* 2000;18(1):62–65.
48. McElroy AE, Bogler A, Weisbaum D, et al. Uptake, metabolism, mutant frequencies and mutational spectra in [lambda] transgenic medaka embryos exposed to benzo[[alpha]] pyrene dosed sediments. *Mar Environ Res.* 2006;62(Suppl. 1):S273–S277.
49. Winn RN, Norris MB, Brayer KJ, et al. Detection of mutations in transgenic fish carrying a bacteriophage lambda cII transgene target. *Proc Natl Acad Sci USA.* 2000;97(23):12655–12660.
50. Stephens TD, Bunde CJW, Fillmore BJ. Mechanism of action in thalidomide teratogenesis. *Biochem Pharmacol.* 2000;59(12):1489–1499.
51. OECD 414. OECD guideline for testing of chemicals. Test No. 414: Prenatal Developmental Toxicity Study. Available at www.oecd.org. 2000.
52. OECD 421. OECD guideline for testing of chemicals. Test No. 421: Reproduction/ Developmental Toxicity Screening Test. Available at www.oecd.org. 2000.
53. Bailey J, Knight A, Balcombe J. The future of teratology research is in vitro. *Biogen Amines.* 2005;19(2):97–146.
54. Spielmann H, Seiler A, Bremer S, et al. The practical application of three validated in vitro embryotoxicity tests – The Report and Recommendations of an ECVAM/ ZEBET Workshop (ECVAM Workshop 57). *ATLA.* 2006;34(5):527–538.
55. Jensen GE, Niemelä JR, Wedebye EB, Nikolov NG. QSAR models for reproductive toxicity and endocrine disruption in regulatory use – a preliminary investigation. *SAR and QSAR in Environmental Research.* 2008;19(7):631–641.
56. Klopman G, Dimayuga ML. Computer Automated Structure Evaluation (CASE) of the teratogenicity of retinoids with the aid of a novel geometry index. *Journal of Computer-Aided Molecular Design.* 1990;4(2):117–130.
57. Vijay KG, Borgstedt H, Enslein K et al. A QSAR Model of Teratogenesis. *Quantitative Structure-Activity Relationships.* 1991;10(4):306–332.
58. Langheinrich U. Zebrafish: A new model on the pharmaceutical catwalk. *BioEssays.* 2003;25(9):904–912.
59. Bachmann J. *Entwicklung und Erprobung eines Teratogenitäts-Screening-Testes mit Embryonen des Zebrabärblings Danio rerio* [doctoral thesis], TU Dresden; 2002.
60. Nagel R. DarT. The embryotest with the zebrafish *Danio rerio* – a general model in ecotoxicology and toxicology. *ALTEX Alternativen zu Tierexperimenten.* 2002;19 (Suppl 1/02):38–48.
61. Ito T, Ando H, Suzuki T, et al. Identification of a Primary Target of Thalidomide Teratogenicity. *Science.* 2010;327(5971):1345–1350.

62. Stigson M, Kultima K, Jergil M, et al. Molecular targets and early response biomarkers for the prediction of developmental toxicity in vitro. *Altern Lab Anim.* 2007;35(3):335–342.
63. Busquet F, Nagel R, von Landenberg F, et al. Development of a new screening assay to identify proteratogenic substances using zebrafish Danio rerio embryo combined with an exogenous mammalian metabolic activation system (mDarT). *Toxicol Sci.* 2008;104(1):177–188.
64. Iwamatsu T. Stages of normal development in the medaka Oryzias latipes. *Mech Devel.* 2004;121(7–8):605–618.
65. Berman DM, Karhadkar SS, Hallahan AR, et al. Medulloblastoma growth inhibition by hedgehog pathway blockade. *Science.* 2002;297(5586):1559–1561.
66. Chen JK, Taipale J, Young KE, et al. Small molecule modulation of smoothened activity. *PNAS.* 2002;99(22):14071–14076.
67. Incardona J, Gaffield W, Kapur R, et al. The teratogenic Veratrum alkaloid cyclopamine inhibits sonic hedgehog signal transduction. *Development.* 1998;125(18):3553–3562.
68. Ferrari S, Yanega R. Effect of cyclopamine on medaka (*Oryzias latipes*) embryos. Course Experiment, Developmental Biology, Franklin & Marshall College. Retrieved from http://www.swarthmore.edu/NatSci/sgilber1/DB_lab/Student/Medaka_cyclo.html. 2000.
69. Büttner A, Seifert K, Cottin T, et al. Synthesis and biological evaluation of SANT-2 and analogues as inhibitors of the hedgehog signaling pathway. *Bioorg Med Chem.* 2009;17(14):4943–4954.
70. Yap YG, Camm AJ. Drug induced QT prolongation and torsades de pointes. *Heart.* 2003;89(11):1363–1372.
71. EMEA. ICH Topic S7B: The nonclinical evaluation of the potential for delayed ventricular repolarization (QT interval prolongation) by human pharmaceuticals. Retrieved from http://www.emea.europe.eu. 2005.
72. Kimmel CB, Ballard WW, Kimmel SR, et al. Stages of embryonic development of the zebrafish. *Developmental Dynamics.* 1995;203(3):253–310.
73. Chan PK, Lin CC, Cheng SH. Noninvasive technique for measurement of heartbeat regularity in zebrafish (*Danio rerio*) embryos. *BMC Biotechnol.* 2009;9:11.
74. Senior JR. Drug Hepatotoxicity from a Regulatory Perspective. *Clinics in Liver Disease.* 2007;11(3):507–524.
75. FDA. Nonclinical assessment of potential hepatotoxicity in man. Retrieved from http://www.fda.gov. 2000.
76. McGrath P, Li C-Q. Zebrafish: A predictive model for assessing drug-induced toxicity. *Drug Discov Today.* 2008;13(9–10):394–401.
77. Vanparys P, Spanhaak S, Steemans M, et al. Larvae of the zebrafish as test organism for hepatotoxicity testing. EPAA (The European partnership for alternative approaches to animal testing) 2007 Annual Conference. Poster. Retrieved from http://ec.europe.eu. 2007.
78. Foster WR, Chen S-J, He A, et al. A retrospective analysis of toxicogenomics in the safety assessment of drug candidates. *Toxicol Pathol.* 2007;35(5):621–635.
79. FDA. Memorandum of understanding between the United States Department of Health and Human Services, National Institutes of Health, National Institute on Aging, Laboratory of Neurosciences and the United States Department of Health and Human Services, Food and Drug Administration. MOU number: 225–94–3001. Retrieved from http://www.fda.gov. 1994.
80. Richards FM, Alderton WK, Kimber GM, et al. Validation of the use of zebrafish larvae in visual safety assessment. *J Pharmacol Toxicol Methods.* 2008;58:50–58.
81. Berghmans S, Butler P, Goldsmith P, et al. Zebrafish based assays for the assessment of cardiac, visual and gut function – Potential safety screens for early drug discovery. *J Pharmacol Toxicol Methods.* 2008;58:59–68.

82. Ton C, Parng C. The use of zebrafish for assessing ototoxic and otoprotective agents. *Hearing Res.* 2005;208(1–2):79–88.
83. Chiu L, Cunningham L, Raible D, et al. Using the zebrafish lateral line to screen for ototoxicity. *J Assoc Res Otolaryngol.* 2008;9(2):178–190.
84. Winter MJ, Redfern WS, Hayfield AJ, et al. Validation of a larval zebrafish locomotor assay for assessing the seizure liability of early-stage development drugs. *J Pharmacol Toxicol Methods.* 2008;57(3):176–187.
85. Giacomini NJ, Rose B, Kobayashi K, et al. Antipsychotics produce locomotor impairment in larval zebrafish. *Neurotoxicol Teratol.* 2006;28(2):245–250.
86. Milan DJ, Peterson TA, Ruskin JN, et al. Drugs that induce repolarization abnormalities cause bradycardia in zebrafish. *Circulation.* 2003;107(10):1355–1358.
87. Langheinrich U, Vacun G, Wagner T. Zebrafish embryos express an orthologue of HERG and are sensitive toward a range of QT-prolonging drugs inducing severe arrhythmia[star, open]. *Toxicol Appl Pharmacol.* 2003;193(3):370–382.
88. Mittelstadt SW, Hemenway CL, Craig MP, et al. Evaluation of zebrafish embryos as a model for assessing inhibition of hERG. *J Pharmacol Toxicol Methods.* 2008;57(2):100–105.
89. Hentschel DM, Park KM, Cilenti L, et al. Acute renal failure in zebrafish: A novel system to study a complex disease. *Am J Physiol Renal Physiol.* 2005;288(5):F923–929.
90. Herbomel P, Thisse B, Thisse C. Ontogeny and behaviour of early macrophages in the zebrafish embryo. *Development.* 1999;126(17):3735–3745.
91. van der Sar AM, Appelmelk BJ, Vandenbroucke-Grauls CM, et al. A star with stripes: Zebrafish as an infection model. *Trends Microbiol.* 2004;12(10):451–457.
92. Pressley ME, Phelan PE, Witten PE, et al. Pathogenesis and inflammatory response to *Edwardsiella tarda* infection in the zebrafish. *Dev Comp Immunol.* 2005;29(6):501–513.
93. Watzke J, Schirmer K, Scholz S. Bacterial lipopolysaccharides induce genes involved in the innate immune response in embryos of the zebrafish (*Danio rerio*). *Fish Shellfish Immunol.* 2007;23:901–905.
94. Alder AC, Bruchet A, Carballa M, et al. Consumption and occurrence. In: Ternes T, ed. *Human Pharmaceuticals, Hormones and Fragrances: The Challenge of Micropollutants in Urban Water Management.* London: IWA Publ.; 2006:15–54.
95. Heberer T. Occurrence, fate, and removal of pharmaceutical residues in the aquatic environment: a review of recent research data. *Toxicol Lett.* 2002;131(1–2):5–17.
96. Fent K. Effects of pharmaceuticals on aquatic organisms. In: Kümmer K, ed. *Pharmaceuticals in the Environment – Sources, Fate, Effects and Risks.* Berlin: Springer; 2008:175–203.
97. Sumpter JP. Environmental effects of human pharmaceuticals. *Drug Inf J.* 2007;41(2):143–147.
98. Jones OAH, Voulvoulis N, Lester JN. Aquatic environmental assessment of the top 25 English prescription pharmaceuticals. *Water Res.* 2002;36(20):5013–5022.
99. Zwiener C, Glauner T, Frimmel FH. Biodegradation of pharmaceutical residues investigated by SPE- GC/ITD-MS and on-line derivatization. *Hrc-J High Res Chromat.* 2000;23(7–8):474–478.
100. EMEA/CHMP. Guideline on the environmental risk assessment of medicinal products for human use. EMEA/CHMP/SWP/4447/00; 2006.
101. FDA. Guidance for industry – environmental assessment of human drug and biologics applications. US Department of Health and Human Services, Food and Drug Administration, CMC6, revision 1. 1998.
102. Scholz S, Schirmer K, Altenburger R. Pharmaceutical contaminants in urban water cycles – A discussion of novel concepts for environmental risk assessment. In: Kassinos F, Bester K, K ümmerer K, eds. *Xenobiotics in the Urban Water Cycle: Mass Flows, Environmental Processes and Mitigation Strategies.* Vol 16. Heidelberg: Springer; 2010.

103. OECD 210. OECD guideline for testing of chemicals. Test No. 210: Fish, early life stage toxicity test. 1992.
104. Renshaw SA, Loynes CA, Trushell DM, et al. A transgenic zebrafish model of neutrophilic inflammation. *Blood.* 2006;108(13):3976–3978.
105. Burns CG, Milan DJ, Grande EJ, et al. High-throughput assay for small molecules that modulate zebrafish embryonic heart rate. *Nat Chem Biol.* 2005;1(5):263–264.
106. Carvan MJr, Dalton TP, Stuart GW, et al. Transgenic zebrafish as sentinels for aquatic pollution. *Ann N Y Acad Sci USA.* 2000;919:133–147.
107. Russell W, Burch R. *The Principles of Humane Experimental Technique.* London: Methuen; 1959.
108. Yang L, Kemadjou J, Zinsmeister C, et al. Transcriptional profiling reveals barcode-like toxicogenomic responses in the zebrafish embryo. *Genome Biol.* 2007;8(10):R227.
109. Garner RC. Less is more: the human microdosing concept. *Drug Discov Today.* 2005;10(7):449–451.

14 The role of genetically modified mouse models in predictive toxicology

Glenn H. Cantor

14.1 OVERVIEW

14.1.1 Introduction

Genetically modified mouse models (genetically engineered mice, GEMs), a standard tool in biology for many years, are increasingly used in toxicology studies. At an early stage of pharmaceutical discovery and development, GEMs are used to validate novel targets. If safety issues emerge later, GEMs are widely used for mechanistic investigations to determine if the liability is on or off target. Newer models now incorporate specific human genes into the mouse system to better predict toxicities that are relevant to humans. GEMs have also been developed to enhance the rate of carcinogenesis, facilitating mouse carcinogenesis studies that can be done in six months instead of two years.

14.1.2 Importance of mouse strains and background genetics

One complication of GEMs is that the phenotype is often due to the interaction of many genes and is therefore strain dependent. A knockout in one strain of mice may have a specific phenotype, yet the same knockout in another strain may have a different phenotype.[1,2] Differences among strains with the same knocked-out gene are particularly notable with phenotypes that are polygenic, such as diabetes mellitus.[3,4] For example, mice that are heterozygous for knockout of both the insulin receptor and the insulin receptor substrate-1 (IRS-1) on a C57Bl/6J genetic background have a high incidence of diabetes (85 percent at 6 months of age), whereas those on a 129Sv background do not become diabetic.[3] In some cases, especially if the knockout is on a mixed genetic background, the knockout phenotype disappeared upon further breeding, much to the consternation of the investigators.[5] To have replicable results, it is important to use GEMs of specific and documented strains of inbred mice, rather than outbred mice or mice of mixed strains.

Unfortunately, the technology of making knockout mice leads to mice with mixed genetic backgrounds. Most knockouts have been made in embryonic stem cells of various 129/Sv strains of mice, and then these embryonic stem cells are implanted into blastocysts of C57Bl/6 mice of various substrains, such as C57Bl/6J or C57Bl/6N. This results in GEMs that are chimeric and include genes from both parental strains. The most common approach to obtaining GEMs with a well-defined genetic background is to backcross the mice to the desired strain for multiple generations. The gold standard is ten generations, although, because of the expense and time required, many studies have been done with fewer backcrosses.

A faster alternative to achieving congenicity is known as speed congenics.[6–8] With each generation of backcrossing, there is variability among the progeny. Specific marker loci on each chromosome that vary between two strains are amplified by PCR to determine their strain of origin. Then, individual animals that are the most similar to the desired genotype are selected for further breeding. Using speed congenics, backcrossing for approximately five generations can achieve what would otherwise require ten generations by conventional selection and breeding.

An alternative to time-consuming backcrossing is to use embryonic stem cells from the same strain as the desired genetic background. Some vendors are currently able to use C57Bl/6J embryonic stem cells, which avoids the need to backcross the mice into a C57Bl/6J background.[9]

The subject of mouse nomenclature has been reviewed extensively[10] and will not be discussed here, other than to emphasize the importance of knowing the full details of the mouse strain that is used and of using correct nomenclature to document the strain. For example, the C57Bl/6N strain diverged from the C57Bl/6J strain in 1951, when The Jackson Laboratory transferred mice to the National Institutes of Health. Due to random mutations and genetic drift, a number of genes are known that differ between the C57Bl/6J and C57Bl6/N strains. To further complicate matters, various vendors have their own colonies that are reproductively isolated from the colonies of other vendors and evolve independently. So, for example, C57Bl/6NCrl mice, which are bred by Charles River Laboratory, are genetically different from C57Bl/6NTac mice, which are bred by Taconic. Clearly, it is insufficient to refer to mice as only "C57Bl/6."

14.1.3 GEM breeding technology

GEM breeding technology has been reviewed extensively elsewhere,[11,12] so only a few salient aspects are discussed here.

Genomic versus cDNA transgenics

Mice with the identical transgenes can differ based on the regulatory elements that are included in the construct. At the simplest, cDNA of the gene of interest is cloned downstream of an exogenous transgenic promoter and injected into embryonic stem cells. Integration into the host genome occurs randomly, such that the transgene is under the influence of adjacent host enhancers and other regulatory elements, as well as host chromosomal factors. Alternatively, the gene of interest can be cloned as a complete genomic cassette, including its native exons and introns, or the gene of interest can be cloned along with flanking sequences. In those cases, provided that the flanking sequences are long enough to include the relevant regulatory elements, the transgene may be regulated in a completely different manner.

Cre-Lox system, including temporal and spatial conditional mice

The ability to create knockout mice that express genes only in specific tissues or at specific times or under specific circumstances has revolutionized biology.[13] Specific DNA sequences, termed loxP are introduced to flank the gene of interest. These sequences are recognized by the enzyme Cre recombinase, which excises the gene that is flanked by the lox sites. Key to this system is that mice can be generated in which Cre expression is under the control of tissue-specific or inducible promoters. The Cre-expressing mice are crossed with the mice in which a gene of interest is flanked by lox, resulting in deletion of the gene in the progeny. For example, if Cre is under the control of the albumin promoter, *alb*, then the gene of interest will only be knocked out in hepatocytes. In addition Cre can be fused to a mutated ligand-binding domain of the human estrogen receptor (ER), resulting in Cre expression that is activated at a specific time when the investigator gives the mice the synthetic estrogen receptor ligand, tamoxifen.[14,15] A useful database of Cre mouse lines is available electronically.[16,17]

14.1.4 Breeding timelines

An important consideration in design of GEM mice for use in predictive toxicology is the time required to generate and propagate the mice, relative to the timelines of the project. Development of the initial line of knockout mice can take one to two years, depending on the complexity of the model. After that, it must be considered that the gestation period of mice is three weeks and that mice should be approximately eight weeks old for breeding. Thus, each generation requires a minimum of eleven weeks or, more practically, three months. To expand a line of founders to sufficient numbers to do a reasonably sized study may require two or three generations (even without backcrossing to congenicity, as discussed earlier), that is six to nine months. Because of these long timelines, it is often prudent to begin work on knockout or transgenic mice as early as possible so that mice are available when needed.

14.1.5 Mouse phenotyping

Whether trying to understand the function of a gene or to validate a new target, thorough phenotyping is essential. A wide variety of phenotyping tools is available, spanning essentially all biological methods.[12,18–22] Some vendors and academic core facilities now offer quite comprehensive phenotyping packages.[23–27] Common techniques include gross, microscopic, and clinical pathology; radiography; behavioral observations and tests; physiological measurements; and immunological assays. More recently, some investigators are using metabonomics to assess GEM strains.[28,29] Any of these techniques also can be used with animals that are challenged in a variety of ways. For example, many researchers do oral glucose tolerance tests as part of routine phenotyping of knockouts. Others have measured phenotypic behavioral endpoints after exposure to behavioral stressors[30,31] or evaluated cardiovascular phenotypes after exercise.[32]

If one is routinely phenotyping a number of GEM strains, it is important to develop an organized, consistent, yet flexible strategy. In general, one only finds what one looks for, so it is desirable to use as comprehensive an approach as possible. On the other hand, every researcher is constrained by economic limitations, so an appropriate balance must be achieved. One widely used approach is to have a core battery of tests that is done on all new knockout strains and then to have flexible batteries of tests that are specific to the project or therapeutic area.[19]

14.1.6 Value of heterozygotes or hypomorphs

A limitation of knockout mice as a model of the effects of an inhibitory drug is that the gene of interest is entirely eliminated in the GEM, yet many drugs only partially inhibit the function of their target. Sometimes, the heterozygote knockout, in which there may be partial expression of the gene of interest, can be a more accurate model. Heterozygotes are also of potential value when the homozygous knockout is embryonically lethal; the heterozygotes may be viable and allow the investigation to proceed.[33] Hypomorphs, which have reduced expression of the gene of interest, can also be generated. Insertions of the *Neo* cassette into introns[34,35] or upstream regions[36,37] have been used to interfere with transcription and reduce gene expression. Some researchers have generated a hypomorphic series, a set of GEM mice in which expression is graded. For example, Lin et al.[38] inserted a *Neo* cassette to develop a hypomorphic strain of mouse with reduced expression of the aryl hydrocarbon receptor-associated protein-9, Ara9, termed Ara9(*fxneo/fxneo*A). They then crossed *Ara9* wild type (+/+), null (–/–), and hypomorphic (Ara9(*fxneo/fxneo*)) mice. This resulted in mice with a series of genotypes, including +/+, +/*fxneo*, +/–, *fxneo/fxneo*, and the –/– control. Among these five lines of mice, expression of Ara9 was 100 percent, 60 percent, 50 percent, 10 percent, and nil, respectively. The advantages of this sophisticated approach are that a full dose-response relationship can be explored and the effects of an inhibitory drug may be better modeled, although the expense of developing these cohorts of mice may preclude widespread use.

14.1.7 Knockdowns (siRNA, shRNA, antisense)

An alternative method to reduce gene expression without eliminating it ("knockdown") is to use antisense or siRNA (small interfering RNA).[39,40] This can either be delivered systemically at the beginning of the experiment, or the mice can be genetically engineered to express inheritable shRNA (small hairpin RNA), which is then converted to siRNA.[41] Considerable commercial interest has built around exogenous delivery of siRNA and antisense, and that topic will not be reviewed here. The genetic approach is increasingly popular. An advantage of this approach is that knockdowns often can be prepared much faster than conventional GEMs.[39,42] As with knockouts, shRNA-driven knockdowns can be temporally inducible. Seibler et al. have reported development of mice that express inducible shRNA (short hairpin RNA) to knockdown expression of the insulin receptor, resulting in mice with type 2 diabetes.[43] In that model, the authors used a modified tetracycline resistance repressor that was inducible upon the administration of doxycycline. Upon withdrawal of doxycycline, the diabetic phenotype reversed.

Of perhaps great future promise for toxicology, transgenic rats that express inducible shRNA to inhibit a gene of interest, in this case the insulin receptor, have recently been generated.[44] This approach circumvents a major difficulty of generating knockouts in rats, the lack of embryonic stem cells for gene targeting by homologous recombination (see Section 14.1.6).

14.2 USE OF GEMS IN TARGET SAFETY VALIDATION

One of the major uses of GEMs in drug discovery is validation of the safety of a proposed target. A mouse that lacks a particular protein can be a model for a patient in whom that protein is inhibited by a drug. One can then ask in the mouse model if there are any unexpected phenotypic abnormalities or adverse effects that might predict side effects in humans who are dosed with the drug.

As an example, when beta-secretase (BACE1) was proposed as a target for Alzheimer's disease, several groups phenotyped the BACE1 knockout mouse. The mice had normal phenotypes, thus providing more confidence in the safety of compounds designed to inhibit BACE1.[45,46]

If unexpected phenotypic abnormalities are discovered, there are multiple strategic options. One option is to decide that, based on the GEM phenotyping data, the risk of adverse effects is too great and the decision is made to immediately drop the project. An alternative option is to first verify the observed phenotypic effect in the mouse model and then, if positive, investigate the potential liability. Sometimes, the observed phenotype, upon further investigation, proves to be spurious. For example, in an initial phenotypic screen to validate a novel target, one of four individual knockouts was identified with reduced bone density in a vertebra, by micro-CT imaging (Figure 14.1). This initial observation caused us to initiate a larger study to confirm the initial observations. Six groups of nine mice per group were compared (wild type, heterozygous, and homozygous knockouts of both genders), and thirteen morphometric measures of cortical and trabecular bone architecture were made. There were no significant differences between the knockouts and wild type in quantitative measurements of bone architecture, and the study was unable to confirm the initial observations. To pursue the issue, we performed a second study to test potential interactions of the knockout with a well-established model of bone loss, gonadectomy. In that study, we compared wild type versus

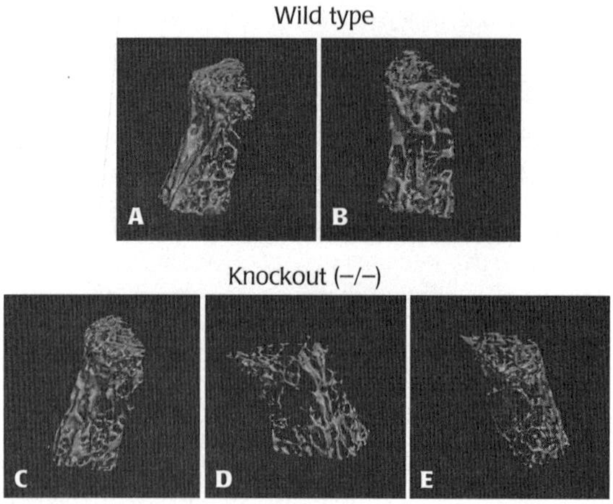

Figure 14-1: Fifth lumbar vertebra of wild type mice (A and B) versus knockout mice (C, D, and E). Micro-CT image. Note reduced bone density in D.

knockout mice of each gender, either intact or gonadectomized (eight mice/group). While gonadectomy produced profound changes in bone architecture in both genders, the knockout did not contribute to the observed changes. From that study, we concluded that bone density loss was not a great risk, and chemistry efforts continued to identify a suitable compound.

Identification of phenotypic abnormalities in knockout mice at the early stage of target validation is also valuable in guiding the safety assessment program. The abnormality may be one that is not routinely assessed in early toxicology testing (e.g., bone density, as discussed previously); knowing that it may be a liability is valuable in tailoring the toxicology studies to fit the specific program. Also, an early alert can help in designing appropriate biomarkers for clinical assessment.

A critical question is whether the adverse effect is likely to occur in humans. To answer this, genetic and mechanistic understanding is important. Obviously, the biology of mice and humans differ, and for many reasons, effects in the mouse may not validly predict effects in humans. Humanized GEMs are discussed more in Section 14.5. Another consideration is whether the effect is due to early embryonic or prenatal effects in the GEM model. Since it is likely that a drug that inhibits the target of interest will be given to adult humans, early embryonic or prenatal effects may be irrelevant, except as they may predict reproductive toxicity (Section 14.7). It is also necessary to consider the effects of partial inhibition. Many inhibitory drugs do not inhibit the target completely or may block only some functions of the target without complete abrogation, and in that sense, a knockout model can be misleading (see Section 14.1.6).

Failure of a GEM model to predict human risk can also be due to technical reasons. One is that the mouse knockout may delete not only the gene of interest but other genes as well, which may not be relevant to humans. Alternative splicing may result in a particular exon being used to encode multiple proteins, including ones that are not even known. Knockout of that exon can simultaneously delete expression not only of the protein of interest but also of other proteins encoded by that exon, and the phenotypic effect may be due to lack of those proteins, rather than the one of interest. That is, the "specific" knockout may not be as specific as the investigator thinks.

Broader issues also should be considered. One is the severity and impact of the effect and how easy it would be to monitor and reverse the toxicity in clinical trials. The therapeutic indication is important, particularly when assessing if the toxicity is tolerable for the disease indication. For example, a low-grade toxicity may be acceptable as a side effect of a cancer drug, yet it may be completely intolerable with a drug designed to control obesity. More broadly, the company's overall portfolio balance and how much risk the company is prepared to accept for the particular project come to bear on decision making.

These issues are discussed in more detail in Chapter 12.

14.3 USE OF GEMS IN ON- OR OFF-TARGET LIABILITY ASSESSMENT

If toxicity is seen early in drug development, it is important to determine whether the toxicity is on- or off-target. On-target toxicity is when inhibiting (or stimulating) the molecular target not only has the intended therapeutic effect but also causes adverse effects. This can be due to altering a target with multiple biological functions or a target that is distributed in various tissues other than the intended ones. In contrast, off-target toxicity, also called compound-specific toxicity, is due to adverse effects caused by interaction of the compound with other, unintended targets.

The importance of determining whether toxicity is on or off target lies in the different approaches taken to mitigate the toxicity. If the toxicity is on target, then the considerations discussed in Section 14.2 are important. If the toxicity is off target, the solution is often to design a different molecule or chemotype. There is great economic advantage to identifying off-target toxicities as early as possible in the drug discovery and development process so that resources are not wasted and can be diverted to more successful molecules. In this respect, it is quite helpful if the mechanism of off-target toxicity can be identified. For example, if toxicity is due to interaction of a compound with another receptor, then a molecular counterscreen can be designed to exclude future compounds that interact with that receptor.

GEM models can be useful in identifying off-target toxicities (Figure 14.2). If a knockout does not have an adverse phenotype, but the compound has an adverse effect, then the compound can be tested in the knockout model. If the adverse effect is seen in the knockout, that is, in the absence of the intended target, then the effect must be off target.

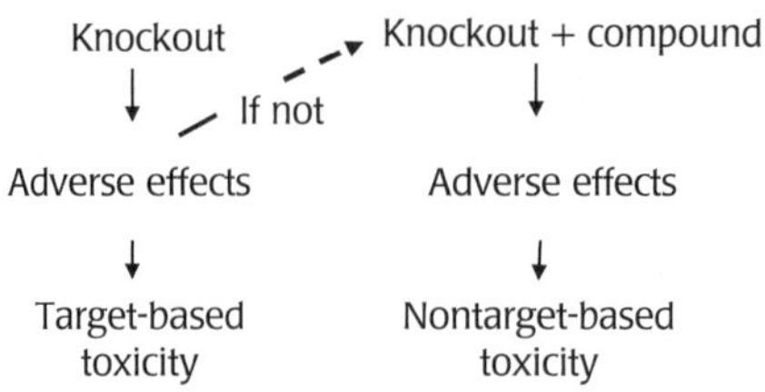

Figure 14-2: Use of GEM models to evaluate on- or off-target toxicity.

14.4 GEMS FOR MORE RAPID CARCINOGENESIS STUDIES

Two-year carcinogenesis studies in rats and mice are a significant time and resource barrier to drug development. Accordingly, there has been considerable work to reduce these timelines by using rodents that are already more prone to carcinogenesis. Using these models, mouse carcinogenicity studies can be conducted in six months instead of two years. Because of the impact of the results on human health and on corporate economics, extensive formal validation,[47] as well as acceptance by regulatory agencies, was essential before these models could be used. Currently, the mouse models are considered supplemental to the conventional two-year rat carcinogenicity study.[48] Because the focus of this book is the earlier stages of drug development, carcinogenesis models will be reviewed only briefly here.

Presently, three GEM models are in use for accelerated (six-month) carcinogenicity testing and their utility has been reviewed.[49,50] The p53 heterozygotic ($p53^{+/-}$) mouse, in which one allele of the p53 tumor suppressor gene has been deleted, is used for genotoxic compounds,[51] the Tg.RasH2 mouse, which contains multiple transgenic copies of the human c-Ha-ras oncogene, is used for genotoxic or nongenotoxic compounds,[52–54] and the Tg.AC mouse,which has multiple copies of a zeta-globulin promoter-driven v-Ha-ras oncogene, is used for dermal genotoxins.[55,56] Of these, the $p53^{+/-}$ has been the most extensively used in the U.S. pharmaceutical industry.[50]

14.5 HUMANIZED GEMS

14.5.1 Mouse versus human targets

A weakness of any GEM model is that the mouse system does not always faithfully replicate human biology. This is a particular problem when a compound only interacts with the human target and not with the rodent target. Guided mainly by the need for efficacy models, a number of mouse models have been generated which express the human target. Typically, the mouse target is first knocked out and then the human target is added (referred to as "knockout–knock-in"). As a spin-off from efficacy testing, humanized models are also quite useful in early safety testing. This is particularly important for the development of biologicals such as monoclonal antibodies, which often are human specific. Some biologicals cross-react with chimpanzee target molecules, but chimpanzees are an endangered species and pharmaceutical testing is necessarily limited.

As an example, Herzyk et al.[57] used mouse CD4 knockout–human CD4 transgenic mice to examine the immunomodulatory properties of a therapeutic CD4 antibody. As part of the safety investigation, they demonstrated that it altered the immune system in specific ways but did not cause general immunosuppression.

One risk in generating humanized knockout–knock-in models is that even though they express the human target protein, they may not express the appropriate intracellular signaling or regulatory proteins that are necessary for the biological effect. As a way around this problem, some investigators have chosen to express chimeric molecules, which have the extracellular portion of the human molecule and the intracellular portion of the mouse molecule.[58] Of course, this strategy depends on which part of the target molecule the drug interacts with and how the target molecule interacts with other host molecules to transduce a signal.

Another weakness is that, even though the specific human target gene is expressed, there may be other human genes that are not expressed that could mediate off-target toxicity. Accordingly, these off-target toxicities might be missed in the humanized knockout–knock-in model. Another potential problem is that transgenics can overexpress the gene of interest, due to insertion of multiple copies of the transgene into the host genome, and this may alter the biology of the humanized target protein.

14.5.2 Humanized metabolism models

Some toxicities are driven by metabolism. Drug metabolites can be more toxic or can have effects that were not predicted by the behavior of the parent drug. Drug-induced up- or down-regulation of nuclear hormone receptors such as PXR and CAR can alter cytochrome P450 levels, resulting in altered metabolism of many exogenous and endogenous compounds.[59–61] Drug-induced changes in hepatocyte or biliary transporters can be instrumental in driving toxicities.[62]

A variety of GEM models are now available in which aspects of mouse metabolism have been replaced by their human counterparts. Mice with knocked-out mouse pregnane X receptor (mPXR) and knocked-in human PXR (hPXR) have been available for some time. Now, mice with knocked-out mouse constitutive androstane receptor (mCAR) and knocked-in human CAR (hCAR) and mice with both hPXR and hCAR have been generated.[63]

Another interesting and novel set of GEM models has linked regulatory elements of relevance to toxicology to genes encoding secreted reporter proteins. For example, the antioxidant response element (ARE) has been linked to the human chorionic gonadotropin (hCG) beta chain gene to produce a urinary marker that is detectible with an antibody in an ELISA format.[64] Mice with this construct are presently under development.

14.5.3 Humanized liver models

Although not strictly a genetically engineered mouse model, mice have been developed in which mouse hepatocytes have been replaced by human hepatocytes. These mice have been used for metabolism and toxicity testing,[65–69] although perhaps their most valuable application is for focused mechanistic *in vivo* studies.

The mice are immunodeficient (*scid/scid*) so that they can receive engraftment, and they express the transgene *alb-uPA* (urokinase-type plasminogen activator, driven by the albumin promoter).[70] The urokinase-type plasminogen activator, when expressed in hepatocytes, kills the hepatocytes by apoptosis, and the *alb* promoter drives expression in the relevant cell, the hepatocyte.[71] The advantage of this model is that the hepatocytes die shortly after birth, but the architecture of the liver, including portal areas, central veins, the reticulin network, and the biliary tree, is preserved. Then, cryopreserved human hepatocytes are injected into the spleen, from which they are taken up by the splanchnic circulation and carried home to the liver. A weakness of the model is that occasional mouse hepatocytes remain and regrow, presumably under the influence of mouse hepatocyte growth factor. Accordingly, the livers are a mixture or chimera of human and mouse hepatocytes. The quantitative nature of the mixture can be determined by measuring human versus mouse serum albumin. Presently, mice are available in which the livers contain up to 95 percent human hepatocytes.[72] The mice produced by a company in Japan (PhoenixBio) are not available in the United States or Europe; studies using the mice are done at the company, which operates a contract research organization to perform studies using the mice.[72]

14.6 GENETICALLY ENGINEERED RATS

Rats are a species of choice for many toxicologists, due to the large historical toxicology database, personal and institutional experience, and the ability to draw multiple blood samples from individual animals. A barrier to developing knockout rats has been the lack of suitable rat embryonic stem cells. Transgenic rats, including ones with human genes under the control of tissue-specific promoters, have been used for a number of studies[73–75] and are available from vendors.[76] One drawback, however, of making knock-in rats that express human genes of interest is that the transgenic rat still expresses the rat orthologous gene. In some cases, this may complicate the biology or toxicology of the experiment. More recently, knockout rats have become available,[76–78] and this allows the construction of true knockout–knock-in rats that only express the human gene of interest and do not express the rat orthologue. An alternative method to reduce expression of a gene of interest in rats is to use shRNA. Recently, an shRNA targeted to the insulin receptor was introduced as a transgene to rats, resulting in dramatic knockdown of the insulin receptor and development of marked hyperglycemia.[44]

One feature to consider with rat models is that, in general, the rat host is outbred. For example, the Sprague-Dawley rat has been used commonly for transgenesis. This can be either an advantage or a disadvantage. It could be argued that the genetically modified outbred host is robust and perhaps more representative of the population as a whole, but genetic manipulation of animals of mixed genetic backgrounds can make it difficult sometimes to replicate results.

14.7 GEM PITFALLS AND CAVEATS

A major pitfall with GEM models is the complex network of modifier and regulatory genes, a network that can vary among different strains. Accordingly, the phenotype of a mouse with a particular knockout may vary depending on the strain of mouse into which the knockout is introduced. A further complexity is introduced by the use of embryonic stem cells of the so-called "129 strain," which actually consists of numerous strains,[10] and the interbreeding that follows as mouse lines are developed. One recent improvement is the development of C57Bl/6J embryonic stem cells, which allows much more rapid development of mice with a uniform genetic background.

In addition to specific modification of the gene of interest by strain-specific aspects of the mouse genome, it is also important to consider the normal phenotypic features of the background strain. Each mouse strain carries its own attributes. For example, mice of the C57Bl/6J strain often exhibit excessive grooming, sometimes of one particular spot on the skin, or barbering (grooming of other mice), resulting in focal hair loss or even chronically inflamed skin. This inflammation can result in amyloidosis, to which C57Bl/6J mice are also susceptible.[5,19] Since the excessive grooming, hair loss, and focal skin inflammation are only sporadic, the traits sometimes can be seen just by chance only in the genetically modified individuals in a study and not in the control mice. This should not be interpreted as a phenotype caused by the gene of interest, without additional work to verify the assertion. Other traits that are prevalent in C57Bl/6J mice include hydrocephalus, microphthalmia, corneal opacities or corneal mineralization, deafness, and melanosis of the spleen and organs. Phenotyping of GEM models can be quite tricky, and, to avoid embarrassing errors, the participation of a qualified comparative pathologist is critically important.[79–81]

Other caveats of interpreting GEM results stem from the biology itself. With conventional knockouts, the gene of interest is absent from the embryonic stage onward. Clearly, this does not mimic the onset of drug therapy by an adult patient. In the absence of the gene of interest, the developing knockout mouse may adapt alternative endogenous biochemical pathways to make up for the insufficiency. One may need to knock out the gene of interest only at particular times of the mouse lifecycle, using temporally inducible knockouts.

Another caveat is the specificity of the GEM model. A "specific" knockout may not be as specific as claimed, if deletion of a key exon, for example, results in the loss of other proteins that rely on alternative splicing. With transgenics, if the gene of interest is inadvertently inserted into another gene, the expression of that gene may be abrogated, resulting in a phenotypic effect unrelated to the gene of interest.

14.8 CONCLUSIONS

Clearly, GEM models can be highly useful in predictive toxicology. Recognition of pitfalls and caveats is important to avoid being misled by results. With the availability of more advanced models, including humanized models and models that use reporter genes, the use of GEM models will only increase in the field of toxicology and pharmacology.

REFERENCES

1. Harvey M, McArthur MJ, Montgomery CA, Jr., et al. Genetic background alters the spectrum of tumors that develop in *p53*-deficient mice. *FASEB J.* 1993;7:938–943.
2. Donehower LA, Harvey M, Vogel H, et al. Effects of genetic background on tumorigenesis in *p53*-deficient mice. *Molec Carcinogen.* 1995;14:16–22.
3. Kulkarni RN, Almind K, Goren HJ, et al. Impact of genetic background on development of hyperinsulinemia and diabetes in insulin receptor/insulin receptor substrate-1 double heterozygous mice. *Diabetes.* 2003;52:1528–1534.
4. Goren HJ, Kulkarni RN, Kahn CR. Glucose homeostasis and tissue transcript content of insulin signaling intermediates in four inbred strains of mice: C57Bl/6, C57BLK/6, DBA/2, and 129X1. *Endocrinology.* 2004;145:3307–3323.
5. Barthold S. "Muromics": Genomics from the perspective of the laboratory mouse. *Comp Med.* 2002;52(3):206–223.
6. The Jackson Laboratory. Speed congenic development service. 2010. Retrieved from http://jaxservices.jax.org/speedcongenic.html.
7. Wakeland E, Morel L, Achey K, et al. Speed congenics: A classic technique in the fast lane (relatively speaking). *Immunol Today.* 1997;18(10):472–477.
8. Markel P, Shu P, Ebeling C, et al. Theoretical and empirical issues for marker-assisted breeding of congenic mouse strains. *Nat Genet.* 1997;17:280–284.
9. Taconic Artemis. Model generation. 2010. Retrieved from http://www.taconic.com/wmspage.cfm?parm1=1474.
10. Simpson EM, Linder CC, Sargent EE, et al. Genetic variation among 129 substrains and its importance for targeted mutagenesis in mice. *Nat Genet.* May 1997;16(1):19–27.
11. Tymms MJ, Kola I. *Gene knockout protocols.* Totawa, NJ: Humana Press; 2001.
12. Ward JM, Mahler JF, Maronpot RR, et al. *Pathology of Genetically Engineered Mice.* 1st ed. Ames: Iowa State University Press; 2000.
13. Orban PC, Chui D, Marth JD. Tissue- and site-specific DNA recombination in transgenic mice. *Proc Natl Acad Sci USA.* 1992;89:6861–6865.
14. Metzger D, Chambon P. Site- and time-specific gene targeting in the mouse. *Methods.* 2001;24:71–80.
15. Feil S, Valtcheva N, Feil R. Inducible Cre mice. In: K ühn R, Wurst W, eds. *Gene Knockout Protocols.* 2nd ed. New York: Humana Press; 2009:343–363.
16. Nagy Laboratory. CreXmice database. 2010. Retrieved from http://www.mshri.on.ca/nagy/.
17. Nagy A, Mar L, Watts G. Creation and use of a Cre recombinase transgenic database. In: K ühn R, Wurst W, eds. *Gene knockout protocols.* 2nd ed. New York: Humana Press; 2009:365–378.

18. Sundberg JP, Boggess D. *Systematic Approach to Evaluation of Mouse Mutations*. 1st ed. Boca Raton, FL: CRC Press; 2000.
19. Brayton C, Justice M, Montgomery CA. Evaluating mutant mice: Anatomic pathology. *Vet Pathol*. 2001;38(1):1–19.
20. Crawley JN. *What's Wrong with My Mouse: Behavioral Phenotyping of Transgenic and Knockout Mice*. 2nd ed. Wilmington, DE: Wiley-Liss; 2007.
21. Papaioannou VE, Behringer RR. *Mouse Phenotypes: A Handbook of Mutation Analysis*. 1st ed. Cold Spring Harbor, NY: Cold Spring Harbor Laboratory Press; 2004.
22. de Angelis MH, Brown S, Chambon P. *Standards of Mouse Model Phenotyping*. Hoboken, NJ: John Wiley & Sons; 2006.
23. Taconic. Phenotypic characterization: Phenotac™. 2010. Retrieved from http://www.taconic.com/wmspage.cfm?parm1=3726.
24. The Jackson Laboratory. Phenotyping services. 2010. Retrieved from http://jaxservices.jax.org/phenotyping/index.html.
25. Charles River. Phenotyping Services. 2010. Retrieved from http://www.criver.com/en-US/ProdServ/ByType/Discovery/Pages/PhenotypingServices.aspx.
26. Frimorfo. Services and products. 2010. Retrieved from http://www.frimorfo.com/services_products/servicesproducts.shtml.
27. Taconic. Phenotyping services. 2010. Retrieved from http://www.taconic.com/wmspage.cfm?parm1=1640.
28. Zhen Y, Krausz KW, Chen C, et al. Metabolomic and genetic analysis of biomarkers for peroxisome proliferator-activated receptor alpha expression and activation. *Molec Endocrinol*. 2007;21:2136–2151.
29. Pears MR, Cooper JD, Mitchison HM, et al. High resolution 1H NMR-based metabolomics indicates a neurotransmitter cycling deficit in cerebral tissue from a mouse model of Batten disease. *J Biol Chem*. 2005;280:42508–42514.
30. Burne TH, Johnston AN, McGrath JJ, et al. Swimming behaviour and post-swimming activity in Vitamin D receptor knockout mice. *Brain Res Bull*. 2006;69:74–78.
31. Karl T, Duffy L, Herzog H. Behavioural profile of a new mouse model for NPY deficiency. *Eur J Neurosci*. 2008;28:173–180.
32. Bernstein D. Exercise assessment of transgenic models of human cardiovascular disease. *Physiol Genom*. 2003;13:217–226.
33. Holzenberger M, Dupont J, Ducos B, et al. IGF-1 receptor regulates lifespan and resistance to oxidative stress in mice. *Nature*. 2003;421:182–187.
34. Walisser JA, Bunger MK, Glover E, et al. Patent ductus venosus and dioxin resistance in mice harboring a hypomorphic *Arnt* allele. *J Biol Chem*. 2004;279:16326–16331.
35. Trotman LC, Niki M, Dotan ZA, et al. Pten dose dictates cancer progression in the prostate. *PLoS Biol*. 2003;1(3):385–396.
36. McDevitt MA, Shivdasani RA, Fujiwara Y, et al. A "knockdown" mutation created by cis-element gene targeting reveals the dependence of erythroid cell maturation on the level of transcription factor GATA-1. *Proc Natl Acad Sci USA*. 1997;94:6781–6785.
37. Morita M, Ohneda O, Yamashita T, et al. HLF/HIF-2α is a key factor in retinopathy of prematurity in association with erythropoietin. *EMBO J*. 2003;22:1134–1146.
38. Lin BC, Nguyen LP, Walisser JA, et al. A hypomorphic allele of *Aryl Hydrocarbon Receptor-Associated Protein-9* produces a phenocopy of the *Ahr*-null mouse. *Molec Pharmacol*. 2008;74:1367–1371.
39. Seibler J, Küter-Luks B, Kern H, et al. Single copy shRNA configuration for ubiquitous gene knockdown in mice. *Nucleic Acids Res*. 2005;33:e67.
40. Tiscornia G, Singer O, Ikawa M, et al. A general method for gene knockdown in mice by using lentiviral vectors expressing small interfering mRNA. *Proc Natl Acad Sci USA*. 2003;100:1844–1848.
41. Hitz C, Steuber-Buchberger P, Delic S, et al. Generation of shRNA transgenic mice. In: K ühn R, Wurst W, eds. *Gene Knockout Protocols*. 2nd ed. New York: Humana Press; 2009:101–129.

42. Taconic. Gene knock down *in vivo* by RNAi. 2010. Retrieved from http://www.taconic.com/wmspage.cfm?parm1=1799.
43. Seibler J, Kleinridders A, Küter-Luks B, et al. Reversible gene knockdown in mice using a tight, inducible shRNA expression system. *Nucleic Acids Res.* 2007;35:e54.
44. Herold MJ, van den Brandt J, Seibler J, et al. Inducible and reversible gene silencing by stable integration of an shRNA-encoding lentivirus in transgenic rats. *Proc Natl Acad Sci USA.* 2008;105:18507–18512.
45. Luo Y, Bolon B, Kahn S, et al. Mice deficient in BACE1, the Alzheimer's beta-secretase, have normal phenotype and abolished beta-amyloid generation. *Nat Neurosci.* 2001;4(3):231–232.
46. Roberds SL, Anderson J, Basi G, et al. BACE knockout mice are healthy despite lacking the primary beta-secretase activity in brain: implications for Alzheimer's disease therapeutics. *Human Molec Genet.* 2001;10(12):1317–1324.
47. Robinson DE, MacDonald JS. Background and framework for ILSI's collaborative evaluation program on alternative models for carcinogenicity assessment. *Toxicol Pathol.* 2001;29S:13–19.
48. Food and Drug Administration. Guidance for Industry S1B: Testing for carcinogenicity of pharmaceuticals; 1997:1–10.
49. Alden C, Smith P, Morton D. Application of genetically altered models as replacement for the lifetime mouse bioassay in pharmaceutical development. *Toxicol Pathol.* 2002;30:135–138.
50. McDonald J, French JE, Gerson RJ, et al. The utility of genetically modified mouse assays for identifying human carcinogens: A basic understanding and path forward. *Toxicol Sci.* 2004;77:188–194.
51. Storer RD, French JE, Haseman J, et al. p53+/– hemizygous knockout mouse: Overview of available data. *Toxicol Pathol.* 2001;29S:30–50.
52. Tamaoki N. The rasH2 transgenic mouse: Nature of the model and mechanistic studies on tumorigenesis. *Toxicol Pathol.* 2001;29S:81–89.
53. Tamaoki N. The rasH2 transgenic mouse: Nature of the model and mechanistic studies on tumorigenesis. *Toxicol Pathol.* 2001;29S:81–89.
54. Morton D, Alden CL, Roth AJ, et al. The Tg rasH2 mouse in cancer hazard identification. *Toxicol Pathol.* 2002;30:139–146.
55. Tennant R, Stasiewicz S, Eastin WC, et al. The Tg.AC (v-Ha-ras) transgenic mouse: Nature of the model. *Toxicol Pathol.* 2001;29S:51–59.
56. Eastin WC, Mennear JH, Tennant R, et al. Tg.AC genetically altered mouse: Assay working group overview of available data. *Toxicol Pathol.* 2001;29S:60–80.
57. Herzyk DJ, Gore ER, Polsky R, et al. Immunomodulatory effects of anti-CD4 antibody in host resistance against infections and tumors in human CD4 transgenic mice. *Infec Immun.* 2001;69:1032–1043.
58. Ohno S, Ono N, Seki F, et al. Measles virus infection of SLAM (CD150) knockin mice reproduces tropism and immunosuppression in human infection. *J Virol.* 2007;81:1650–1659.
59. Nelson SD. Drug-drug interactions: Toxicological perspectives. In: Rodrigues AD, ed. *Drug–Drug Interactions.* 2nd ed. New York: Informa Healthcare; 2008:687–708.
60. Reschly EJ, Krasowski MD. Evolution and function of the NR1I nuclear hormone receptor subfamily (VDR, PXR, and CAR) with respect to metabolism of xenobiotics and endogenous compounds. *Curr Drug Metab.* 2006;7:349–365.
61. Parkinson A, Ogilvie BW. Biotransformation of xenobiotics. In: Klaasen CD, ed. *Casarett & Doull's Toxicology: The Basic Science of Poisons.* 7th ed. New York: McGraw Hill Medical; 2008:161–304.
62. Lehman-McKeeman LD. Absorption, distribution, and excretion of toxicants. In: Klaasen CD, ed. *Casarett and Doull's Toxicology: The Basic Science of Poisons.* 7th ed. New York: McGraw Hill Medical; 2008:131–159.

63. Scheer N, Ross J, Rode A, et al. A novel panel of mouse models to evaluate the role of human pregnane X receptor and constitutive androstane receptor in drug response. *J Clin Invest.* 2008;118:3228–3239.
64. CXR Biosciences. Tox Reporter models. 2010. Retrieved from http://www.cxrbiosciences.com/page/CXR_Biosciences_Toxicity_Reporter_models_99.html.
65. Tateno C, Yoshizane Y, Saito N, et al. Near completely humanized liver in mice shows human-type metabolic responses to drugs. *Am J Pathol.* 2004;165:901–912.
66. Aoki K, Kashiwagura Y, Horie T, et al. Characterization of humanized liver from chimeric mice using coumarin as a human CYP2A6 and mouse CYP2A5 probe. *Drug Metab Pharmacokinet.* 2006;21:277–285.
67. Nishimura M, Yoshitsugu H, Yokoi T, et al. Evaluation of mRNA expression of human drug-metabolizing enzymes and transporters in chimeric mouse with humanized liver. *Xenobiotica.* 2005;35:877–890.
68. Katoh M, Watanabe M, Tabata T, et al. In vivo induction of human cytochrome P450 3A4 by rifabutin in chimeric mice with humanized liver. *Xenobiotica.* 2005;35:863–875.
69. Katoh M, Matsui T, Okumura H, et al. Expression of human phase II enzymes in chimeric mice with humanized liver. *Drug Metab Disposit.* 2005;33:1333–1340.
70. Sandgren EP, Palmiter RD, Heckel JL, et al. Complete hepatic regeneration after somatic deletion of an albumin-plasminogen activator transgene. *Cell.* 1991;66:245–256.
71. Rhim JA, Sandgren EP, Palmiter RD, et al. Complete reconstitution of mouse liver with xenogeneic hepatocytes. *Proc Natl Academy of Sci USA.* 1995;92:4942–4946.
72. PhoenixBio. PXB mouse services. 2010. Retrieved from http://www.phoenixbio.co.jp/en/activities/pxb/index.html.
73. Herrara A, Oberdorf-Maass S, Rother T, et al. Overexpression of the sarcolemmal calcium pump in the myocardium of transgenic rats. *Circ Res.* 1998;83:877–888.
74. Roebuck BD, Johnson DN, Sutter CH, et al. Transgenic expression of aflatoxin aldehyde reductase (AKR7A1) modulates aflatoxin B1 metabolism but not hepatic carcinogenesis in the rat. *Toxicol Sci.* 2009;109:41–49.
75. Zhang W, Purchio AF, Coffee R, et al. Differential regulation of the human Cyp3A4 promoter in transgenic mice and rats. *Drug Metab Disposit.* 2003;32:163–167.
76. GenOway. GenOway. 2010. Retrieved from http://www.genoway.com/.
77. Transposagen. 2010. Transposagen. Retrieved from http://www.transposagenbio.com/.
78. Ostertag EM, Madison BB, Kano H. Mutagenesis in rodents using the L1 retrotransposon. *Genome Biol.* 2007;8(Suppl 1):S16.11–S16.19.
79. Bolon B, Brayton C, Cantor GH, et al. Editorial: Best pathology practices in research using genetically engineered mice. *Vet Pathol.* 2008;45:939–940.
80. Ince TA, Ward JM, Valli VE, et al. Do-it-yourself (DIY) pathology. *Nat Biotechnol.* 2008;26:978–979.
81. Cardiff RD, Ward JM, Barthold S. 'One medicine – one pathology': Are veterinary and human pathology prepared? *Lab Invest.* 2008;88:18–26.

15 Toxicogenomic and pathway analysis

Bin Lu, Ying Jiang, and Chester Ni

Toxicogenomics is the use of genomic technology for evaluating toxic potential of chemicals. It allows for large-scale study of gene expression changes associated with toxicity endpoints. While toxicogenomics brings greater access to information of chemical effects on gene expression than ever before, it presents unprecedented challenges to data analysis and interpretation, which is crucial if we want to turn the new available information into risk assessment knowledge that helps decision making.

In this chapter, we start with background information of toxicogenomics and its applications, challenges, and progress. We then focus on toxicogenomics data analysis by first highlighting the impact of study design, followed by a review of biological pathway and network, including their application to data analysis. Finally we discuss some case study by pathway approach. Even though this chapter largely focuses on transcription-based technologies, the study of toxicogenomics covers a far broader scope, including proteomics, metabonomics, and, by a broad definition, pharmacogenetics that links underlying genetics to different susceptibilities to toxicants. Indeed, an integral analysis of toxicity often calls for incorporating other 'Omics such as proteomics and metabonomics.

15.1 INTRODUCTION TO TOXICOGENOMICS

With the advance of genome sequencing and availability of chip technology in the late 1990s, study of the genome-wide effect of toxicants become possible. Spawning the field of toxicogenomics is a drive from applied genomics. Whereas it began with cDNA arrays custom designed for toxicology,[1] commercial whole genome chip for toxicologically important species such as rat, mouse, or dog soon become available and is being used in a variety of toxicogenomics studies. As a result, a wealth of information has been generated at academic research labs and chemical and pharmaceutical companies.

Toxicogenomics is being increasingly applied to a wide range of fields from drug discovery to environmental health surveillance, and its reported reference has witnessed a rapid growth over the past decade as shown in Figure 15.1, compared

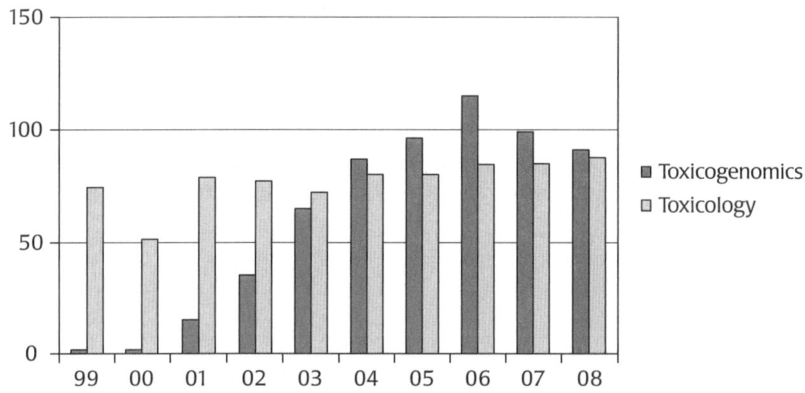

Figure 15-1: Toxicogenomics literature has shown a rapid increase over the last decade. PubMed (http://www.ncbi.nlm.nih.gov) literature number was surveyed per year over the past decade using the key term "toxicogenomics" and "toxicology," respectively. The number from "toxicology" is divided by a factor of 50 to be normalized with that of "toxicogenomics" as the absolute count for "toxicology" paper is still bigger.

with the relative flat number of general toxicology studies over the same period. At the same time, a number of database initiatives in both public and private sectors serve as repositories for toxicogenomics data. For example, public effort includes chemical effects in biological systems (CEBS)[2] by the National Institute of Environmental Health Sciences (NIEHS) and ArrayTrack[3] championed by Food and Drug Administration (FDA)'s National Center for Toxicological Research (FDA/NCTR). Both ArrayExpress at EBI and Gene Expression Omnibus (GEO) by National Center of Biological Information (NCBI) host substantial toxicogenomics data, though they are for microarray data of general purpose. In the commercial arena, GeneLogic's ToxExpress and Entelo's DrugMatrix are the two major proprietary databases.

Toxicogenomics promises to deliver a revolutionary impact on safety assessment, especially in pharmaceutical industry, where resource-intensive animal study accompanied by a usual histopathology reading remains standard in preclinical research. Application of toxicogenomics is expected to improve efficiency in the existing workflow. By monitoring drug-induced gene changes, toxicogenomics data could also help to achieve a greater understanding of mechanism and better detection of organ toxicity.

In 2005, the pharmcogenomcis guideline is published by the U.S. Food and Drug Administration (FDA).[4] Since then there have been a number of voluntary genomics data submissions in support of regulatory filing as well as facilitating dialogues with the agency. To influence regulatory authorities to embrace toxicogenomics and its related technologies is an important step. Under the auspices of independent parties like Predictive Safety Testing Consortium (PSTC), part of the Critical Path initiative (leveraging technology to medical product development), scientists from academia, industries are working to positively impact drug development through a collaborative effort on toxicogenomics data and safety biomarkers.[5]

15.2 TOXICOGENOMICS APPLICATIONS AND CURRENT CHALLENGES

Data from a toxicogenomics study essentially consist of one or more snapshots of transcript profiles of the cells or tissues. These snapshots turn out to be a powerful tool that enables researchers to ask prospectively of what is going to happen, concurrently of what is going on, or retrospectively of what had happened. Predicting late toxicities, identifying safety biomarkers, and improving mechanistic understanding of adverse events are three main areas that toxicogenomics is making impacts.

Prediction of adverse drug reaction is where toxicogenomics holds an early promise. It is assumed that toxicants that elicit similar late pathology would likely exhibit common patterns of gene expression profiles early on. Even though phenotypic anchoring that correlates patterns of gene expression to specific endpoints comes as an inherent power of toxicogenomics,[6] characteristic in expression could be recorded before toxic lesion is evident. In contrast to toxicity evaluation with histopathology and clinical pathology that often demands prolonged period of dosing, predictive toxicogenomics offers a great advantage as an early readout from it could reduce the cycle time. If integrated successfully into the early drug screen, a gene expression-based approach could enhance the efficiency in compound selection by uncovering safety liability early rather than at a costly late phase.

To build a model, expression data from a group of compounds positive for an endpoint of interest, along with those of negative controls form the training set that serves as the input to a prediction algorithm such as support vector machine[7] or partial least square, which in turn identifies patterns of expression profile correlated with the desired endpoint. When such pattern is matched by a future test compound, the test compound likely shares the same effect with those used to build the model and could be expected to produce a similar endpoint. It is noted that prediction is usually driven by statistics not mechanism; a gene picked up by a computational algorithm to be a classifier may or may not yield any mechanistic knowledge.

Effort over the years to use genomics for predictive toxicology is representatively summarized (see Table 15.1). By no coincidence, two major proprietary prediction systems Toxshield and DrugMatrix also come from two main database vendors Genelogic and Entelos. In addition, most big pharmaceutical companies and many academic labs have participated the effort. However, to date reported success is quite underwhelming compared with initial promise of the approach. Besides a fair share of early skepticism, genomics prediction faces a high bar of proving its usefulness as either cross validation or independent forward validation could prove inadequate and an ultimate proof might only come from a retrospective analysis. But baring a few exceptions,[8] a thorough and unbiased retrospective analysis in drug discovery is difficult as the experimental data are usually not complete, and the input, especially the input that requires a long-term study, is more or less biased because only selected compounds will be resourced to a late phase study. However, sustained effort is needed for toxicogenomics prediction to prove itself over time. Its impact on pharmaceutical

Table 15-1. Use toxicogenomics for predictive toxicology

Training set	Prediction outcome	High-throughput screen(HTS)	Advantages and disadvantages	Examples
In vitro (e.g., human or rat primary hepatocytes)	*In vivo* toxicity	Yes	Relatively low cost including low drug amount requirement, but cell line consistency and lack of contextual biology for metabolism and multicellular system are major concerns.	Use primary rat hepatocytes to predict hepatotoxicity[9]
Surrogate tissues that are accessible like blood	Target tissues that are inaccessible	Possible	Enable safety monitoring through noninvasive approach. It is more valuable if translation to the clinic could be achieved.	Gene expression from blood to predict liver toxicity[15]
Short-term (a few days or less) studies	Long-term toxicity	No	Prediction performance is crucial to show advantages over standard clinical chemistry and histopathology endpoints and gain regulatory acceptance.	DrugMatrix; 5 -day signatures predict 30-day nephrotoxicity[10]
Preclinical animal studies	Human toxicity	No	An ultimate goal of preclinical safety assessment. However, retrospective analysis is difficult as a proper data set takes very long to acquire.	Gene Logic ToxShield

R&D won't be felt until its wider acceptance by scientists who could apply the technology in a routine screen process.

Accompany the shift from early enthusiasm to a more reasonable expectation comes some lesson learned. First, the prediction model cannot be applied as black boxes. A good understanding of the underlying models and algorithms is necessary to judge the quality of the prediction and the appropriateness of its interpretation. For example, an *in vitro* prediction system brings a number of advantages (see Table 15.1), but its application needs to be carefully evaluated as inappropriate extrapolation of its reading to *in vivo* outcome could result in compromised science. Second, it is important to recognize limitations of using genomics for prediction. A good understanding of the biology of an endpoint often helps though modeling is statistically driven. A lesion endpoint

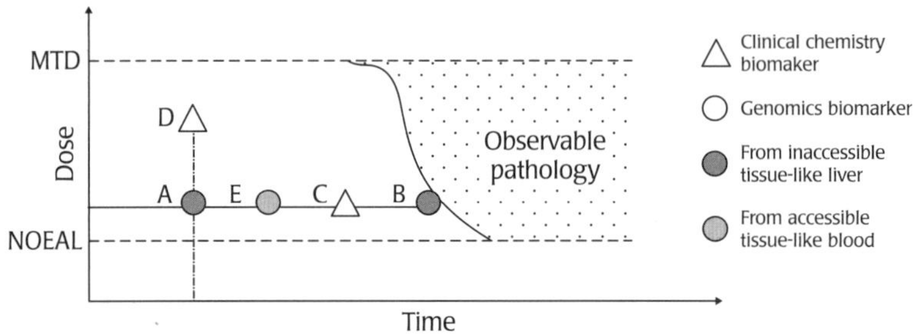

Figure 15-2: Schematic illustration of potential advantages of genomic biomarkers in a dose–time plot of toxicological study. Histopathology lesion is expected to occur when an animal is dosed between MTD (maximum tolerated dose) and NOEAL (no observed adverse effect level). The triangles and circles indicate where a biomarker can be detected or applied to indicate late injury. Genomic marker A is more predictive than clinical chemistry marker C because it can be detected earlier under the same dose treatment and is more sensitive as it works at a lower dose compared to another presumed clinical chemistry marker D.

that involves multiple sequential steps like necrosis could be more difficult to model than a clearly defined one like hytropophy; a pathology that implicates multicellular processes might be beyond complexity that an *in vitro* system is capable to predict. Third, prediction success might be achieved for a specific purpose. For example, while it is ideal to derive prediction from structurally diverse compounds, a model built from only limited chemotypes is expected to be less robust but might still serve its defined needs. Another instance is that it is possible to sacrifice sensitivity to build a model with high specificity. Such model that enables chemists to avoid true positive toxic compounds with relatively high confidence could be useful in early drug discovery.

Safety biomarker discovery is another important application of toxicogenomics. Large-scale exploration of biomarker candidates becomes possible as databases from Gene Logic or Novartis GeneAtlas allow selecting genes by ranking expression in the target tissue – disease or toxicant dosed – over the other tissues, which often is the first step to isolate tissue-specific probes. Moreover, technologies such as robotics or multiplex greatly increase the assay throughput for biomarker validation and application. The proposed advantage of a genomic biomarker could be illustrated by a diagram (see Figure 15.2) showing where a biomarker can be applied in a time–dose plot. Genomic marker A is more predictive than clinical chemistry marker C as it can be detected earlier under the same dose treatment and is more sensitive as it works at a lower dose compared to another presumed clinical chemistry marker D.

Genomic biomarkers have been reported for a variety of tissues such as kidney.[11] Among those identified markers, many can be deemed as mechanistic biomarkers as they are not merely correlated to, but biologically linked to, the underlying toxicity. For example, Kim-1, one of the nephrotoxicity biomarkers submitted to FDA by PSTC is an endogenous ciliary flow-sensing protein that responds to kidney malfunction.[12]

Markers that are concurrent with toxic lesion are diagnostic, whereas those indicative of late pathology are predictive. The latter is of greater value as it demands less exposure time for a study. For example in Figure 15.2, at a dose that produces later organ injury, genomic biomarker A is predictive whereas biomarker B is merely diagnostic. Biomarker Kim-1 is predictive as it is up-regulated within 1 day under the condition that takes much longer to develop kidney injury.[13] By an extended definition, predictive biomarkers could also include genomics signatures used in previously discussed predictive models.

Genomics biomarkers in target organ tissues have one obvious limitation as they often cannot be monitor by a noninvasive approach, hampering their clinical applications. To develop biomarkers in surrogate tissues like blood is of great interest.[14] In Figure 15.2, assuming genomic biomarker A is from an inaccessible target tissue like liver and biomarker E is from blood, E is not necessarily more predictive or more sensitive, but it offers obvious advantages for monitoring safety in a testing subject. In rat, one reported success is that gene expression signatures derived from peripheral blood are found to be a good marker for liver toxicity following administration of acetaminophen.[15] If validated in the human population, such safety biomarkers are expected to enable better longitudinal measurements and further impact clinical study design.

Toxicogenomics also proves to be extremely useful to study and understand the mechanisms of toxicant action. While quantitative information at the transcription level provides a rich insight that is unparalleled by any traditional toxicological measurement, to organize such information often relies on interconnected biological networks and pathways, which are discussed later in this chapter. Besides being biologically intuitive, pathway approach provides a more robust measurement compared to single-gene assessments.[16] It is worth noting that toxicogenomics usually is not the end game; rather, an initial global expression survey is often a good starting point to formulate hypotheses from which further mechanistic studies including cellular and biochemical assays could be designed to confirm such hypotheses that are related to the etiology of toxicities.

The assessment by microarray is targeted at the mRNA and may not reflect changes at the protein level. When for example, treatment of 1-aminobenzotriazole (ABT) was monitored for hepatic metabolizing enzyme induction, cytochrome P450 (CYP) was found to be suppressed in a biochemical assay but up-regulated in microarray study.[17] The seemingly conflicting data actually reveal a feedback loop in which CYP enzyme inhibition activated its transcription. On the other hand, gene expression–based query is probably not best applied to study any posttranscriptional mechanisms.

As the amount of data from toxicogenomics study on large numbers of chemicals and exposure conditions is huge, data standardization and downstream analysis could become the biggest challenge. To collect such data in a reliable and consistent manner and organize them, along with traditional toxicology information in curated databases is a daunting task probably on the similar scale of human genome sequencing, but it must be undertaken to unlock the vast potential of this new field which could only become ever more valuable as the knowledge base grows.

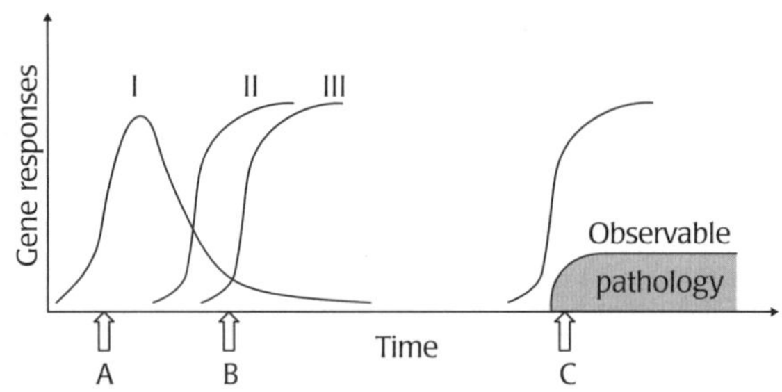

Figure 15-3: Temporal transcriptional responses to toxicities. For the temporal study, ED_{50}, chosen from the dose–gene response data, could be used to avoid overt toxicity and lethality in a longer term study. A biomarker derived from time point A is predictive for late pathology, whereas a biomarker from late point C is diagnostic.

Progress so far has been measurable. It has been learned that data consistency could be improved by using commercially manufactured chips.[18] And a centralized toxicogenomics repository also provides increased consistency, thereby attaining greater confidence in generated data. It is impossible to provide a comprehensive review of all the possible solutions regarding toxicogenomics data management and analysis. We devote the following discussion to highlighting some information gleaned from our past effort in exploring toxicogenomics data.

15.3 TOXICOGENOMIC STUDY DESIGN

It is only logical for data analysts to examine how the data are generated, which invariably involves experimental design. Because toxicogenomics data, even for one compound study can be collected at a variety of different species, doses, and time points, how an experiment is conducted could have a sizable impact on the downstream data analysis.

It might be helpful to understand the temporal transcriptional response that is likely to occur in a toxicology study. In Figure 15.3, a very simplified diagram, curve I represents genes that are activated rapidly and transiently in response to toxic substances. Many of the genes in this group are expected to be transcriptional factors that would further the downstream cascade. Curve II and III represent the secondary and tertiary responses, respectively. Assuming there is a threshold to trigger toxic action,[19] it is plausible that at a certain point the balance of gene expression could be tipped from an overall adaptive response toward a toxic response, a shift theoretically intersected with point of departure (POD) in the context of toxicological dosing.[20] At late time, genes involved in necrosis or apoptosis, represented by curve IV are expected to turn on accompanying the appearance of histopathological lesions.

As previously discussed, a snapshot of expression profile is taken at the time when target organ or tissue is collected for study; such result is expected to be time specific. In Figure 15.3, snapshots taken at time point A and B are likely to generate two distinct profiles. In a real experiment where expression dynamics

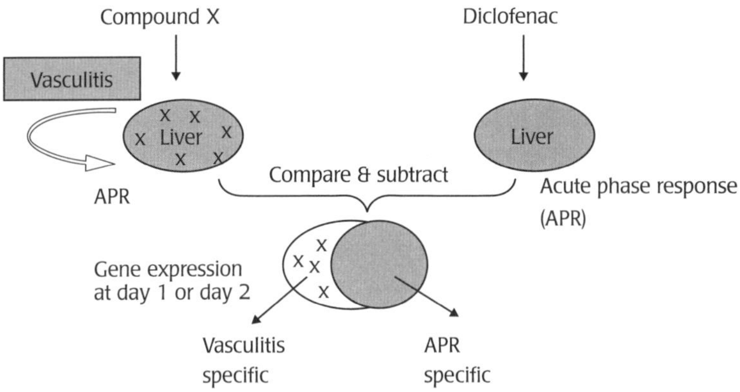

Figure 15-4: *In silico* subtraction method for mechanistic study to compare the hepatic gene expression profile induced by compound X to other compounds that induce hepatic APR secondary to inflammation at sites other than the liver. In the proposed simple model, compound X-induced gene expression change has two components. One is vasculitis specific; the other is acute phase response (APR) specific. By subtracting the APR specific component, we might select candidate genes that are specifically associated with the hepatic vascular lesion; Diclofenac known to induce APR without triggering vasculitis in liver is used to subtract genes activated by hepatic APR from the compound X response.

is far more complicated, particularly in transcriptionally active organs such as liver, a toxicogenomics endpoint is probably more time dependent than those that are traditionally monitored in clinical pathology or histopathology.

This brings an important consideration to toxicogenomics experiment design. An initial time course study could be as informative as a dose-range-finding experiment. For mechanistic inquiry, a plan designed to cover all crucial time points increases the odds of investigation success.[16] For class prediction to achieve the optimal result, it is advised to follow the conditions used to building the initial model. For instance, models in ToxShield (Gene Logic) are built with data mostly from 1-day exposure, whereas those derived from DrugMatrix (Entelos) are using data of 1-, 3-, or 5-day exposure.

However, because of constraint of resources, sometimes toxicogenomics is not necessary if the sole purpose is to run a study in preclinical safety assessment; it is more likely to piggyback on other toxicology conducts. At other times, a microarray study happens to run because of leftover of interested frozen tissues, a mere afterthought rather than a planned experiment. Such practice might confound the data interpretation and limit the future reference value of the study. As discussed earlier, the incremental value of toxicogenomics lies in the ever-expanding reference data of quality.

Comparative toxicogenomics is another example that experiments could be strategically designed to facilitate studies of compound-specific effects, cross-species differences,[21] or safety advantage over competitor drugs. One such approach depicted in Figure 15.4 is *in silico* subtraction method.

Even though the concept probably could trace back to the early differential screening in which desired cDNA clones could be enriched by subtracting against a separate source of undesired clones, the principle remains the same

Table 15-2. Cases of using *in silico* subtraction for mechanistic study

Study object	Target toxicity	Target compound	Subtraction compound	Example
Early toxic action vs. late general inflammation responses	Vasculitis	Compound X	Diclofenac or other NSAIDs that induce an acute phase response but not vasculitis in liver	Lu et al.[22]
Compound-specific effects vs. class effects or	Microvesicular steatosis	Cyclopropane carboxylic acid (CPCA)	Butyrate, structurally similar to CPCA, but does not cause microvesicular steatosis	Jolly et al.[23]
toxic vs. nontoxic isomer	Hepatocellular toxicity	Acetaminophen (APAP)	Nonhepatotoxic APAP isomer *N*-acetyl-*m*-aminophenol	Beyer et al.[24]
On-target effects vs. off-target effects	Cardiomyopathy	Doxorubicin/ Epirubicin	Etoposide with similar pharmacology to Doxorubicin but does not cause cardiomyopathy	Unpublished study

except now it is done through *in silico* subtraction. As in Figure 15.4, Compound X induces hepatic vasculitis as well as the subsequent acute phase response. To differentiate genes in these tandemly linked but different processes, expression profile by compound X is compared to Diclofenac, which induces only an acute phase response in liver. Subtraction between the two enables *in silico* selection of candidate genes that are involved in the hepatic vasculitis rather than in the acute phase response that occurs secondary to vasculitis.

Several applications of subtraction method are listed in Table 15.2. The method is probably best employed when one has an initial hypothesis so that the subtraction can be designed to isolate genes that are responsible for the postulated effect. To achieve an effective subtraction, not only is the selection of compound for subtraction critical, but the pair of compounds of study should also be applied at an equipotent dose, of which an accurate determination could require additional studies. In a comparative study of two hepatotoxicants TCDD and TCDF,[25] the equipotent dose issue has been elegantly explored by using toxic equivalency factors (TEFs) based on endpoint-specific relative potencies.

15.4 PATHWAYS AND NETWORKS

The importance of biological pathways and networks for predicting xenobiotic toxicity via toxicogenomics profiles has been demonstrated with various degree of success in recent years.[26] Although the terms "pathway" and "network" sometimes are used interchangeably in 'Omics data analyses, there are key differences between these two concepts. According to the definition from National Human Genome Research Institute (http://www.genome.gov), a biological pathway is "a series of actions among molecules in a cell that leads to a certain product or a change in a cell." By this definition a pathway has a well-defined function in a cell. A well-known resource for pathway information is the Boehringer-Mannheim/Roche Applied Science wall charts of "Biochemical Pathways" (electronic forms are accessible from the ExPASy Web site http://www.expasy.ch/tools/pathways).[27] For the last few decades these wall charts have improved over time and provided a relatively comprehensive overview of most known metabolic and regulatory pathways. Another good resource for pathway information is KEGG (http://www.genome.jp/kegg), which has richer contents and is updated more frequently.[28]

Contrary to pathways' inherent association with biological functions, biological networks carry broader definitions in scope. Types of biological networks range from interconnected biological pathways,[27,28] protein–protein interaction networks,[29–31] co-expression networks,[32–34] and Bayesian networks.[35–37]

There are many public and commercial databases and applications for pathway and network information. Many of them are summarized at the Pathguide Web site.[38] Currently it contains information from 294 biological pathway resources. Among them, 240 are free to academic users, and there are 20,988,152 nodes (genes/proteins) and 34,986,532 edges (interactions/reactions). Data quality of this rich "interactome" information varies among these resources. On the commercial side, major pathway analysis tools include Ingenuity's Pathway Analysis suite, Ariadne's Pathway Studio, and GeneGo's MetaCore and MetaDrug.

Although integrating large volume of 'Omics data within the context of biological networks has provided insights of underlying biological phenomena in various disciplines, its application in toxicogenomics is still in its infancy and has great potential in identifying molecular mechanisms of various drug-induced toxicity. This is evident in the study of functional gamma secretase inhibitors (FGSIs) induced gastrointestinal (GI) toxicity characterized as goblet cell metaplasia. It is known that signals transduced from the intracellular domain of Notch (NICD) play an essential role in the intestinal cell fate decisions, cell growth, and cell differentiation, evidenced by Hes-1 and Math-1 (Rath-1 in Rat) KO experiments.[39] Inhibition of Notch processing will switch off the Hes-1 transcriptional repressor, which in turn increases the expression of Math-1, causing intestinal progenitor cells to differentiate into secretory lineage, which includes goblet cells.[40] A toxicogenomic profiling study of FGSIs identified the dysregulation of a number of genes indicating the perturbation of notch signaling.[40] Given that FGSIs can inhibit Notch processing, the perturbation of Notch signaling by FGSIs is thus implicated as the molecular mechanism of FGSIs mediated GI toxicity – goblet cell metaplasia.

The National Academy of Sciences put together a symposium entitled "Toxicity Pathway-Based Risk Assessment: Preparing for Paradigm Change." Presentations from this symposium highlighted the importance of and challenges in applying pathway and network analysis for toxicity and risk assessments.[41]

15.5 INTEGRATIVE PATHWAY AND NETWORK ANALYSIS FOR 'OMICS DATA

Among the 405 "'Omics" listed under omics.org – including lipidomics and glycomic – transcriptomics, proteomics, and metabolomics/metabonomics are the most relevant 'Omics for drug safety studies. While applying multiple 'Omics technologies to study potential drug-induced injury in preclinical species and clinical subjects, a typical work flow as summarized in Figure 15.5 can be assumed.

Typically, a biological system of interest will be identified for a specific project (e.g., a dose-range-finding study for a discovery compound in canine). The next step is to select appropriate 'Omics technology to meet the study requirements and to design proper experiment protocols for project execution. Each 'Omics technology has its advantages and limitations. These technology-specific characteristics, such as throughput and precision, need to be taken into consideration while designing experiments that could include selection of sample size and sample collection/processing protocols, and so on.

Another important factor to be taken into account while applying multiple 'Omics technologies is the informatics infrastructure. Given the high-throughput, high-content characteristics of most 'Omics technologies, a high performance computing infrastructure is essential to handle issues like data capture, QA/QC, data storage, data access, data report and data integration. Finally

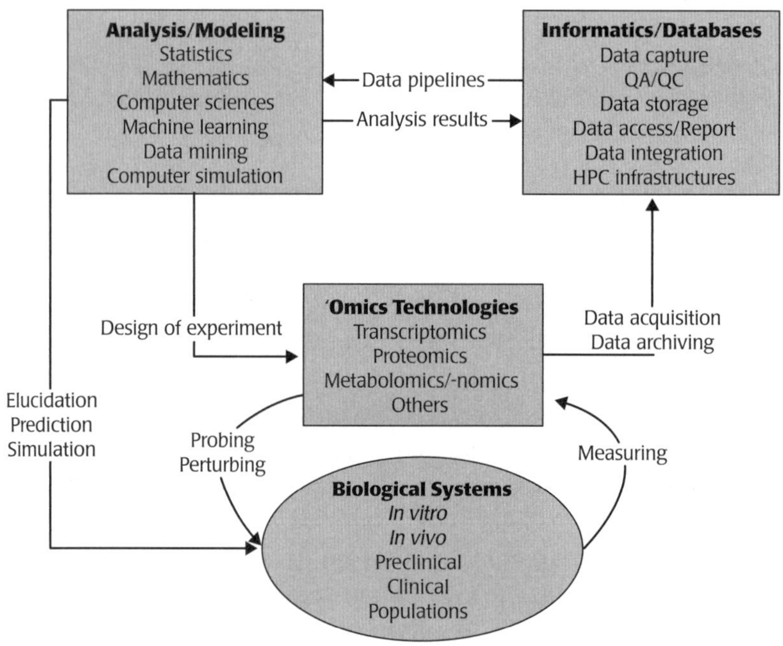

Figure 15-5: A typical work flow in applying multiple 'Omics technologies.

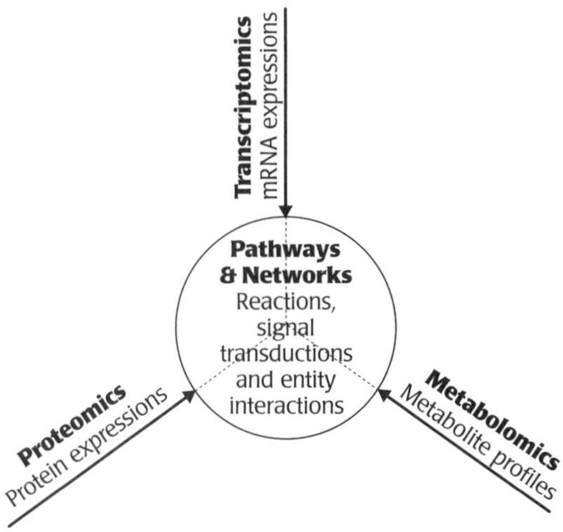

Figure 15-6: Pan-omics study: the orthogonal relationship of transcritomics, proteomics, metabolomics/metabonomics, and their confirmatory effect on pathway analysis.

robust data analysis pipelines need to be developed to analyze multiple 'Omics data from each and every technology, and then integrative analyses must be performed across technologies.

There are generally two types of approaches for data integration. One is knowledge driven, and the other is statistics driven. The knowledge-driven approach relies on mechanism or biology knowledge in which the orthogonal relationship of transcritomics, proteomics, metabolomics/metabonomics, and pathways/networks can be demonstrated in Figure 15.6. An integrative analysis of multiple 'Omics data, combined with traditional toxicology endpoint data, often bring confirmatory result. The statistics-driven approach is usually based on algorithms such as Random Forests or partial least square. We will exemplify each of the approach in the following discussion.

15.6 PATHWAY ANALYSIS SCENARIO I: KNOWLEDGE-DRIVEN INTEGRATED 'OMICS

An integrated 'Omics approach increases confidence in study by bridging gene expression to intra- or extracellular protein or metabolites in bodily fluid at the pathway or network level. Proteomics or metabolomics can also help identify accessible biomarkers, and their data are often easy to interpret.

A knowledge-driven integrated 'Omics approach was applied to understand those human neuroendocrine (NE) cancers with poor prognosis.[42] Genomic profiling of various prostate neuroendocrine cell lines and genetic models lead to the identification of genomic signature,which best distinguished good and poor prognosis NE cancer groups. Through genomics-directed metabolomics, reconstructed metabolic maps in KEGG revealed a metabolic signature indicative of poor-prognosis human NE tumors. Focused metabolomics profiling further validated such metabolic pathway and a final metabolomic signature and its corresponding enzymes in polyamine metabolism were thus identified to define poor prognosis in human neuroendocrine cancers. It is only reasonable that such an approach can be readily applied in xenobiotics toxicology.

The activation of deleterious pathways itself is a risk indicator of safety liability for xenobiotics. Sustained proliferation poses tumorigenesis risk, inflammation is often associated with tissue damage, and DNA damage has been the major subject of genotoxicity studies. Similarly, oxidative stress or damage has been implicated in much drug-induced toxicity.[43,44] To identify xenobiotic-induced oxidative stress, a biochemical anchoring or metabolomics-directed genomics approach could be very useful. Various metabolites have been measured to indicate cellular damages by free radicals, such as F2-isoprostanes for lipid oxidation, 8-OH-dG for DNA damage, or nitrotyrosine for protein oxidation.[45] A genomic study could be guided by such metabolomic data so as to identify genomic signature correlates with the changes in metabolites of oxidative damage. Identifying oxidative stress before tissue injury could predict risk of potential safety liability. In the absence of tissue injury, metabolites, which are indicative of oxidative stress, were measured to anchor the genomic-profiling studies for the discovery of a real oxidative stress signature rather than a signature associated with tissue injury.

15.7 PATHWAY ANALYSIS SCENARIO II: RANDOM FORESTS CLASSIFICATION

We previously applied Random Forests (RF), a tree-based classification and regression method to pathway analysis of gene expression data.[46] The proposed methods allow researchers to rank the significance of biological pathways as well as discover important genes in the same process.

The dataset derives from a study designed to find out the yet unknown molecular mechanism of vascular injury triggered by adenosine receptor agonist CI-947 in coronary arteries of dogs. The study included twenty-four animals in two dose groups (low and high), and two time points (6 and 16 h). Lesion was scored by histopathology, and expression data were obtained of left extramural coronary arteries from all dogs.[46]

Random Forests classification requires two inputs: expression data from the study and pathway information. The latter includes 441 KEGG and BioCarta-derived pathways each consisting of between 3 and 151 genes. Each pathway was scored based on its ability to distinguish between dogs with lesion and those without. Pathways were then ranked by misclassification error rate. We found the most significant pathways from the analysis also yield biologically informative results, confirming the relevance of Random Forest (RF)-based classification. The top three pathways (see Table 15.3) are (a) LDL pathway during atherogenesis, (b) Msp-Ron receptor signaling pathway, and (c) Hypoxia and p53 in the cardiovascular system. They are all related to vascular injury: Pathway (a) contains a collection of key signaling molecules in arterial blood and endothelial

Table 15-3. Pathways ranked by RF-based classification error rate[46]

Pathway	Error rate (%)	Number of genes
LDL pathway during atherogenesis	3.4	4
Msp-Ron receptor signaling pathway	3.4	6
Hypoxia and p53 in the cardiovascular system	3.4	14
Role of Ran in mitotic spindle regulation	6.9	8
Granzyme A mediated apoptosis pathway	6.9	5
CTCF first multivalent nuclear factor	6.9	18
CDK regulation of DNA replication	6.9	10
Sumoylation by RanBP2 reg. trans. repression	6.9	8
Circadian rhythm	6.9	9
Nitric oxide signaling pathway	6.9	14
Aminosugars metabolism	6.9	19
Wnt signaling pathway	6.9	68
Aminoacyl-tRNA biosynthesis	6.9	19
Pertussis toxin-insensitive CCR5 signaling in macrophage	6.9	15
Leukocyte adhesion	6.9	59

cells; pathway (b) plays a part in inflammation and tissue injury; pathway (c) is a collection of genes induced by hypoxic stress.[46]

Results from RF-based pathway analysis also helped to identify potential biomarkers that would otherwise be difficult. Output for every pathway also included a list of genes, each with its own significant score calculated in a way similar to that for pathways. If a gene repeatedly showed up in a group of top-ranked pathways, it could be of interest. For example, CCL2, chemokine (C–C motif) ligand 2 also known as MCP-1 is a common gene shared by four pathways: leukocyte adhesion, LDL pathway, MSP, and pertussis toxin pathway (see Table 15.3). It turns out that CCL2 is directly related to vascular injury and is one of those strongly up-regulated in endothelial microvascular injury. However, this gene would be ranked No.187 in the two-sample *t*-test, a standard data processing step comparing treated versus control samples. CCL2 would be difficult to identify without RF-based pathway analysis. Protein kinase C alpha PRKCA is another example that was found in three pathways (i.e. WNT signaling, NO signaling, and pertussis toxin pathways). PRKCA was previously found to form a complex with RhoA, which is involved in vascular inflammation.[46]

15.8 A COMPREHENSIVE VIEW MORE THAN SNAPSHOTS

What started as snapshots of transcript profiles has profoundly changed the study of toxicology. Researchers use them to make prediction of likely future

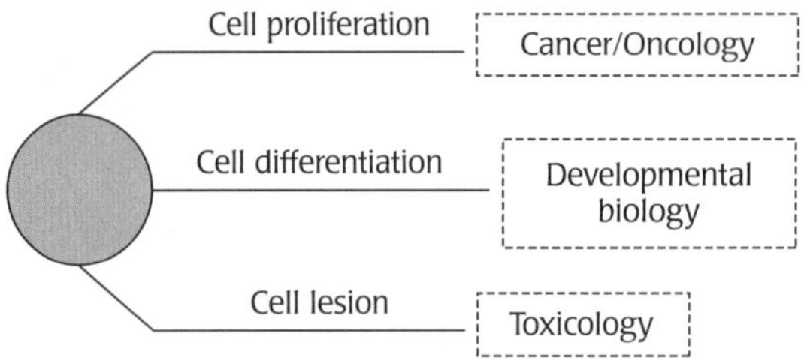

Figure 15-7: Analysis of cellular events at the pathway level enables a cross-disciplinary understanding of cancer, development biology, and toxicology.

toxic events, in the same way doctors use X-ray film for diagnosis; novel genomic biomarkers of toxicity come out from a comparative study of these snapshots. Information pieced together from snapshots taken at different conditions would offer some clue of what was transpiring behind toxic lesions. With additional pathway information and network models, a comprehensive view that is more than snapshots emerges rendering a dynamics picture of cellular responses.

Pathway and network analyses have also opened new vistas in bridging toxicology to other areas of biosciences such as developmental biology and cancer research. At the outset, they take on opposite directions toward their research. Toxicology studies effects from chemicals, an exogenous influence, while developmental biology and cancer research focus on more endogenous events: The former studies programmed development that is largely genetically controlled, and the latter mainly deals with events that cannot be controlled. Yet they converge on a unifying theme anchored by biological pathways (see Figure 15.7). The same pathway that is responsible for cell proliferation or differentiation, triggered by external influences, could also be the one that pushes cell to lesion. In the previous gamma secretase inhibitor example, hunting down GI pathologies led us to the pathway of Notch, which has long been known in early animal development as the controller of cell fate and is also implicated in cancer.[47] In a comparative toxicogenomics study of acetaminophen (APAP) and its nonhepatotoxic isomer, c-Myc-centered interactome is the most significant network associated with liver injury. c-Myc, as a large body of literature could attest to, is a master transcriptional factor regulating switch between proliferation and differentiation.[48]

Understanding the contextual biology of toxicity could now draw upon previous hard-won knowledge from other disciplines such as cancer research, which in turn will benefit the quest of mechanistic biomarkers for safety monitoring. In the gamma secretase example, unraveling the pathways underlying the toxicity also helped to identify mechanism-based biomarkers (e.g., adipsin) that could be deployed to monitor the toxicity during drug development.[40] It is believed in the near term that the most promising use for toxicogenomics would be to clarify pathways for different types of toxicity and identify their corresponding biomarkers to enable better nonclinical assessment and future toxicodynamic monitoring.[49]

As we gain a better understanding of network and pathway data across different species, integration of molecular toxicology would help to close the knowledge gap between preclinical safety and clinic adverse findings, potentially bringing down the high attrition rate in late drug development. The ultimate value of toxicogenomics resides in improving relevance and confidence of risk extrapolation to the clinical study.

Despite of challenges such as handling a tsunami of data or evaluation for regulatory purposes, toxicogenomics and pathway analysis have made headway over the past decade and are poised to advance further into the future. A broader understanding at the molecular, pathway, and network level would remain the pillars on which we expect to build continued success in deciphering chemical toxicity, and its successful application in clinical practice would help to ensure future patients in drug therapy judiciously monitored and relieved of undue harm.

REFERENCES

1. Pennie WD. Custom cDNA microarrays; Technologies and applications. *Toxicology.* 2002;181–182:551–4.
2. Fostel J, Choi D, Zwickl C, et al. Chemical effects in biological systems – data dictionary (CEBS-DD): A compendium of terms for the capture and integration of biological study design description, conventional phenotypes, and 'omics data. *Toxicol Sci.* 2005; 88(2):585–601.
3. Tong W, Harris S, Cao X, et al. Development of public toxicogenomics software for microarray data management and analysis. *Mutat Res.* 2004;549(1–2):241–253.
4. U.S. Food and Drug Administration. Guidance for Industry: Pharmacogenomic data submissions. FDA White Paper 2005.
5. Mattes WB. Public consortium efforts in toxicogenomics. *Methods Mol Biol.* 2008;460:221–238.
6. Paules R. Phenotypic anchoring: Linking cause and effect. *Environ Health Perspect.* 2003;111(6):A338–A339.
7. Jiang Y, Gerhold DL, Holder DJ, et al. Diagnosis of drug-induced renal tubular toxicity using global gene expression profiles. *J Transl Med.* 2007;5:47.
8. Foster WR, Chen SJ, He A, et al. A retrospective analysis of toxicogenomics in the safety assessment of drug candidates. *Toxicol Pathol.* 2007;35(5):621–635.
9. Hultin-Rosenberg L, Jagannathan S, Nilsson KC, et al. Predictive models of hepatotoxicity using gene expression data from primary rat hepatocytes. *Xenobiotica.* 2006;36(10–11):1122–1139.
10. Fielden MR, Eynon BP, Natsoulis G, et al. A gene expression signature that predicts the future onset of drug-induced renal tubular toxicity. *Toxicol Pathol.* 2005;33(6):675–683.
11. Wang EJ, Snyder RD, Fielden MR, et al. Validation of putative genomic biomarkers of nephrotoxicity in rats. *Toxicology* 2008;246(2–3):91–100.
12. Kuehn EW, Hirt MN, John AK, et al. Kidney injury molecule 1 (Kim1) is a novel ciliary molecule and interactor of polycystin 2. *Biochem Biophys Res Commun.* 2007;364(4):861–866.
13. Rokushima M, Fujisawa K, Furukawa N, et al. Transcriptomic analysis of nephrotoxicity induced by cephaloridine, a representative cephalosporin antibiotic. *Chem Res Toxicol.* 2008;21(6):1186–1196.
14. Rockett JC, Burczynski ME, Fornace AJ, et al. Surrogate tissue analysis: Monitoring toxicant exposure and health status of inaccessible tissues through the analysis of accessible tissues and cells. *Toxicol Appl Pharmacol.* 2004;194(2):189–199.

15. Bushel PR, Heinloth AN, Li J, et al. Blood gene expression signatures predict exposure levels. *Proc Natl Acad Sci USA* 2007;104(46):18211–18216.
16. Yu X, Griffith WC, Hanspers K, et al. A system-based approach to interpret dose- and time-dependent microarray data: Quantitative integration of gene ontology analysis for risk assessment. *Toxicol Sci.* 2006;92(2):347–348.
17. Fasulo LM, Schomaker SJ, Ryan AM, et al. Comparison of biochemical analysis to gene expression and laser scanning cytometry for the assessment of rat hepatic cytochrome P450 (CYP) enzyme induction. *Toxicol. Sci.* (suppl.) 2009;108:56.
18. Bammler T, et al. Members of the Toxicogenomics Research Consortium. Standardizing global gene expression analysis between laboratories and across platforms *Nat Methods.* 2005;2(5):351–356.
19. Waters KM, Tan R, Opresko LK, et al. Cellular dichotomy between anchorage-independent growth responses to bFGF and TPA reflects molecular switch in commitment to carcinogenesis. *Mol Carcinog.* 2009; 48(11):1059–1069.
20. Burgoon LD, Zacharewski TR. Automated quantitative dose-response modeling and point of departure determination for large toxicogenomic and high-throughput screening data sets. *Toxicol Sci.* 2008;104(2):412–418.
21. Mattes WB. Cross-species comparative toxicogenomics as an aid to safety assessment. *Expert Opin Drug Metab Toxicol.* 2006; 2(6):859–874.
22. Lu B, Nelms L, Floyd G, et al. Using correlation analysis and hierarchical clustering to discriminate genes associated with hepatic vasculitis from subsequent hepatic inflammation. *Toxicol. Sci.* (suppl.) 2004;78:412.
23. Jolly, RA, Ciurlionis R, Morfitt D, et al. Microvesicular steatosis induced by a short chain fatty acid: effects on mitochondrial function and correlation with gene expression. *Toxicol Pathol.* 2004;32(Suppl. 2),19–25.
24. Beyer RP, Fry RC, Lasarev MR, et al. Multicenter study of acetaminophen hepatotoxicity reveals the importance of biological endpoints in genomic analyses. *Toxicol Sci.* 2007;99(1):326–337.
25. N'Jai A, Boverhof DR, Dere E, et al. Comparative temporal toxicogenomic analysis of TCDD- and TCDF-mediated hepatic effects in immature female C57BL/6 mice. *Toxicol Sci.* 2008;103(2):285–297.
26. Ganter B, Zidek N, Hewitt PR, et al. Pathway analysis tools and toxicogenomics reference databases for risk, *Pharmacogenomics.* 2008;9(1):35–54.
27. Michal G. *Biochemical Pathways: An Altlas of Biochemistry and Molecular Biology.* Hoboken, NJ: Wiley; 1998.
28. Kanehisa M, Araki M, Goto S, et al. KEGG for linking genomes to life and the environment. *Nucleic Acids Res.* 2008;36,D480–D484.
29. Rual JF, et al. Towards a proteome-scale map of the human protein–protein interaction network. *Nature.* 437, 1173–1178.
30. Stelzl U, Worm U, Lalowski M, et al. A human protein–protein interaction network: A resource for annotating the proteome. *Cell.* 2005;122(6):957–968.
31. Gavin A C, et al. Proteome survey reveals modularity of the yeast cell machinery. *Nature.* 2006;440,631–636.
32. Stuart JM, Segal E, Koller D, et al . A gene-coexpression network for global discovery of conserved genetic modules. *Science.* 2003;302,249–255.
33. Obayashi T, Hayashi S, Shibaoka M, et al. COXPRESdb: A database of coexpressed gene networks in mammals. *Nucleic Acids Res.* 2008;36:D77–D82.
34. Jun Zhu, et al. Integrating large-scale functional genomic data to dissect the complexity of yeast regulatory networks, *Nat Genet.* 2008;40,854–861.
35. Friedman N, et al. Using Bayesian networks to analyze expression data. *J. Comput Biol.* 2000;7:601–620.
36. Werhli AV, et al. Comparative evaluation of reverse engineering gene regulatory networks with relevance networks, graphical gaussian models and bayesian networks. *Bioinformatics.* 2006;22:2523–2531.

37. Margolin A, et al. ARACNE: An algorithm for the reconstruction of gene regulatory networks in a mammalian cellular context. *BMC Bioinformat.* 2006;7(Suppl 1):S7.
38. Bader GD, Cary MP, Sander C. Pathguide: A pathway resource list., *Nucleic Acids Res.* 2006;34(Database issue):D504–D506.
39. Searfoss GH, Jordan WH, Calligaro DO, et al. Adipsin, a biomarker of gastrointestinal toxicity mediated by a functional gamma-secretase inhibitor. *J Biol Chem.* 2003;278(46):46107–46116.
40. Brittan M, Wright NA. Gastrointestinal stem cells. *J Pathol.* 2002;197(4):492–509.
41. Symposium on Toxicity Pathway-Based Risk Assessment: Preparing for Paradigm Change, The National Academy of Sciences, Washington, DC, May 11–13, 2009. Retrieved from http://dels.nas.edu/best/risk_analysis/symposium.shtml.
42. Ippolito JE, Xu J, Jain S, et al. An integrated functional genomics and metabolomics approach for defining poor prognosis in human neuroendocrine cancers. *Proc Natl Acad Sci USA.* 2005;102(28):9901–9906.
43. Yen HC, Oberley TD. Vichitbandha S, et al. The protective role of manganese superoxide dismutase against adriamycin-induced acute cardiac toxicity in transgenic mice. *J Clin Invest.*1996;98(5):1253–1260.
44. Masutani J. Oxidative stress and redox imbalance in acetaminophen toxicity. *Pharmocogenom J.* 2001;1(3):165–166.
45. Kadiiska MB, Gladen BC, Baird DD, et al. Biomarker of oxidative stress study: II. Are oxidation products of lipids, proteins and DNA markers of CCL4 poisoning. *Free Radical Biol Med.* 2005;38:698–710.
46. Pang H, Lin A, Holford M, et al. Pathway analysis using random forests classification and regression. *Bioinformatics.* 2006; 22(16):2028–2036.
47. Purow B. Notch inhibitors as a new tool in the war on cancer: a pathway to watch. *Curr Pharm Biotechnol.* 2009;10(2):154–160.
48. Demeterco C, Itkin-Ansari P, Tyrberg B, et al. c-Myc controls proliferation versus differentiation in human pancreatic endocrine cells. *J Clin Endocrinol Metab.* 2002; 87(7):3475–3485.
49. Jacobs A. An FDA perspective on the nonclinical use of the X-omics technologies and the safety of new drugs. *Toxicol Lett.* 2009;186(1):32–35.

16 **Drug safety biomarkers**

David Gerhold and Frank D. Sistare

16.1 SCOPE

There is growing impetus to develop improved biomarkers for drug safety: to make medicines safer, to reduce the growing costs of drug development, and to catalyze improved disease diagnosis and patient care. Even though we have largely relied on the same biomarkers for decades, we now have new technologies for biomarker discovery and development such as inexpensive genome sequence analyses, and gene expression technologies, multiplexed protein analytics, and multiple imaging modalities. The history of safety biomarker development illustrates the current state of affairs, and the opportunities and challenges for additional biomarkers.

We will address the nature of safety biomarkers, the current status of these tools, the difficulties and recent successes in biomarker development, and the outlook for qualifying new safety biomarkers for utility in regulated phases of drug development. To limit the scope of this discussion, we define safety biomarkers as measurable molecules or characteristics that provide information regarding the health and physiological function of an organism following exposure to a drug or drug candidate. Biomarkers may be indicators of injury (e.g., proteins released into serum), of exposure (e.g., DNA adducts), or of susceptibility (e.g., a DNA polymorphism). This review will focus on safety biomarkers that describe active responses to injury, as well as the passive consequences of injury such as loss of organ function and release of contents from dying cells. Focus will be on safety biomarkers as molecules or images that indicate adverse events in drug-treated animals or patients, rather than models as surrogates. For example this leaves out of scope: the Ames Assay bacterial model for mammalian mutagenicity, the tabulation of tumors from rodent carcinogenicity studies as surrogate predictors of human carcinogenicity, and the phospholipidosis assays performed in cultured human cells.

Biomarker responses to chemical toxicities in animals are often replicated in disease responses, promising future clinical applications of these biomarkers for diagnosing disease and for monitoring therapeutic mitigation of progression. Unintended responses to drugs are expected to be nearly synonymous with responses to pesticides and environmental toxicants, and also to shed light on disease responses in many cases. Toxicity and disease overlap in that both can (a) damage and kill cells, releasing cellular contents; (b) trigger adaptive responses including regeneration, repair, inflammation, and tissue fibrosis; (c) erode tissue functions acutely or chronically; and (d) change the structure and therefore image of an organ, or the behavior of an animal. Conversely, biomarkers of disease may be more complex than preclinical animal toxicities due to the complex interplay between disease and organismal development, host–pathogen interactions, or our ignorance of the time of onset and etiology of a disease. Nevertheless, there are many examples of biomarkers that illuminate disease progression and toxicant injury alike, and new biomarkers should and will continue to be evaluated in both applications. For example, liver enzymes released to blood, such as alanine aminotransferase (ALT), are used to monitor toxicant injury (e.g., alcoholic cirrhosis), as well as injury from diseases such as viral hepatitis or genetic syndromes (e.g., hemochromatosis).[1] Importantly, such toxicant-injury biomarkers may also be applied to assess efficacy of drugs in ameliorating disease progression.

Much progress in discovering biomarkers of response to toxicant injury has been made since the 1995 advent of gene expression microarray technology.[2] This technology has enabled genome-wide surveys of how animal or human tissues respond to injury. This work has also been accelerated by elucidation of the genomic sequences of man, mouse, rat, and other model organisms, particularly by the near-comprehensive "gene catalogs" that have emerged for each organism.[3] Gene transcripts, or more recently micro-RNAs (miRNAs), are themselves useful biomarkers, although the utility of messenger RNAs mRNAs or miRNAs is generally limited to controlled animal studies, or to circulating cells or tissue biopsies.[4] From these transcriptional data, candidate biomarkers have then been identified in the form of secreted proteins or organic metabolite products (e.g., References 5, 6). In general, the more immediately useful and practical safety biomarkers to transform medicine will be *accessible biomarkers*, readily available and easily measurable in blood, urine, or cerebrospinal fluid and by noninvasive imaging techniques.[7] These accessible biomarkers will be emphasized in this chapter.

16.2 CURRENT STATUS

In the standard practice of drug development, well-characterized and widely accepted biomarkers are used early to support histopathology to diagnose toxicities and adverse events in preclinical studies. Such accessible safety biomarkers are used to establish whether adverse findings are monitorable, could trigger mitigating intervention decisions, and allow full reversibility in preparation for clinical safety studies and to assess the time course of adverse events. If a drug candidate causes an adverse event with a moderate window of safety in animals, a biomarker that renders the event monitorable and helps establish reversibility in animals could enable cautious testing of this candidate in man to assess human relevance.[8] Toxicities seen in drug development often do not translate between common test species and humans.[9] Safety biomarkers in current practice include a mix of biomarkers that were identified and characterized in animals prior to evaluation in clinical practice and biomarkers that were characterized directly in man and have been "reverse-translated" into preclinical studies.[10]

Safety biomarkers in current use may be classified as *injury biomarkers per se* in the case of molecules that leak from injured cells, as *injury–response biomarkers*, or as organ *function biomarkers*. Widely used safety injury biomarkers include measurements of proteins or enzyme activities leaked from injured cells such as cardiac troponins, ALT, Aspartate Aminotransferase, and Creatine Kinase (AST, and CK, respectively). Injury–response biomarkers may include small molecule hormones or other proteins actively secreted by cells such as steroid hormones or Brain-Derived Natriuretic Peptide (BNP), inflammatory mediators such as chemokines or other inflammatory cytokines, proteins participating in regenerative responses such as Kim-1 and fibrotic or other adaptive and intended protective responses such as extracellular matrix components, Clusterin, and Neutrophil Gelatinase-Asociated Lipocalin (NGAL). Organ function biomarkers include small molecules that may accumulate in fluids revealing altered production, impaired uptake or decreased clearance (e.g., bilirubin, bile acids, Cystatin C, or serum creatinine), or secreted proteins (e.g., albuminuria). Noninvasive imaging can be performed for example to assess kidney function, heart structure and function, or cardiac electrical activity. Existing biomarkers are limited in many ways: in ability to diagnose toxicity to specific cell types within major organs, insight to pathogenesis, specificity to distinguish injury from benign events, ability to grade progressive injury and fibrosis, and sensitivity to diagnose toxicity early and to monitor reversibility. These limitations and the availability of new technological approaches have provoked a surge in biomarker qualification efforts.

Some excellent work has been performed to discover earlier safety biomarkers that may *predict* an adverse event, for example.[11–16] Biomarkers that can accurately predict a common toxicity by one or several weeks to months would be a boon to drug development. Such predictive biomarkers have been established for narrow mechanistic cases, cases in which a known target of the drug causes the adverse event, such as References 17–19. Prediction has also been successful in the case of a polymorphic drug metabolizing gene; for example, polymorphic *VKORC1* and *CYP2C9* variants can lead to poor metabolism of warfarin-predicting hemorrhage or the need for more accurate dosing to avoid hemorrhage.[20]

Without knowledge of the mechanism that leads to an adverse event, it has proven more difficult to predict broadly defined drug-induced adverse events such as hepatocellular necrosis or renal tubular toxicity. Since single genes have not proven reliably predictive, groups of genes are being tried in conjunction with predictive algorithms. Such multigene approaches demand large sample sizes in independent training and test sets in order to overcome the multiplicity problem inherent in the multiple analyte approach.[21,22] New diagnostic safety biomarker panels are being successfully developed, whereas the challenges and practicality of identifying robust predictive biomarkers for unknown toxicity mechanisms are still in an exploratory phase.[23] Some reviewers have suggested that biomarkers could "predict" drug adverse events in man based on their effects in animal preclinical studies. One approach is to identify biomarkers of general biochemical, physiologic, and molecular modes of action associated across many diverse classes of toxic agents. If such approaches can "predict" histopathology in animal preclinical studies at later time points, then they may prove useful for similarly predicting drug adverse events in humans. Although hemodynamic or atherogenic biomarkers may provide some utility in this regard, in general, accessible biomarkers are currently reporters of histopathologic and physiologic alterations, and so are unlikely to outperform histopathology. Instead, accessible biomarkers are likely to serve as reporters of concurrent histopathology and physiological alterations in human studies, where these endpoints are unavailable for ethical reasons. Biomarkers that could detect early histologic changes when mild injuries remain fully reversible, represent a practical goal.

Cardiac injury and cardiac dysfunction biomarkers have shown noteworthy advancements in recent years. Several drugs or drug candidates were found to prolong the cardiac QT interval, increasing the risk of Torsade de pointes arrhythmias and sudden death from heart failure.[24] The QT interval is thus a biomarker that is commonly measured in dogs, or nonhuman primates, to evaluate drug candidates. The human ion channel *Ether-a-go-go*, or hERG was found to be the unintended target of drug candidates and certain approved drugs including antibiotics, antimalarials, antiemetics, antipsychotics, and cardiovascular drugs. The subsequent identification, cloning, and expression of the hERG target have enabled screening of drug candidates *in vitro* at earlier stages in drug development.[24] Naturally, the accuracy of these *in vitro* systems has limitations. Furthermore, questions relating to how much QT prolongation, and whether all mechanisms of QT prolongation or hERG channel perturbations represent relevant equivalent risk for Torsades remain unresolved.[25]

Cardiac Troponins have become among the most effective safety biomarkers in preclinical and clinical use. Troponin proteins I, T, and C form abundant triplexes in cardiac myocytes. These subunits leak from cardiac myocytes upon injuries that include cardiac ischemic and toxicant cellular necrotic injuries.[26] The cardiac Troponins I and -T are effective interspecies translational safety biomarkers for myocardial injury Troponin.[26,27] The availability of superior antibodies to cardiac-specific isoforms of Troponin I and Troponin T, along with very low background circulating levels in the absence of any ischemic injury provide the Troponins with a strong signal-to-noise ratio and practical advantages. Creatine kinase MB is a heterodimer that is specifically formed in the heart and has also served as a leakage biomarker for myocyte damage.[28] Creatine kinase-MB isoenzyme (CK-MB) is a specific biomarker of cardiac myocyte necrosis since the heart is the only major organ that produces the MB heterodimer. This organ specificity would be expected to make CK-MB a useful biomarker in animal studies of drug-induced acute heart toxicity. However, perhaps because circulating background levels render a poor signal-to-noise, or because the analytical tools directed at this biomarker are inferior, it remains a relatively insensitive biomarker for clinical myocardial infarction.[29] BNP and various fragments of this pre-pro-hormone have been shown clinically to be of value for diagnosis of the cardiac hypertrophy response.[27] It will be important to investigate its versatility to assess hypertrophy arising from diverse causes such as cardiac valve dysfunction, intrinsic failure of the musculature, or prolonged excessive afterload. Evaluation of its value in animal test species is hampered by the lack of a sufficiently sensitive and robust analytical assay. Imaging approaches are also beginning to be deployed and evaluated in drug development test species in this regard.

Vascular injury and associated inflammation originating from disease or as a result of drug toxicity have generated a need for accessible biomarkers, and many promising candidates have been proposed that await fuller evaluation.[27,29,30] These include markers of endothelial injury or dysfunction such as E-selectin and P–selectin, von Willebrand factor, soluble intercellular adhesion molecule 1 (or ICAM-1), L-arginine and assymetric- or symmetric-dimethylarginine, and nitric oxide metabolites. Inflammatory signals may also serve as biomarkers, such as C-reactive protein (CRP), and cytokines, or vasoactive hormones such as endothelin or angiotensin II. Vascular injury may also be signaled by remodeling proteins originating from vasculature or heart, such as procollagen type III amino terminal peptide (PIIINP); D-dimer, matrix metalloproteinases-1, -2, -7, -8, and -9; or tissue inhibitors of metalloproteinases-1, -2, or -4.[29,31] Evaluation of such a large menu of candidate biomarkers will require a systematic method of identifying and developing good assays and applying them to well-defined study sample sets across preclinical test species and in appropriate clinical contexts. The detailed qualification of such biomarkers may be expected to help evaluate and resolve concerns that vascular injury and inflammation seen in a test species may present a risk for an acute thrombus or hemorrhagic event, or serve as a prolonged stimulus for atherogenesis progression.

Much research progress is also being made in safety biomarkers for renal toxicities. Current clinical practice relies heavily on buildup of serum creatinine to determine whether the kidneys are functionally impaired. Since serum creatinine does not change until kidney function is reduced by over 50 percent, more sensitive biomarkers revealing subtle injury are needed.[32]

Albuminuria has been evaluated in a variety of clinical situations and found to be a useful diagnostic particularly for diabetic nephropathy and other conditions and toxicants that harm the glomerular membrane or the podocytes that support it. Glomerulopathy results in massive leakage of plasma components into the glomerular filtrate resulting in marked albuminuria and proteinuria. Whereas the small amount of albumin that passes into the filtrate is normally absorbed by the proximal tubule epithelial cells, massive proteinuria injures these cells and impairs their ability to absorb these proteins. Direct toxicity or injury to proximal tubule epithelial cells also blocks protein absorptive function, resulting in a moderate albuminuria. Clinically, "macroalbuminuria" resulting from glomerular dysfunction is generally defined as >300 mg albumin per gram creatinine, whereas proximal tubule dysfunction results in "microalbuminuria" of 30–300 mg albumin per gram creatinine in urine.[33] Kidney injury molecule 1 (called Kim-1, HAVCR-1, or TIM1), has accumulated evidencse in rat and human studies of being a sensitive and reliable indicator of proximal tubule cell injury and the regenerative process associated with injury.[34,35] Efforts in the last few years have also compared diverse panels of renal biomarkers across a variety of rat acute kidney toxicant studies and in several clinical groups with risk of acute kidney injuries (see References 35, 36). In rats, urinary biomarkers Kim-1, Albumin, TFF3, and Clusterin were shown to be useful markers relative to serum creatinine for tubular injuries. Similarly, urinary Cystatin C, beta-2-microglobulin, and total protein were found to be useful as markers of glomerular toxicity. These biomarkers were recently qualified for preclinical use by the Predictive Safety Testing Consortium (PSTC) Nephrotoxicity Working Group, and specific claims of the utility were accepted by the FDA and European Medicines Agency (EMEA).[36] In humans, Vaidya et al. evaluated nine biomarkers in a set of patients, identifying gradations in ability to distinguish acute kidney injury from comorbidities associated with hospital intensive care. Kim-1 and NGAL, for example, showed greater specificity for acute kidney injury patients, whereas Hepatocyte Growth Factor and Vascular Endothelial Growth Factor (HGF and VEGF) tended to be nonspecific, and Cystatin C, Interleukin 18, chemokine interferon-inducible protein 10, N-acetyl-beta-D-glucosaminidase, (IL-18, IP10, and NAG, respectively) and total protein, were intermediate.[35] Evaluation of Kim-1, NAG, and other urinary biomarkers in various clinical populations has begun to identify complementary information resulting from each of the biomarkers assessed as components of a panel. Clinical qualification of renal biomarkers is limited by the need to assess performance according to the insensitive biomarker, serum creatinine. Paradoxically, an insensitive endpoint such as serum creatinine will cause more sensitive biomarker responses to be classified as putative false positives. Well-designed longitudinal clinical studies are needed to understand the thresholds associated with biologically meaningful alterations in such promising new biomarkers of renal safety.

A number of well-established biomarkers are widely used for monitoring liver safety. Hepatocyte injury is typically assessed as serum or plasma ALT enzyme activity increase relative to AST increase. Although ALT and AST are released from multiple organs following injury, ALT fold-increases that exceed AST fold-increases have been found empirically to indicate liver injury.[37] There are apparent false positive exceptions to this rule in which ALT increases occur absent histologic liver injury.[37] In these exceptions, additional hepatocyte leakage enzymes, such as sorbitol dehydrogenase, glutamate dehydrogenase, lactate dehydrogenase, and arginase may distinguish between incipient injury and events unrelated to injury. Biliary injury, liver hypertrophy, and other liver alterations may occur without producing marked ALT/AST changes. Biliary injury and cholestasis may be associated with the the release of alkaline phosphatase into blood, but alkaline phosphatase activities can derive from other tissues as well.

Liver function biomarkers include unconjugated bilirubin, which can rise in serum due to hepatocyte dysfunction, or glucuronide-conjugated bilirubin often resulting from bile duct injury, obstruction, or other source of cholestasis.[38] Biliary injury and cholestasis may be diagnosed as increased bilirubin, bile acids, or alkaline phosphatase, in blood. Potentially confounding these biomarkers, hemolysis can also increase plasma-free bilirubin, and plasma unconjugated bilirubin levels can be increased by drug inhibition of bilirubin-to-glucuronide conjugation via uridine diphosphate-glucuronosyltransferase 1A1 (UGT1A1), or by drug inhibition of specific hepatocyte-to-bile duct transporters. Additional liver biomarkers may be useful to complement ALT activity. Such complementary liver biomarkers could distinguish situations where ALT increases may represent benign excursions that return to normal despite continued dosing, from situations where ALT increases result from pathological changes that presage fibrosis or liver failure.

Several multianalyte diagnostic methods have been marketed to assess the level of liver fibrosis, such as Fibroscan and Fibrotest.[39] These tests may leave room for improved biomarkers; however, the accuracy of the biopsy method has also been questioned as a source of error in evaluation of these studies. Additional liver biomarkers are needed that improve on the specificity of ALT to differentially diagnose injury severity, or improve on the sensitivity of serum bilirubin or serum albumin and clotting factors to help assess liver function.

16.3 NEEDS FOR IMPROVED SAFETY BIOMARKERS

The current status of biomarkers may be summarized as a collection of tools that have been progressively characterized and used for decades, with new examples added at a snail's pace. The availability of genomics technology and the stagnation in drug development efficiency and success rate have spurred calls for novel safety biomarkers. There are expectations that new biomarkers can spur development of safer drugs. Complete genome sequences and gene catalogs are available for man and preclinical species rat, mouse, dog, rhesus, and cynomolgous monkeys. Gene expression microarrays and other genomics techniques enable the enumeration of genes that are expressed selectively in tissues of interest and genes that are induced by toxic, but not benign, drug treatments. The FDA has published the Critical Path initiative, including a call to arms for new safety biomarker development,[40] and established the Biomarker Qualification Review Teams to evaluate qualification claims in new biomarker submissions.[41] The Critical Path Institute and International Life Sciences Institute are sponsoring collaborative work advancing safety biomarkers.[42] The European Commission has similarly catalyzed support for biomarker development through the formation of the Innovative Medicines Initiative.[43] Why then are new qualified biomarkers trickling into practice at such a slow pace?

Novel biomarkers are often identified using gene expression profiling for proteins encoded by genes that are transcriptionally induced by injury.

Alternatively, proteomic profiling approaches can identify induced proteins, or protein biomarkers that leak from damaged cells. Small molecules (e.g., nucleosides, nitric oxide metabolites, eicosanoids, and hormones) may be implied by gene expression changes or identified directly using metabonomic profiling. Gene expression profiling is limited to induced genes, is high throughput, and is relatively comprehensive covering nearly all the ~20,000 genes in the genome, whereas proteomics and metabonomics are relatively laborious and limited to hundreds of abundant proteins or metabolites. Extensive searches for truly novel biomarkers are now feasible; however, identifying those biomarkers that are complementary or that can be superior to existing biomarkers requires extensive and laborious experiments to evaluate their performance.

There are many promising examples of candidate safety biomarkers for liver, kidney, and cardiovascular toxicities, for example, which are lacking sufficient experimental data to support broad use and regulatory acceptance in drug development. The bottleneck for implementing new biomarkers into common practice is thus the laborious preclinical and clinical qualification needed to evaluate performance simultaneously and compare the relative utility of these promising biomarkers. The logical approach is to target "fit-for-purpose" biomarker qualification to establish that a very specifically defined adverse event is monitorable in a preclinical animal model. Then further qualification of this biomarker can proceed in the clinic, using standard of care therapeutic agents whose use is associated with the same expected and specifically defined adverse event observed in animal studies. Such a targeted fit-for-purpose initial specific safety biomarker qualification may spur additional broader qualification efforts on successful biomarkers in wider contexts of toxicities and disease. Biomarker qualification could also be accelerated by closer communication, cooperation, and collaboration between preclinical and clinical teams, by more systematic opportunistic collections of patient samples, and by establishing panels of validated biomarker assays.

A significant portion of the current time needed to develop a new drug is consumed in two-year carcinogenicity testing of drugs in rats and/or mice. Accessible biomarkers that reliably diagnose or precede tumor development would speed this process markedly. The polygenic nature of tumor development makes this an important need for future efforts. Promising recent results with the discovery of detectable levels of circulating miRNA's from patients presenting with tumors is encouraging in this regard.[44]

Collective experience suggests that it will be difficult to identify biomarkers that exceed the sensitivity of ALT for hepatotoxicity, or the sensitivity and specificity of cardiac troponins for myocyte injuries. Nevertheless, new biomarkers that are complementary to these biomarkers should enable diagnosis of a wider variety of toxicities to these tissues or provide more specific diagnoses regarding the nature of the injury, the region of the organ effected, or the cell type that is injured. A liver biomarker that is not inducible and is expressed solely in liver could provide improved specificity over ALT. An additional cardiac-specific biomarker that persists longer in serum than the short half-life cardiac troponins would be more practical for routine deployment in animal toxicology testing studies. Thus, additional biomarkers can add value without exceeding the sensitivities of existing biomarkers.

A variety of biomarkers have been shown to be valuable individually for one or several toxicant or disease situations. Few of these biomarkers have been systematically evaluated for the plethora of situations that might provoke false positive responses. Acceleration of the current pace of biomarker evaluation and qualification demands (a) the availability of panels of biomarker–assays that can be comparatively evaluated on well-defined common sample sets, (b) fit-for-purpose performance evaluation in controlled animal studies with carefully benchmarked histological endpoints and samples from well-defined focused clinical trial cohorts, and (c) ready availability of banked blood and urine sample archives from clinical trial populations with carefully documented morbidities such as the Framingham Heart Study,[45] or the Drug-Induced Liver Injury Network (DILIN) prospective study,[46] to name a few. Availability of such panels of validated biomarker assays and well-documented preclinical and clinical samples, as well as increased cooperation between animal model researchers and clinical researchers will enable individual biomarkers to be qualified for sensitivity of specifically defined adverse events, qualified for appropriate specificity using samples of defined benign events, and collected into panels that yield complementary information about the health and safety of animals and patients.

16.4 QUALIFYING NEW SAFETY BIOMARKERS TO FOSTER REGULATORY ACCEPTANCE

New safety biomarkers cannot be used to improve clinical drug evaluation without gaining acceptance from regulatory authorities. The FDA, EMEA, and Pharmaceutical and Medical Devices Agency (PMDA), have recently established review teams in the United States, Europe, and Japan, respectively, to formally evaluate proposed novel safety biomarkers. The pace of biomarker qualifications could be improved by establishing global consensus on fit-for-purpose minimal evidentiary standards, and by improving the collaborative infrastructure for biomarker qualification research across industry, within government, and by cooperation with academic and medical centers. Improvement in the infrastructure shows encouraging signs as evidenced by the creation of biomarker consortia such as the PSTC within the Critical Path Institute, by several biomarker initiatives in ILSI/HESI, by the Innovative Medicines Initiative through the European Commission, and by the Foundation for the NIH Biomarker Consortium. Such consortia are proving that even though qualification of biomarkers for regulatory decision making may be too onerous and expensive for any single pharmaceutical or biotechnology company, progress establishing safety biomarkers is in the common interest, and is possible and effective through cooperation and collaboration. By working together and through close dialog with appropriate representatives from regulatory agencies, critical questions can be approached by such consortia to define how much data are needed to support qualification claims, what threshold of change for a biomarker is clinically meaningful, and in what specific contexts it is appropriate to rely on measurement of a new biomarker.

REFERENCES

1. Sikorska K, Stalke P, Jaskiewicz K, et al. Could iron deposits in hepatocytes serve as a prognostic marker of HFE gene mutations? *Hepatogastroenterology*. 2008;55:1024–1028.
2. Schena M, Shalon D, Davis RW, et al. Quantitative monitoring of gene expression patterns with a complementary DNA microarray. *Science*. 1995;270:467–470.
3. Collins FS, Haseltine WA. Of genes and genomes: What lies between the base pairs. *J Investig Med*. 2000;48:295–301.
4. Ahmed FE. Role of miRNA in carcinogenesis and biomarker selection: a methodological view. *Expert Rev Mol Diagn*. 2007;7:569–603.
5. Lee HJ, Wark AW, Corn RM. Microarray methods for protein biomarker detection. *Analyst*. 2008;133:975–983.
6. Peng Y, Li W, Liu Y. A hybrid approach for biomarker discovery from microarray gene expression data for cancer classification. *Cancer Inform*. 2007;2:301–311.
7. Lonneborg A. Biomarkers for Alzheimer disease in cerebrospinal fluid, urine, and blood. *Mol Diagn Ther*. 2008;12:307–320.
8. Wagner JA, Williams SA, Webster CJ. Biomarkers and surrogate end points for fit-for-purpose development and regulatory evaluation of new drugs. *Clin Pharmacol Ther*. 2007;81:104–107.
9. Olson H, et al. Concordance of the toxicity of pharmaceuticals in humans and in animals. *Regul Toxicol Pharmacol*. 2000;32:56–67.
10. Wagner JA. Overview of biomarkers and surrogate endpoints in drug development. *Dis Markers*. 2002;18:41–46.
11. Tugendreich S, Pearson CI, Sagartz J, et al. NSAID-induced acute phase response is due to increased intestinal permeability and characterized by early and consistent alterations in hepatic gene expression. *Toxicol Pathol*. 2006;34:168–179.
12. Fielden MR, et al. A gene expression signature that predicts the future onset of drug-induced renal tubular toxicity. *Toxicol Pathol*. 2005;33:675–683.
13. Fielden MR, Brennan R, Gollub J. A gene expression biomarker provides early prediction and mechanistic assessment of hepatic tumor induction by nongenotoxic chemicals. *Toxicol Sci*. 2007;99:90–100.
14. Oguri T, et al. MRP7/ABCC10 expression is a predictive biomarker for the resistance to paclitaxel in non-small cell lung cancer. *Mol Cancer Ther*. 2008;7:1150–1155.
15. Dehdashti F, et al. PET-based estradiol challenge as a predictive biomarker of response to endocrine therapy in women with estrogen-receptor-positive breast cancer. *Breast Cancer Res Treat*. 2009;113:509–517.
16. Dagues N, et al. Investigation of the molecular mechanisms preceding PDE4 inhibitor-induced vasculopathy in rats: tissue inhibitor of metalloproteinase 1, a potential predictive biomarker. *Toxicol Sci*. 2007;100: 238–247.
17. Kim DH, et al. Elevation of sphinganine 1-phosphate as a predictive biomarker for fumonisin exposure and toxicity in mice. *J Toxicol Environ Health A*. 2006;69: 2071–2082.
18. Costa LG, et al. Paraoxonase (PON 1) as a biomarker of susceptibility for organophosphate toxicity. *Biomarkers*. 2003;8:1–12.
19. Nantermet PV, et al. Identification of genetic pathways activated by the androgen receptor during the induction of proliferation in the ventral prostate gland. *J Biol Chem*. 2004;279:1310–1322.

20. Palacio L, et al. Pharmacogenetic Impact of VKORC1 and CYP2C9 Allelic Variants on warfarin dose requirements in a Hispanic population isolate. *Clin Appl Thromb Hemost.* 2009; 16: 83–90.
21. Tibshirani R. A simple method for assessing sample sizes in microarray experiments. *BMC Bioinformat.* 2006;7:106.
22. Tong T, Zhao H. Practical guidelines for assessing power and false discovery rate for a fixed sample size in microarray experiments. *Stat Med.* 2008;27:1960–1972.
23. Mattes WB, Walker EG. Translational toxicology and the work of the predictive safety testing consortium. *Clin Pharmacol Ther.* 2009;85:327–330.
24. Recanatini M, Poluzzi E, Masetti M, et al. QT prolongation through hERG K(+) channel blockade: Current knowledge and strategies for the early prediction during drug development. *Med Res Rev.* 2005;25:133–166.
25. Olson S, Robinson S, Giffin R, rapporteurs. *Forum on Drug Discovery, Development, and Translation*; Institute of Medicine 100. National Academies Press; Washington DC 2009.
26. O'Brien PJ. Cardiac troponin is the most effective translational safety biomarker for myocardial injury in cardiotoxicity. *Toxicology* 245, 206–218 (2008).
27. Boswood A. Biomarkers in cardiovascular disease: beyond natriuretic peptides. *J Vet Cardiol* 11 Suppl 1, S23–32 (2009).
28. Collison, PO. Cardiac markers. *Br J Hosp Med (Lond).* 70, M84–87 (2009).
29. Menown IB, et al. Prediction of recurrent events by D-dimer and inflammatory markers in patients with normal cardiac troponin I (PREDICT) study. *Am Heart J.* 2003;145:986–992.
30. Kerns W, et al. Drug-induced vascular injury – a quest for biomarkers. *Toxicol Appl Pharmacol.* 2005;203:62–87.
31. Brott D, et al. Biomarkers of drug-induced vascular injury. *Toxicol Appl Pharmacol.* 2005;207:441–445.
32. Devarajan P. Emerging biomarkers of acute kidney injury. *Contrib Nephrol.* 2007;156:203–212.
33. Sawicki PT, Heinemann L, Berger M. Comparison of methods for determination of microalbuminuria in diabetic patients. *Diabet Med.* 1989;6:412–415.
34. Vaidya VS, Bonventre JV. Mechanistic biomarkers for cytotoxic acute kidney injury. *Expert Opin Drug Metab Toxicol.* 2006;2:697–713.
35. Vaidya VS, et al. Urinary biomarkers for sensitive and specific detection of acute kidney injury in humans. *Clin Transl Sci.* 2008;1:200–208.
36. Dieterle F et al. Renal biomarker qualification submission: a dialog between the FDA-EMEA and Predictive Safety Testing Consortium. *Nat Biotechnol.* 2010; 5:455–462.
37. Amacher DE. Serum transaminase elevations as indicators of hepatic injury following the administration of drugs. *Regul Toxicol Pharmacol.* 1998;27:119–130.
38. Burtis, CA, ed. Fundamentals of Clinical Chemistry, Vol. 6. Philadelphia: W. B. Saunders; 2001.
39. Poynard T, et al. Assessment of liver fibrosis: Noninvasive means. *Saudi J Gastroenterol.* 2008;14:163–173.
40. Williams D. The critical path to medical innovation. *Med Device Technol.* 2004;15:8–10.
41. Woodcock J. Chutes and ladders on the critical path: Comparative effectiveness, product value, and the use of biomarkers in drug development. *Clin Pharmacol Ther.* 2009;86:12–14.
42. Ratner M. Looking for solid ground along the Critical Path. *Nat Biotechnol.* 2006;24:885–887.
43. Hunter AJ. The Innovative Medicines Initiative: a pre-competitive initiative to enhance the biomedical science base of Europe to expedite the development of new medicines for patients. *Drug Discov Today.* 2008;13:371–373.

44. Metias SM, Lianidou E, Yousef GM. MicroRNAs in clinical oncology: At the crossroads between promises and problems. *J Clin Pathol.* 2009;62:771–776.
45. Kannel WB. Cardioprotection and antihypertensive therapy: the key importance of addressing the associated coronary risk factors (the Framingham experience). *Am J Cardiol.* 1996;77:6B-11B.
46. Fontana RJ, et al. Drug-Induced Liver Injury Network (DILIN) prospective study: Rationale, design and conduct. *Drug Saf.* 2009;32:55–68.

17 **Application of TK/PD modeling in predicting dose-limiting toxicity**

Li J. Yu, Lee Silverman, Carl L. Alden, Guohui Liu, Shimoga Prakash, and Frank Lee

17.1 INTRODUCTION

For the development of cytotoxic anticancer pharmaceuticals, the initial phase 1 clinical trials in patients with advanced cancer disease usually include determining a maximum tolerated dose (MTD) and identifying dose-limiting toxicity (DLT).[1,2] The MTD is usually defined as the dose tolerated by five out of six patients with acceptable levels of DLT and dose levels above which result in unacceptable DLT in two or more patients. The dose–response curve for many pharmaceuticals in this class is steep.[3] Traditionally, the dose recommended for phase 2 trials of cytotoxic agents is based on the MTD determined in phase 1. The inherent assumption in establishing and using an MTD is that the therapeutic effect and the associated toxicities are correlated and that the mechanism of action of both the toxic and therapeutic effects is the same – higher doses result in greater efficacy.[2,4] Therefore, it is not uncommon for the efficacious dose of anticancer pharmaceuticals to be at or near the MTD.[5,6] Predicting the dose and exposure at which DLT will likely occur in humans provides value in designing and conducting the first clinical trial for a cytotoxic anticancer pharmaceutical.

Before testing in patients, the toxicities of these pharmaceutical candidates are studied in nonclinical species in toxicology studies to determine the DLT. Toxicokinetics (TK) represent the assessment of systemic exposure in toxicity studies, in which pharmacokinetic data are generated, either from the same animals used in the main toxicology study (usually for larger species such as dogs or monkeys) or from a satellite group (usually for smaller species such as rats or mice) at each dose level used in the main toxicology study. The primary objective of TK studies is to describe the systemic exposure achieved in animals and its relationship to dose level and to toxicological findings. According to regulatory guidelines,[7] such objectives could be achieved through the derivation of one or more pharmacokinetic parameters from measurements made at appropriate time points during the course of the individual studies. The commonly used TK parameters are maximum plasma concentration (C_{max}), area under the plasma concentration-time curve (AUC), and concentration at a predetermined time point (C_{time}).

Several book chapters and articles have been written on pharmacokinetic and pharmacodynamic (PK/PD) models or modeling and their applications in toxicology, including work by Arie Bruinink,[8] Jurgen Timm,[9] Krishnan and Andersen,[10] and Diack and Bois.[11] It would be redundant and add little value to present that material in this book chapter. Instead, the focus of this chapter is to show some unique approaches and applications of PK/PD modeling for the prediction of oncologic chemotherapeutic candidate DLT in nonclinical toxicology studies during drug discovery and early development. Two case studies will be presented in this chapter to illustrate how simple PK/PD modeling was used for predicting DLT.

17.2 WHAT IS A MODEL AND WHAT IS ITS PURPOSE

In pharmacokinetic-pharmacodynamic modeling, the models are mathematical and statistical in nature, and they attempt to characterize the relationship between dose and some dependent variables. A pharmacokinetic model describes the relationship between dose and drug concentrations, usually in plasma or serum, whereas a pharmacodynamic model relates drug concentration to efficacy, adverse effects, or outcome. A pharmacokinetic-pharmacodynamic model integrates dose with response.

Modeling, especially quantitative modeling based on mathematics and statistics, serves many useful purposes. One is to characterize and summarize a set of data into a cohesive structure. For example, given a set of concentration-time data, a pharmacokinetic model summarizes the data into a few simple parameters (e.g., clearance – a parameter that relates concentration to rate of change in concentration). Second, and most importantly, modeling may allow predictions to be made, a process referred to as simulation. Given a pharmacokinetic-pharmacodymamic model, predictions on outcome or safety can be made regarding projected changes in dose, dose frequency, or the parameters that describe the system, such as the expected increase in exposure in a case in which the clearance pathway is impaired either by coadministration of a metabolic enzyme inhibitor[12,13] or an impediment in a major clearance organ (e.g., liver or kidney[14,15]). The ability to predict makes simulation a very important tool in drug discovery and development[16] because it provides rationale on how to move forward with a compound with potentially challenging attributes.

17.3 GENERAL CONCEPTS AND CONSIDERATIONS

The selection of modeling approaches is heavily dependent on the questions asked and the dataset available. Before the first submission of an investigational new drug (IND) for a first-in-class program, the available dataset is often limited. It is often unrealistic and/or unnecessary to develop a sophisticated mechanism-based PK/PD model before the first IND for a first-in-class program.

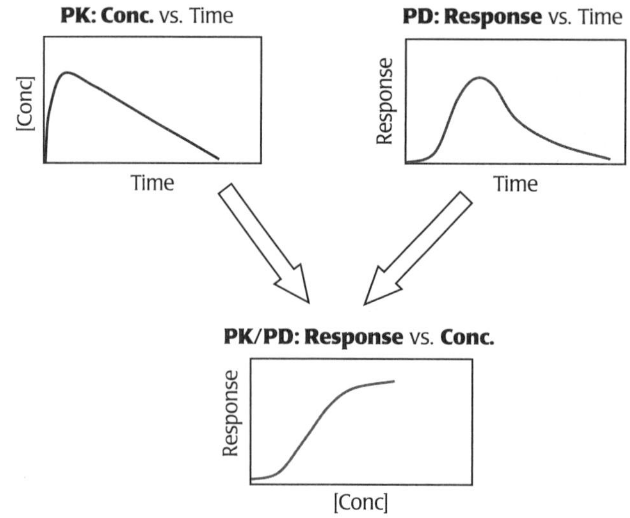

Figure 17-1: General work flow: Key data set needed for PK/PD analysis.

Conventional PK models, which describe a concentration-time profile at a given dose, can be applied either using noncompartmental or compartmental analysis. The most commonly used software is WinNonlin from Pharsight.

The most commonly used pharmacodynamic models are the basic E_{max} model (Equation 1) and the sigmoid E_{max} model (Equation 2) when the concentration–response relationship is direct and immediate. The difference between these two models is the slope factor, gamma, also known as the Hill factor or the sigmoidicity factor. The purpose of adding this single parameter, gamma, to the sigmoid E_{max} model is to modify its steepness to account for concentration–response curves, which are either shallower (gamma < 1) or steeper (gamma > 1) than that captured in the simple E_{max} model.

$$\text{Effect} = \frac{E_{max} * \text{Conc}}{EC_{50} + \text{Conc}} \tag{1}$$

$$\text{Effect} = \frac{E_{max} * \text{Conc}^{\text{gamma}}}{EC_{50}^{\text{gamma}} + \text{Conc}^{\text{gamma}}} \tag{2}$$

In an ideal situation, the PD response is easily measurable, is numerical, and has a direct relationship to the plasma drug level. Therefore, one can apply conventional PK and PD models to predict the dose, time–concentration, and time–effect relationship (Figure 17.1[17,18]).

The difficulty with modeling occurs when dealing with an indirect response or a categorical effect, such as mortality, that may be due to multiple causes. A general workflow to deal with this more difficult scenario is illustrated in Figure 17.2. The first step is to conduct a study using different dosing regimens in animals and monitor for the effect associated with drug treatment. Plasma samples are collected from animals in each dosing group for TK analysis, and

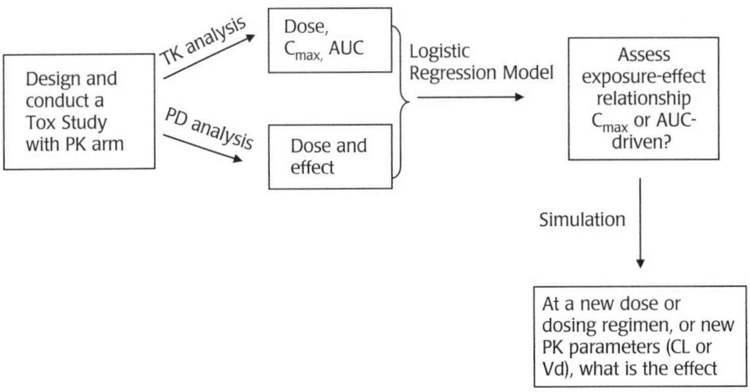

Figure 17-2: Work flow when PD is a categorical or effect-concentration relationship is not easily defined.

exposure parameters (e.g., C_{max} and AUC). The second step is to analyze the correlation between C_{max} and effect versus the correlation between AUC and effect. Ideally, the data are robust enough to show that one correlation is better than the other. In some cases, the effect is known to be C_{max} driven (e.g., QTc[19]) or AUC-driven (e.g., myelosuppression, nephrotoxicity, neutropenia[20,21]). If this is the case, the analysis can be based on prior knowledge. The goal is to determine at what exposure level (either C_{max} or AUC), an effect is expected. Having defined this relationship, one can predict or simulate an effect at a different dose or regimen. Assuming the exposure-effect relationship is consistent among different species, and the only difference between species is the PK, one can predict the effect in another species when the PK parameters are available in the species of interest.

17.4 LOGISTIC REGRESSION MODELS

For many cytotoxic agents, the causes for mortality or DLT may be complex and multifactorial. Understanding the relationship between exposure and each individual toxicity variable (e.g., hematologic toxicity, gastrointestinal disturbance, cardiotoxicity) is important but can be both time and resource consuming. When the first objective is to determine the exposure that is most likely to be associated with mortality or a dose-limiting event in a toxicology study, a logistic regression model is a suitable approach to provide a rapid assessment. This assessment may then be used to compare with the exposure from a pharmacology study at an efficacious dose or from another toxicokinetic study in a different species. Assuming the exposure-effect relationship in the toxicology species is similar to that in humans, the human DLT dose can be predicted based on the targeted AUC and human PK projection with well-described models such as the allometry,[22,23] the Dedrick plot,[24] or the Wajima method.[25]

The toxicity upon pharmaceutical treatment is often described by categorical variables that are either non-ordered (e.g., mortality: dead or alive) or ordered (e.g., severe, moderate, mild, or no effect). The classical PK/PD models (e.g., the linear E_{max} or sigmoid-E_{max} model), which handle measurable quantifiable effects (enzyme inhibition, blood pressure, etc.[26,27]), cannot be applied to describe the relationship between exposure and a categorical variable.

Logistic regression modeling is used for predicting the probability of occurrence of an event by fitting data to a logistic curve.[28] It describes the relationship between the categorical response variable and one or more continuous variables.[29] Such a model can be described in Equation 3:

$$\text{logit}(p) = \log\left(\frac{p}{1-p}\right) \theta + x\beta \tag{3}$$

where p is the probability of an event such as mortality, θ is the intercept, and β is the regression coefficients for variable x. Logistic regression is used extensively in the medical and social sciences for applications such as prediction of survival rate and risk of developing cancer, among others.[30]

When experiments results in ordinate categorical responses, say C categories, a general modeling approach based on logistic regression model can be described as

$$\text{logit}\left(\Pr(Y \le k)\right) = \log\left(\frac{\Pr(Y \le k)}{1-\Pr(Y \le k)}\right) \theta_k + x\beta, \quad k = 1, \dots, C-1 \tag{4}$$

where Y represents the observed response, $\theta_k, k = 1, \dots, C-1$ where ${}_1 < {}_2 < \dots < {}_{C-1}$ represent the cumulative probabilities, $\Pr(Y \le k)$, when no covariates are measured, and β is the regression coefficients for variable x.

As described by the following case studies, logistic regression represents an approach that can sufficiently meet the demands of many real-world pharmaceutical research and development scenarios.[11,31]

17.5 CASE STUDY 1: MODELING TK AND MORIBUNDITY FROM DOG STUDIES

In beagle dog toxicology studies, drug-A (a potent cytotoxic compound synthesized at Millennium Pharmaceuticals, Inc.) was administered either by 5-min IV infusion (6/sex/dose) for two cycles (one cycle consisted of twice weekly dosing for 2 weeks and cycles were separated by a 10-day nondosing period), or by oral gavage (5 males/dose) for one cycle. During these studies, serial plasma samples were collected from each animal on the first and last dosing day in each cycle for toxicokinetic analysis, and subsequently plasma C_{max} and AUC of drug-A were calculated for each animal. Of the total 57 dogs in these studies, 11 either became moribund or died on test because of toxicity (Table 17.1) during the first cycle (8 from the IV treatment groups and 3 from the PO treatment groups).

The correlation between the probability of moribundity (p) and a plasma TK parameter variable (a variable of interest, or VOI, such as C_{max} or AUC) from

Table 17-1. TK and PD data from the dog toxicity studies

Dose (mg/kg)	Route	N (M/F)	Moribundity (No. [%])	Mean Plasma AUC0–24 h (hr·ng/mL)	Mean Plasma C_{max} (ng/mL)
0.10	IV	12 (6/6)	0	512	362
0.10	PO	5 (5/0)	0	492	161
0.14	IV	6 (3/3)	0	547	452
0.20	PO	5 (5/0)	1 (20)	753	220
0.18	IV	12 (6/6)	3 (25)	1080	813
0.30	PO	5 (5/0)	2 (40)	1590	397
0.25	IV	12 (6/6)	5 (42)	1500	856

M, male; F, female.

Table 17-2. Logistic regression model in AUC and C_{max} with moribundity

Route	Variable	Odds ratio	95% confidence interval	P-value
IV	$AUC_{0-24\,h}$ (h·ng/mL)	1.001	(1.0002, 1.0025)	0.019
	C_{max} (ng/mL)	1.004	(1.0011 1.0079)	0.010
IV + PO	$AUC_{0-24\,h}$ (h·ng/mL)	1.001	(1.0004, 1.0025)	0.008
	C_{max} (ng/mL)	1.003	(1.0004, 1.0047)	0.018

individual dogs was assessed using a logistic regression model shown in Equation 5 first on the basis of the IV route alone and then on the basis of IV and PO routes together. In addition, sex was incorporated into the initial model to check whether sex has a significant effect. This analysis was performed using statistical software SAS 9.1 (SAS Institute Inc., Cary, NC).

$$\text{logit}\,(p) = \log\left(\frac{p}{1-p}\right) = \beta_0 + \beta_1 * \text{VOI} + \beta_2 * \text{sex} \tag{5}$$

where p is the probability of mortality, VOI is the PK parameter (AUC or C_{max}), β_0 is the intercept, and β_1 and β_2 are the regression parameters for VOI and sex, respectively.

The initial analysis showed that sex had no significant effect on either TK or dose-limiting toxicity, and subsequently sex was excluded from the model. Table 17.2 summarizes the statistical analysis for correlation between mortality and plasma AUC or C_{max}. The logistic model shown in Table 17.2 was fitted

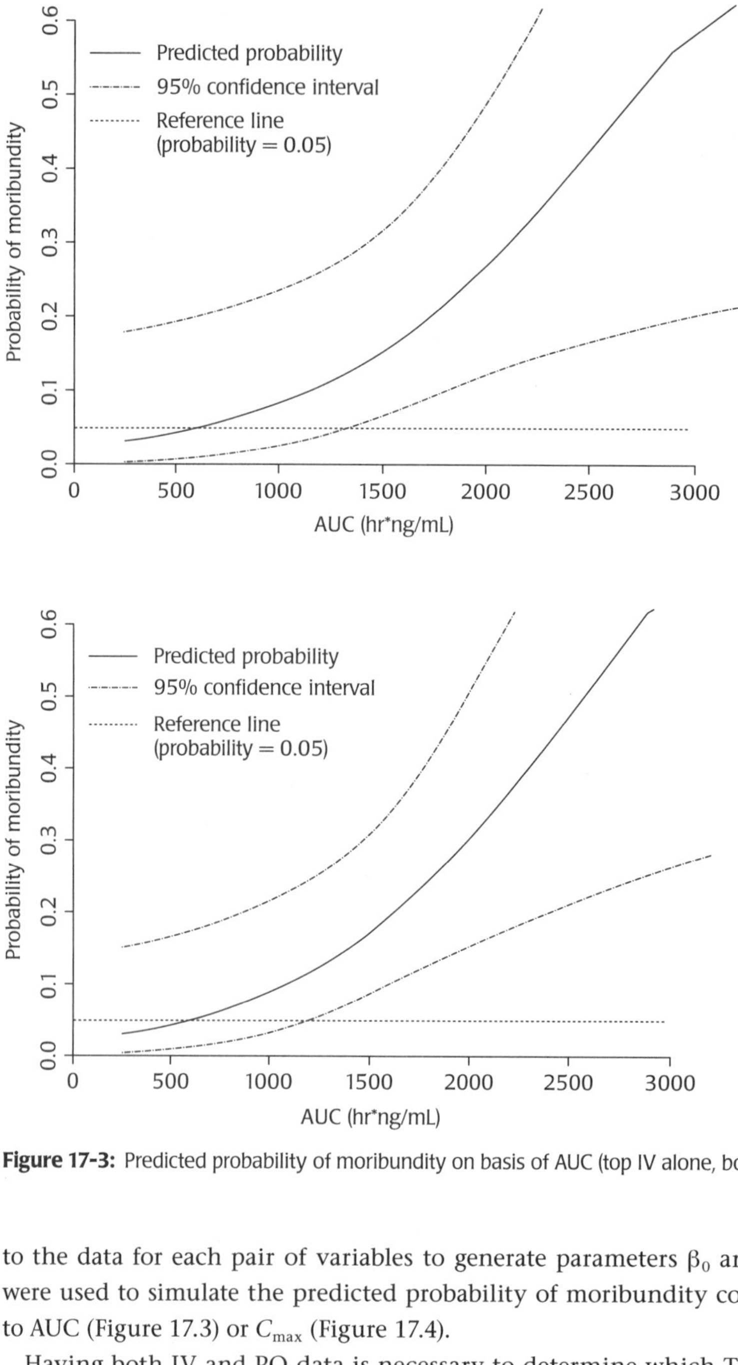

Figure 17-3: Predicted probability of moribundity on basis of AUC (top IV alone, bottom IV + PO).

to the data for each pair of variables to generate parameters β_0 and β_1, which were used to simulate the predicted probability of moribundity corresponding to AUC (Figure 17.3) or C_{max} (Figure 17.4).

Having both IV and PO data is necessary to determine which TK parameter has a higher association with DLT, when DLT is independent of route of administration. If we only had IV data, it would be impossible to determine which parameter (AUC or C_{max}) is more closely correlated with moribundity since AUC and C_{max} correlate with each other within one route. When the IV and PO data were put together as in Table 17.1, one can easily see, without doing any modeling, that there appeared to be a correlation between moribundity and AUC, but

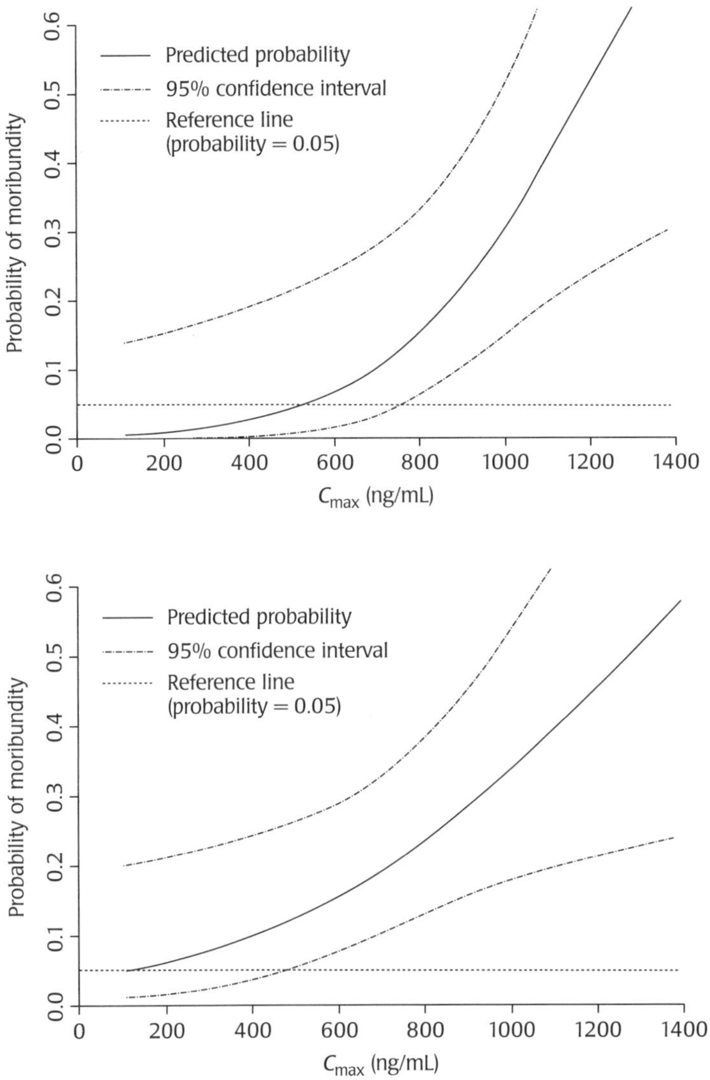

Figure 17-4: Predicted probability of moribundity on basis of C_{max} (top IV alone, bottom IV + PO).

the correlation was not as obvious for C_{max}. The correlation analysis alone on the basis of P-value from both IV and PO data only indicates a better correlation for AUC (P-value = 0.008) than C_{max} (P-value = 0.018). However the simulated probability of mortality graphs shown in Figures 17.3 and 17.4 demonstrate a consistent relationship between moribundity and AUC regardless of route of administration, especially when the AUC value is < 2,000 h·ng/mL. On the other hand, there is no consistent relationship between moribundity and C_{max}. Hence, AUC is a more reliable predictor for moribundity than C_{max}.

The emphasis of this data analysis was to illustrate a simple modeling approach for handling binary response data. This model can provide a quantitative description of exposure–effect relationships. The predicted probability of dose-limiting toxicity corresponding to AUC is a particularly valuable result as it allows one to take the preclinical data, where sample size is limited and data are noncontinuous, and predict for probability of events in the clinical setting, where the larger sample size leads to a more continuous dataset. Using a group mean TK parameter, one of the most conventional methods of analysis, cannot explain why within the same dosing group some dogs became moribund and some did not. By examining individual dog TK and response data using this logistic regression model approach, a very strong correlation between mortality and AUC was demonstrated (*P*-value = 0.008). Thus, we allow for projection of the dose-AUC-effect relationship in different species on the basis of PK modeling (with correction of plasma protein binding when necessary) and assuming similar pharmacodynamic effects across different species.

17.6 CASE STUDY 2: MODELING TK AND SEVERITY OF LESIONS IN TISSUES FROM A RAT STUDY

One of the challenges in studying the relationship between TK and toxicity from a repeat-dose rat toxicology study is that the toxicological findings in the individual main study animals are not directly related to the actual exposure in the same animal (TK is usually collected from a satellite group), and therefore, it is difficult to explain why at a certain dose level, there is toxicity in some but not all animals. In addition, the number of animals used in a study is often not large enough to capture the distribution of adverse events at limited dose levels. To overcome this challenge, Aarons and Graham took a unique approach on modeling TK and toxicity data of a drug from a 28-day rat toxicology study conducted at Glaxo-Wellcome.[32] In this study, rats were divided into three groups: group 1 = placebo, group 2 = 30 mg/kg, and group 3 = 200 mg/kg. The rats were given the drug orally once a day for 4 weeks. On day 28 of the study, plasma samples were taken from each rat through a sparse sampling scheme for toxicokinetic evaluation. Such limited sampling is unlikely to distress the animals, disturb the conduct of a toxicological study, or affect the outcome of the study. After TK sampling, the rats were sacrificed and dissected to observe the severity of lesions within the rats conjectured to be caused by the drug.

For the pharmacodynamic measurement of the drug, the severity of the lesions (pooled over 20 tissues analyzed) was used. Severity was defined on a five-grade scale, where 0 = no lesion; 1 = very slight lesion; 2 = slight lesion; 3 = moderate lesion; and 4 = marked lesion. A TK analysis was carried out by applying the population PK approach using the nonlinear mixed-effects modeling package NONMEM. The population PK modeling is beyond the scope of this chapter, and the reader can find its details from the references provided.[33–37] The individual AUC for each animal was estimated from the mixed-effects population model. The AUCs and lesion scores are given in Table 17.3. From this table, certain characteristic probabilities can be obtained such as the probability of

Table 17-3. TK and PD data from the rat toxicity study

Rat	Dose (mg/kg)	Gender	AUC	Lesion score category				
				0	1	2	3	4
496	30	Male	11.94	13	4	3	0	0
497			11.85	17	1	2	0	0
498			13.95	16	4	0	0	0
515		Female	11.09	18	2	0	0	0
516			15.62	8	3	7	2	0
522			18.01	11	4	4	0	0
499	200	Male	82.35	2	2	11	7	3
501			80.56	0	7	8	7	3
503			78.04	4	8	10	2	1
518		Female	64.76	4	12	6	1	0
519			64.95	13	6	5	0	0
520			77.17	8	7	6	3	0

having a certain category of lesion by the end of the study for either the 30 or 200 mg/kg dose group. It can be clearly seen that the first six rats (corresponding to the 30 mg/kg dose group) have higher percentages in the lower lesion score compared to the last six rats (corresponding to the 200 mg/kg dose group).

A logistic regression model is used in this case again (Equation 6) to assess the relationship between AUC and severity of lesion. This model, containing five grades of lesions, was fitted to the data. The parameters of the model were estimated by Monte Carlo Markov chain simulation using the BUGS program.[38] Various combinations of covariates taken from dose, gender, and AUC were tried in the model. The results indicate that the AUC describes the toxicity event better than the dose. The model parameters generated are listed in Table 17.4, and the predicted probability of each grade lesion versus AUC is shown in Figure 17.5. There is no strong gender effect on relationship between AUC and probability of a specific lesion severity grade because both β_2 and β_3 had 95 percent confidence interval across zero.

$$\text{logit}\left(\Pr(Y_i \le k \mid b_i)\right) = \theta_k + \beta_1 AUC_i + \beta_2 \text{gender}_i + \beta_3 \text{AUC}_i\text{gender}_i + b_i, \quad k = 0, 1, 2, 3 \tag{6}$$

where k is the response category scale, β_1, β_2, and β_3 are the regression parameters for AUC, gender, and the interaction term of AUC and gender, respectively.

The key point illustrated in this case is that the individual estimates of the AUCs appeared to be a better predictor of the severity of the lesion than dose and gender. Such a PK/PD model provides a quantitative prediction – at what AUC level a more severe lesion (such as grade 4) is anticipated – without conducting a study with a large number of animals at a highly toxic dose.

Table 17-4. Parameters generated by equation 6

	Mean	S.D.	95% confidence interval
θ_0	1.979	0.619	(0.799, 3.384)
θ_1	3.362	0.638	(2.215, 4.802)
θ_2	5.333	0.687	(4.101, 6.838)
θ_3	7.128	0.786	(5.671, 8.759)
β_1	−0.0544	0.0118	(−0.0776, −0.0313)
β_2	−1.192	0.893	(−2.757, 0.6638)
β_3	0.0348	0.018	(−0.00573, 0.0657)
σ^a	0.7586	0.306	(0.302, 1.453)

[a] *Inter-rat variability.*

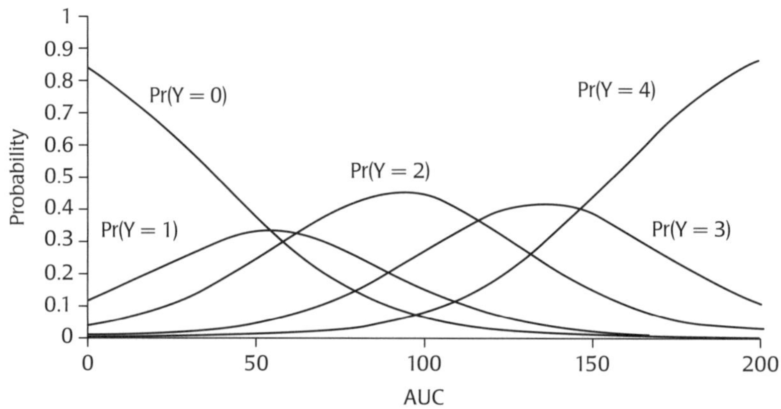

Figure 17-5: Predicted probability of lesion in each category using AUC-based model. Reprinted with permission from Professor Leon Aarons.

17.7 LIMITATION OF THE MODELING APPROACH

Any model has its own inherent utilities and limitations. Determination of what model to use should be dependent on the purpose. The purpose of the models used in these two cases was to determine the exposure that was associated with DLT or severe lesions in the discovery and early development phase when the exposure-based prediction needs to be made as reliably as possible in a short time. Although nonspecific measurements (e.g., DLT or lesion scores) do not scale easily across species, this exposure-based approach should still be better in terms of accuracy of prediction than the conventional dose (mg/m^2)-only based predictions, such as LD_{10} in rodents.[39]

A PK/PD model based on more specific and mechanism-based responses offers some advantages in terms of interpreting data and extrapolating the finding to different species, especially when the species difference is driven by different pharmcodynamics.[40–42] However, mechanism-based modeling usually takes a longer time to be developed and requires a more robust dataset than we normally can obtain in the early phases of a program, especially when the drug is first-in-class for a novel target. A more specific mechanism-based model may be developed over time when more knowledge and data are obtained.

17.8 BRIDGING PRECLINICAL DATA TO HUMANS

The ultimate goal of preclinical PK/PD modeling as an "applied science" tool is to predict safe and efficacious human dose and exposure for drugs progressing into clinical trials. This approach has emerged during the past decades,[43] and some success has been recognized.[44–46] However, not all preclinical models can be successfully extrapolated to the human situation, and many factors should be considered before placing any credibility on the extrapolation.

First, the difference in ADME (absorption, distribution, metabolism, and elimination) properties between preclinical species and human needs to be understood. For example, do animal species generate metabolites that are quantitatively and qualitatively the same as those that occur in human, and are there any active metabolites? Is there any difference in plasma or blood protein binding? If the dosing frequency is the same, do animal species and human have similar $t_{1/2}$ of a pharmaceutical, which dictates the duration of drug exposure within each dosing interval? Efavirenz, a potent nonnucleoside reverse transcriptase inhibitor widely prescribed for the treatment of HIV infection, produces renal tubular epithelial cell necrosis in rats but not in cynomolgus monkeys or humans. The toxicity difference among species is supported by a species-dependent glutathione conjugate metabolite.[47]

Second, the target sensitivity to a pharmaceutical among different species needs to be understood. For example, it was shown that Millennium's proteasome inhibitor, MLN9708 (previously known as MLN2238), had a marked difference in inhibition potency against whole blood proteasome activities in the mouse compared to other species.[48] Troxacitabine is another example in which a species difference was observed in inhibition of cell growth in human tumor compared with murine tumor and normal hemapoietic cell lines.[41] In cases like this, using a qualified mechanism-based biomarker that can be determined across different species will be helpful for bridging to human scenarios (e.g., the model contains species-dependent EC_{50} and E_{max} parameters).

Third, the target expression and pharmacodynamics among different species should be evaluated.[49] Greaves et al.[50] performed a cross-species comparison of adverse effects for forty-five drugs and found that due to differences in target expression and the degree of pharmacodynamic response, species differences in adverse effects are heavily dependent on the target organ or system involved. For example, for the gastrointestinal and bone marrow toxicities induced by antimitotic actives, animal species predict well for humans. On the other hand, skin and neurological toxicities are more difficult to predict based on conventional animal models.

Last but not least, caution should be applied when extrapolating severe DLT or moribundity observed in toxicology studies to human; because in humans intervention/treatment will be immediately applied when DLT is observed to prevent a more serious event. For example, oncologists are very adept in managing the challenge associated with myelosuppression and/or gastrointestinal tract injury that in nonclinical studies would induce a moribund condition.

Within a drug development company, lead compounds that have a PK/PD and/or TK/toxicity model established preclinically and then tested and validated in humans provide a distinctive advantage over those that do not. For example, our knowledge of the PK/PD/toxicity relationship of VELCADE across different species provided the foundation in developing the second generation of proteasome inhibitor, MLN9708.[48,51] As shown by Yu et al.,[48] different species can tolerate similar blood PD responses but not similar doses based on mg/m^2 or plasma AUC basis. Hematological toxicity is often dose limiting for many cytotoxic anticancer agents; therefore, hematological toxicity has been used as the PD for TK/toxicity modeling in different species.[52–55] Establishment of the relationship between pharmacokinetics and nephrotoxicity and myelosuppression for cisplatin, carboplatin, and nedaplatin in rats provided a useful parameter for predicting the degree of toxicity of platinum antitumor compounds.[20] Such an approach adds much-needed rationale into the validity of the model and its extrapolation. Should the lead compound fail and backup compounds having the same mechanism of action need to be created or resurrected from pipeline purgatory, modeling approaches are particularly useful in predicting the probability of success of backup compounds.

17.9 CONCLUSIONS

The TK/PD modeling described in this chapter is an approach that links a TK parameter to a categorical adverse response. Unlike conventional PK/PD modeling used in many pharmacology studies[56] that analyze dose- and time-dependent changes in concentrations and numerical biological responses (e.g., enzyme activities, blood sugar levels), the TK/PD modeling described in this chapter uses binary toxicological findings (e.g., mortality, tissue lesions) as the pharmacodynamic response of interest. For cytotoxics without chemical structure mediated toxicities, the dose-limiting toxicities are mechanism or PD based. In addition, instead of using group mean TK parameters at each dose level, individual TK data, regardless of the dose, was used to directly relate to the toxicological finding in that animal using a logistic regression approach. This TK/PD model is helpful in explaining why, at a certain dose level, there is toxicity in some but not all animals affected, particularly when dealing with cytotoxic pharmaceuticals with steep dose responses. Furthermore, when DLT is used as PD in the model, this model may be used to correlate DLT to a specific TK parameter (e.g., AUC, C_{max}).

REFERENCES

1. Rubinstein LVaS, Richard M. Phase I Clinical Trial Design. In: Budman DR, Calvert AH, Rowinsky EK, Hill BT, eds. *Handbook of Anticancer Drug Development.* Baltimore: Lippincott Williams & Wilkins; 2003:297.
2. Kummar S, Gutierrez M, Doroshow JH, et al. Drug development in oncology: classical cytotoxics and molecularly targeted agents. *Br J Clin Pharmacol.* 2006;62(1): 15–26.
3. Collins JMaEMJ. Measurements of Endpoints in Phase I Drug Design, Toxicity Versus Alternatives. In: Budman DR, Calvert AH, Rowinsky EK, Hill BT, ed. *Handbook of Anticancer Drug Development.* Baltimore: Lippincott Williams & Wilkins; 2003:319.
4. Haines IE. Dose selection in phase I studies: Why we should always go for the most effective. *J Clin Oncol.* 2008;26(21):3650–3652; author reply 3652–3653.
5. Bross PF, Kane R, Farrell AT, et al. Approval summary for bortezomib for injection in the treatment of multiple myeloma. *Clin Cancer Res.* 2004;10(12 Pt 1):3954–3964.
6. Goodman VL, Rock EP, Dagher R, et al. Approval summary: Sunitinib for the treatment of imatinib refractory or intolerant gastrointestinal stromal tumors and advanced renal cell carcinoma. *Clin Cancer Res.* 2007;13(5):1367–1373.
7. FDA. Guideline for Industry – Toxicokinetics: The assessment of Systemic Exposure in Toxicity Studies. March 1995.
8. Bruinink A. In Vitro Toxicokinetics and Dynamics: Modeling and Interpretation of Toxicity Data. In: Gad SC, ed. *Preclinical Development Handbook Toxicology*: Wiley-Interscience; 2008:509–550.
9. Timm J. Mathematical Models for Risk Extrapolation. In: Greim HS, ed. *Toxicology and Risk Assessment A Comprehensive Introduction.* Wiley; Chichester, 2008:479–494.
10. Krishnan KA, Melvin E. Physiologically-based pharmacokinetic modeling in toxicology. In: Hayes AW, ed. *Principles and Methods of Toxicology.* 4th ed. Philadelphia: Taylor & Francis; 2001:193–241.
11. Diack C, Bois FY. Pharmacokinetic-pharmacodynamic models for categorical toxicity data. *Regul Toxicol Pharmacol.* 2005;41(1):55–65.
12. van den Bongard HJ, Sparidans RW, Critchley DJ, et al. Pharmacokinetic drug-drug interaction of the novel anticancer agent E7070 and acenocoumarol. *Invest New Drugs.* 2004;22(2):151–158.
13. Wong CM, Ko Y, Chan A. Clinically significant drug-drug interactions between oral anticancer agents and nonanticancer agents: Profiling and comparison of two drug compendia. *Ann Pharmacother.* 2008;42(12):1737–1748.
14. Chen N, Lau H, Kong L, et al. Pharmacokinetics of lenalidomide in subjects with various degrees of renal impairment and in subjects on hemodialysis. *J Clin Pharmacol.* 2007;47(12):1466–1475.
15. Verbeeck RK. Pharmacokinetics and dosage adjustment in patients with hepatic dysfunction. *Eur J Clin Pharmacol.* 2008;64(12):1147–1161.
16. van Kesteren C, Mathot RA, Beijnen JH, et al. Pharmacokinetic-pharmacodynamic guided trial design in oncology. *Invest New Drugs.* 2003;21(2):225–241.
17. Mandema JW, Sansom LN, Dios-Vieitez MC, et al. Pharmacokinetic-pharmacodynamic modeling of the electroencephalographic effects of benzodiazepines. Correlation with receptor binding and anticonvulsant activity. *J Pharmacol Exp Ther.* 1991;257(1):472–478.
18. Webster R, Allan G, Anto-Awuakye K, et al. Pharmacokinetic/pharmacodynamic assessment of the effects of E4031, cisapride, terfenadine and terodiline on monophasic action potential duration in dog. *Xenobiotica.* 2001;31(8–9):633–650.
19. Chen X, Cass JD, Bradley JA, et al. QT prolongation and proarrhythmia by moxifloxacin: Concordance of preclinical models in relation to clinical outcome. *Br J Pharmacol.* 2005;146(6):792–799.

20. Hanada K, Asano K, Nishimura T, et al. Use of a toxicity factor to explain differences in nephrotoxicity and myelosuppression among the platinum antitumour derivatives cisplatin, carboplatin and nedaplatin in rats. *J Pharm Pharmacol.* 2008;60(3):317–322.
21. Grochow LB, Rowinsky EK, Johnson R, et al. Pharmacokinetics and pharmacodynamics of topotecan in patients with advanced cancer. *Drug Metab Dispos.* 1992;20(5):706–713.
22. Boxenbaum H. Interspecies scaling, allometry, physiological time, and the ground plan of pharmacokinetics. *J Pharmacokinet Biopharm.* 1982;10(2):201–227.
23. Mahmood I. Prediction of clearance, volume of distribution and half-life by allometric scaling and by use of plasma concentrations predicted from pharmacokinetic constants: A comparative study. *J Pharm Pharmacol.* 1999;51(8):905–910.
24. Dedrick R, Bischoff KB, Zaharko DS. Interspecies correlation of plasma concentration history of methotrexate (NSC-740). *Cancer Chemother Rep.* 1970;54(2):95–101.
25. Wajima T, Yano Y, Fukumura K, et al. Prediction of human pharmacokinetic profile in animal scale up based on normalizing time course profiles. *J Pharm Sci.* 2004;93(7):1890–1900.
26. Holford NH, Guentert TW, Dingemanse J, et al. Pharmacodynamics of lazabemide, a reversible and selective inhibitor of monoamine oxidase B. *Br J Clin Pharmacol.* 1994;37(6):553–557.
27. Jann MW, Shirley KL, Small GW. Clinical pharmacokinetics and pharmacodynamics of cholinesterase inhibitors. *Clin Pharmacokinet.* 2002;41(10):719–739.
28. Hosmer DWL, Stanley . *Applied Logistic Regression.* 2nd ed. New York: Wiley; 2000.
29. Agresti A. *Categorical Data Analysis.* New York: Wiley-Interscience; 2002.
30. Nick TG, Campbell KM. Logistic regression. *Methods Mol Biol.* 2007;404:273–301.
31. Ratain MJ. Therapeutic relevance of pharmacokinetics and pharmacodynamics. *Semin Oncol.* 1992;19(Suppl 11):8–13.
32. Aarons L, Graham G. Methodological approaches to the population analysis of toxicity data. *Toxicol Lett.* 2001;120(1–3):405–410.
33. Bonate PL. Nonlinear Mixed Effects Models. In Bonate PL, *Pharmacokinetic-Pharmacodynamic Modeling and Simulation*: Springer; New York, 2006.
34. Ette EI, Williams PJ. Population pharmacokinetics: II. Estimation methods. *Ann Pharmacother.* 2004;38(11):1907–1915.
35. Ette EI, Williams PJ. Population pharmacokinetics: I, Background, concepts, and models. *Ann Pharmacother.* Oct 2004;38(10):1702–1706.
36. Ette EI, Williams PJ, Lane JR. Population pharmacokinetics: III. Design, analysis, and application of population pharmacokinetic Studies. *Ann Pharmacother.* 2004;38(12):2136–2144.
37. Roy A, Ette EI. A pragmatic approach to the design of population pharmacokinetic studies. *Aaps J.* 2005;7(2):E408–420.
38. Spiegelhalter D.J., Best N.G., Gilks W.R., Inskip H. (1995*c*). Hepatitis: a case study in MCMC methods. In *Markov chain Monte Carlo Methods in practice.* (ed.\ W. R. Gilks, S. Richardson, and D. J. Spiegelhalter), pp. 21–43. Chapman and Hall, New York.
39. Goldsmith MA, Slavik M, Carter SK. Quantitative prediction of drug toxicity in humans from toxicology in small and large animals. *Cancer Res.* 1975;35(5):1354–1364.
40. Friberg LE, Freijs A, Sandstrom M, et al. Semiphysiological model for the time course of leukocytes after varying schedules of 5-fluorouracil in rats. *J Pharmacol Exp Ther.* 2000;295(2):734–740.
41. Gourdeau H, Leblond L, Hamelin B, et al. Species differences in troxacitabine pharmacokinetics and pharmacodynamics: implications for clinical development. *Clin Cancer Res.* 2004;10(22):7692–7702.
42. Hassan SB, Haglund C, Aleskog A, et al. Primary lymphocytes as predictors for species differences in cytotoxic drug sensitivity. *Toxicol In Vitro.* 2007;21(6):1174–1181.

43. Hochhaus G, Barrett JS, Derendorf H. Evolution of pharmacokinetics and pharmacokinetic/dynamic correlations during the 20th century. *J Clin Pharmacol.* 2000;40(9):908–917.
44. Cavero I. Using pharmacokinetic/pharmacodynamic modelling in safety pharmacology to better define safety margins: a regional workshop of the Safety Pharmacology Society. *Expert Opin Drug Saf.* 2007;6(4):465–471.
45. Machado SG, Miller R, Hu C. A regulatory perspective on pharmacokinetic/pharmacodynamic modelling. *Stat Methods Med Res.* 1999;8(3):217–245.
46. Rajman I. PK/PD modelling and simulations: utility in drug development. *Drug Discov Today.* 2008;13(7–8):341–346.
47. Mutlib AE, Gerson RJ, Meunier PC, et al. The species-dependent metabolism of efavirenz produces a nephrotoxic glutathione conjugate in rats. *Toxicol Appl Pharmacol.* 2000;169(1):102–113.
48. Yu LJ, Bulychev A, O'Brien L, et al. Pharmacokinetics and Pharmacodynamics of a Selective Proteasome Inhibitor MLN9708 in Nonclinical Species Following either Intravenous or Oral Administration. *Proc Am Assoc Cancer Res.* 2009;50.
49. Aitken MM. Species differences in pharmacodynamics: some examples. *Vet Res Commun.* Dec 1983;7(1–4):313–324.
50. Greaves P, Williams A, Eve M . First dose of potential new medicines to humans: How animals help. *Nat Rev Drug Discov.* 2004;3(3):226–236.
51. Kupperman E, Lee EC, Cao Y, et al. Evaluation of the proteasome inhibitor MLN9708 in preclinical models of human cancer. *Cancer Res.* 2010;70(5): 1970–1980.
52. Simonsen LE, Wahlby U, Sandstrom M, et al. Haematological toxicity following different dosing schedules of 5-fluorouracil and epirubicin in rats. *Anticancer Res.* 2000;20(3A):1519–1525.
53. Schurig JE, Florczyk AP, Bradner WT. The mouse as a model for predicting the myelosuppressive effects of anticancer drugs. *Cancer Chemother Pharmacol.* 1986;16(3):243–246.
54. Karlsson MO, Molnar V, Bergh J, et al. A general model for time-dissociated pharmacokinetic-pharmacodynamic relationship exemplified by paclitaxel myelosuppression. *Clin Pharmacol Ther.* 1998;63(1):11–25.
55. Pessina A, Albella B, Bayo M, et al. Application of the CFU-GM assay to predict acute drug-induced neutropenia: An international blind trial to validate a prediction model for the maximum tolerated dose (MTD) of myelosuppressive xenobiotics. *Toxicol Sci.* 2003;75(2):355–367.
56. Gabrielsson JL, Weiner DL. Methodology for pharmacokinetic/pharmacodynamic data analysis. *Pharm Sci Technol Today.* 1999;2(6):244–252.

18 **Prediction of therapeutic index of antibody-based therapeutics**

Mathematical modeling approaches

Kapil Mayawala and Bruce Gomes

Biologics represent a landmark shift in the pharmaceutical industry. The global market for human medicines was $750 billion and global sales of biologic medicines were $87 billion in 2008.[1] Monoclonal antibodies (mAbs) represented one of the most important classes of biologics with sales of $33 billion. *Remicade* (infliximab; Centocor) for Crohn's disease was the market leader, followed by Rituxan (rituximab; Genentech) for non-Hodgkin's lymphoma, *Herceptin* (trastuzumab; Genentech) for HER2–positive breast cancer, *Avastin* (bevacizumab; Genentech) for colorectal cancer, *Humira* (adalimumab; Abbott) for rheumatoid arthritis, Synagis (palivizumab; Medimmune) for pediatric respiratory disease, and *Erbitux* (cetuximab; Imclone Systems) for colorectal cancer.[2] The growing interest in using mAbs as therapeutics lies in their exquisite specificity for the target antigen. Unlike small-molecule therapeutics, which almost always show off-target effects due to overlapping activities against related members of enzyme families, antibodies can be targeted to individual protein targets. High specificity of antibody–antigen interaction can lead to a desirable therapeutic with high efficacy with minimal nontarget side effects.

18.1 MATHEMATICAL MODELING IN DRUG DISCOVERY

Mathematical modeling in the pharmaceutical industry has been done traditionally in the pharmacokinetic, pharmacodynamics, and drug metabolism groups. Researchers in these groups employ the tools of pharmacokinetic-pharmacodynamic (PKPD) modeling.[3–5] Generally, a model is picked to best fit the animal data, and this model is used for translation from animal to human data for dose predictions based on allometric scaling (i.e., parameters of the models are scaled based on body weights of the species).[6] The PKPD modeling provides practical methods for small-molecule drugs where nonspecificity prohibits complete characterization of the molecular-level interactions between human or animal proteins and small molecules. Furthermore, the absorption, distribution, metabolism, and elimination of small-molecule drugs vary greatly depending on the chemical structure, and these mechanisms are often poorly predictable.[7] However, the utility of PKPD modeling for small-molecule drugs is evident by its inclusion in regulatory application filing.

Pharmacokinetics of mAbs is very different from small-molecule drugs.[8] Within an IgG subclass, therapeutic mAbs differ only in the variable region, which is a small portion of the molecule. The distribution of radiolabeled IgGs has been reported.[9] Any variation from this distribution can be explained by interaction with the target. This alteration in the predicted pattern forms the basis for target-specific mathematical modeling (e.g., References 10–12). The specificity of antibody–antigen interaction is the major driver of the predictive capability of the mechanistic mathematical modeling. Antibody–antigen complex formation occurs in the extracellular space. It might seem that exclusion of the majority of targets that occur inside cells would be a severely limit the application of antibodies as therapeutic agents. However, estimates of the secretome and receptorome suggest that the number of possible targets likely in excess of several thousand proteins, and these proteins contain some of the most important candidates for multiorgan communication and pathology.[13–15] Surprisingly, it is the relatively small set of targets, under conditions that resemble a well mixed solution (the blood) that make mathematical modeling of mAb kinetics tractable. In contrast, mechanistic mathematical modeling of intracellular interactions is much more resource and time consuming than extracellular interactions due to highly interconnected nature of intracellular protein interaction pathways and difficulty in experimental measurements.[16,17] All these features not only make mathematical modeling of mAbs predictive but also practical in an industrial setting.

18.2 MECHANISTIC MATHEMATICAL MODELING OF MAB THERAPEUTIC INDEX

Mechanistic mathematical models describe antibody–protein and protein–protein interactions at the molecular level using experimental data from literature and/or information specifically produced experimentally to inform the model. These interactions can generally be represented in terms of the concentrations of interacting partners, and kinetic (forward and reverse reaction rates) and equilibrium properties (affinity) of their interactions. Using these quantitative properties, a mathematical model represents the underlying biological processes. An important consideration is the appropriate level of details needed to represent a biological system/process in a mechanistic mathematical model.[18] The complexity of the model is governed by the question for which the model is being built; for example, predicting the mAb distribution in the eye after topical administration may require a mathematically intensive spatial model that includes diffusion properties of the mAb molecule, spatial, features and flow patterns in the eye. However, ignoring spatial gradients is often an appropriate assumption if the target is circulating in blood.

Furthermore, it is important to include the mechanism of mAb action. A mAb can be used for therapeutic applications in several ways. Direct modulation of the target antigen has been the mechanism for most of the mAbs in the market today. Triggering cell death using mAb offers another attractive opportunity for oncology therapeutics. The specific mechanisms for cytotoxicity include using mAbs to deliver toxins to cancer cells (e.g., gemtuzumab: Mylotarg) and antibody and complement-dependent cytotoxicity (e.g., alemtuzumab: Campath-1H).

The fundamental concepts used to mathematically represent mechanistic mathematical models are borrowed from chemical reaction kinetics and transport phenomena.[19,20] However, the application of these concepts in biology requires an understanding of the biological literature. The biological data to build a mechanistic model of mAb action typically include

1. Protein expression levels in plasma and clearance half-life from circulation (e.g., high expression and fast clearing targets may need higher dose and more frequent dosing)
2. Site of therapeutic action (if different from plasma circulation): local protein expression and transport rates between the site and blood circulation (e.g., a target in brain will see very small fraction of injected dose due to poor mAb brain penetration, and synovial fluid may have higher concentration of a target inflammation factor than plasma in rheumatoid arthritis)
3. Binding partners and their interaction kinetics (e.g., to bind a receptor antigen, an antagonistic mAb will have to compete with the endogenous ligand)
4. mAb affinity to the target antigen, dose, and dosing frequency.

Extracting the biological data is a time-consuming task that can be made more efficient by using sophisticated text-mining tools.[21] The absence of quantitative data for a subset of these properties does not make mechanistic modeling an unachievable task. However, it limits the predictive capability of a model restricting the types of questions that can be addressed using the model. A typical alternative in the absence of biological data is to explore a suitable range covering the possible values for the unknown property. For example, finding optimal mAb dose and affinity may require exploration over a range of affinities and doses. In the absence of biological data from literature, experimental measurement(s) may be necessary depending on the question.

Finally, an important step is the validation of the mathematical model performed by comparing its predictions to the experimental data from literature or in-house. The data used for validation must be different from the data used to build the model, or it will be a self-fulfilling prediction. Validation using animal or human *in vivo* data, whenever available, will significantly increase confidence in the model.

18.3 MATHEMATICAL MODELING FOR PREDICTING EFFICACY

The application of mechanistic mathematical models for determining the properties of the therapeutic mAbs can help in maximizing the efficacy of the mAb.

In this section, a few examples are used to illustrate the use of mathematical modeling. Keeping in mind the diverse background of readers, simple examples are chosen to avoid mathematical complexity. Consider a target antigen that is freely circulating in the plasma without any plasma-binding proteins. The antigen is elevated in the disease condition. The therapeutic objective might be to knock down the target by 90% and the drug discovery team wants to know the desired mAb affinity and dosing for intravenous (IV) injections. Based on information available in literature and discussing with experts, a mathematical modeler can represent the biological knowledge as

Processes influencing the target concentration:
Secretion and clearance of the target: Source → Target → Sink
Reversible binding to mAb: Target + mAb ↔ mAb.Target complex
Processes influencing the mAb concentration:
Reversible binding to the target: Target + mAb ↔ mAb.Target complex
mAb clearance by fluid phase endocytosis: mAb → Sink

These reactions can be mathematically represented in terms of mass balance of each species using a set of ordinary differential equations as:

$$\begin{aligned}\frac{d[Target]}{dt} &= R_{\text{synthesis}} - k_{\text{TargetClearance}}[Target] - k_{\text{on}}[\text{mAb}][\text{Target}] \\ &\quad + k_{\text{off}}[\text{mAb.TargetComplex}]\end{aligned} \tag{1a}$$

$$\frac{d[mAb]}{dt} = k_{\text{on}}[mAb]\,[\text{Target}] + k_{\text{off}}\,[\text{mAb}\,.\text{TargetComplex}] - k_{\text{mAbCleareence}}[mAb] \tag{1b}$$

[Target], [mAb], and [mAbTargetComplex] are the concentrations of target antigen, free mAb, and mAb-target complex, respectively. Assuming well-mixed plasma, the initial concentration of mAb can be calculated based on dose and plasma volume. $k_{\text{TargetClearance}}$ and $k_{\text{mAbClearance}}$ represent kinetic rate constants of clearance processes. The clearance of the target can occur through a variety of processes (e.g., kidney filtration, proteolysis, receptor-mediated internalization and degradation and fluid phase endocytosis). The clearance through kidneys depends on the protein size, which determines protein's ability to escape or pass through glomerular filtration. Small proteins, <10 kDa, are filtered into urine with almost 100% efficiency resulting in their half-life of about 40 min in human. Large proteins (>100 kDa) (e.g., mAbs) almost escape glomerular filtration. Furthermore, mAbs are also recycled by binding to neonatal Fc receptor (FcRn) in the endosomes significantly reducing their clearance by fluid phase endocytosis.[22] As a result, mAbs can show a long serum half-life of up to ~3 weeks. $R_{\text{synthesis}}$ stands for the rate of synthesis of the target antigen. The synthesis rate should be same as the clearance rate to maintain a steady-state protein level. k_{on} and k_{off} represent the kinetic rate constant for the association and dissociation reactions between therapeutic mAb and target antigen. The binding affinity, measured as K_d, is the ratio of k_{off} and k_{on} ($K_d = k_{\text{off}}/k_{\text{on}}$). For associating proteins in solution, the fastest association rate is determined by the rate of molecular

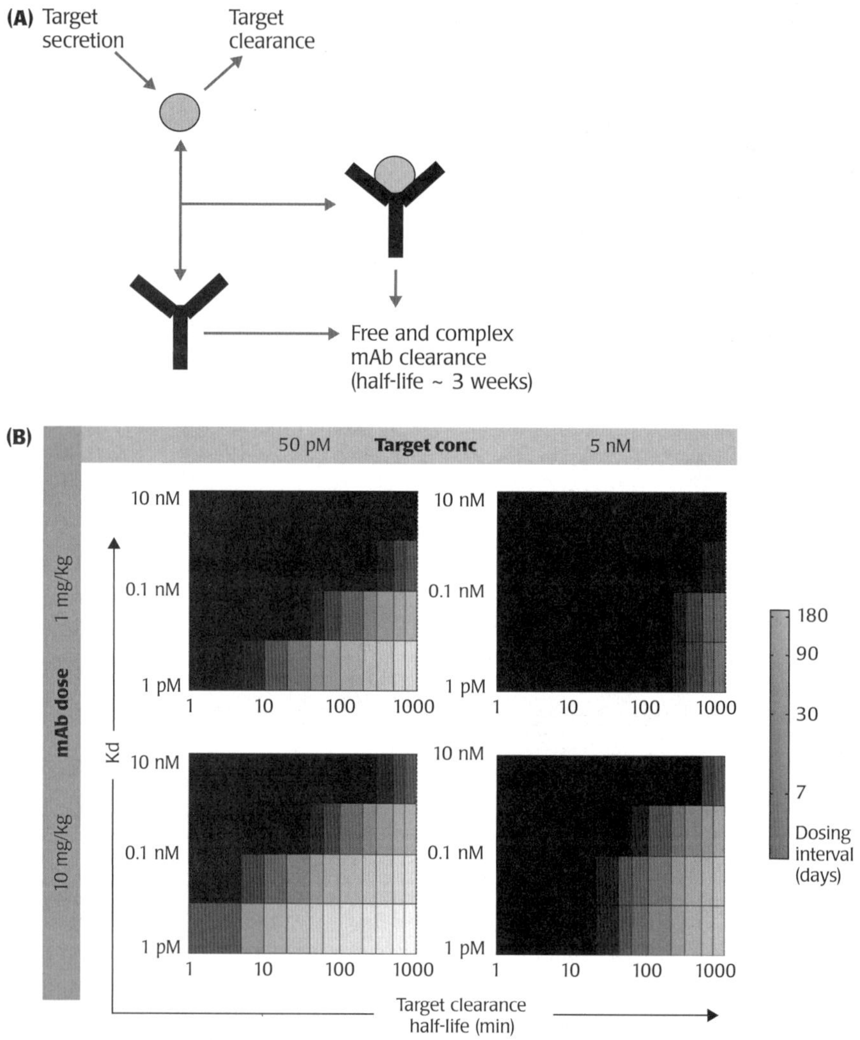

Figure 18-1: Effect of target and mAb properties on dosing interval. Dosing interval is defined as the duration for which the target is knocked down at least 90% of its pre-mAb dose level. (A) Representation of mAb and target interaction. (B) The target clearance half-life is varied over 1–1,000 min at two concentrations of 50 pM and 5 nM. The mAb affinity (K_d) for the target is varied over 1 pM to 10 nM at two doses of 1 mg/kg and 10 mg/kg in a human model. Different shades of gray correspond to different dosing intervals (in days) as indicated on the shading scale. Higher concentration of target, faster target clearance (short half-life), weaker mAb affinity (higher K_d) and lower mAb dose lead to a shorter dosing interval (shown by darker shade of gray).

collisions, which is controlled by the rate of diffusion. Based on typical protein sizes, the diffusion-limited value of k_{on} is around 10^4–10^6 $M^{-1}s^{-1}$ in plasma.

The set of differential equations in Equation 1 relates properties of target and mAb, and its solution will result in concentration changes with time. Figure 18.1 explores the effects of mAb affinity, mAb dose, target synthesis/clearance rate, and target concentration on dosing interval. As expected, mAb with higher dose and higher affinity reduces the plasma concentration of the target for a longer

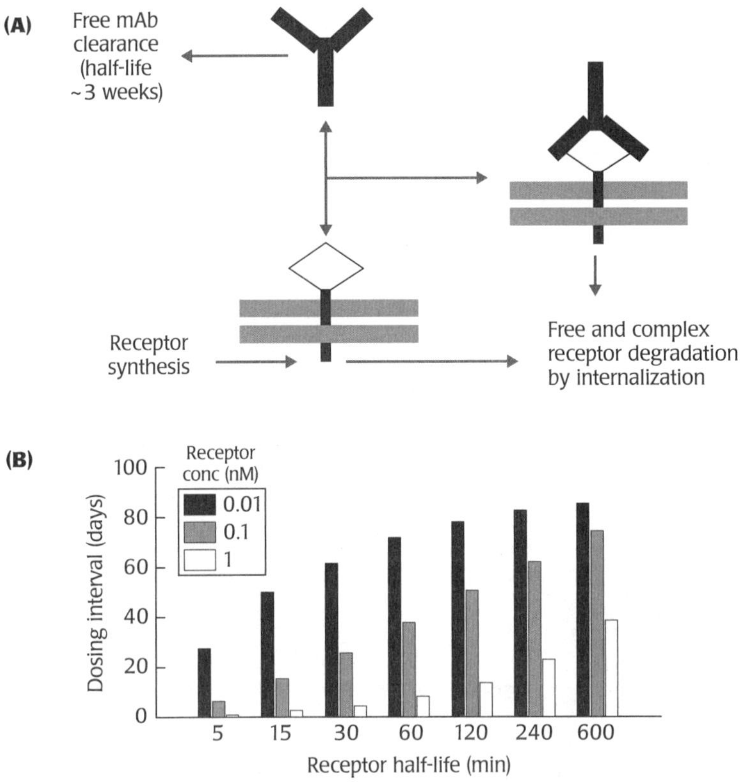

Figure 18-2: Effect of receptor properties on dosing interval of a receptor targeting mAb. Dosing interval is defined as the duration for which the target is knocked down at least 90% of its pre-mAb dose level. (A) Representation of mAb and target receptor interaction. (B) The mAb has an affinity of 1 n*M* for the target receptor and is injected intravenously at a dose of 1 mg/kg in a human model. Three different receptor concentrations are explored: 0.01, 0.1, and 1 n*M*, shown by black, gray and white bars, respectively. The receptor concentration is calculated based on plasma volume assuming well-mixed plasma. The half-life of the receptor degradation by internalization is varied from 5 min to 10 h. The mAb–receptor complex is assumed to degrade with the half-life of the free receptor. Higher receptor expression and faster degradation lead to a lower dosing interval.

duration, and higher expression and faster clearing targets are difficult to knock down. In this example, the qualitative nature of the results is very intuitive. However, value of the modeling lies in quantitative results which can be useful for preclinical team to design mAb properties. Unfortunately (from a drug discovery viewpoint), biology is rarely so simple that therapeutic mAb properties can be determined based on Figure 18.1. The properties of the specific biological target lead to significant deviations from Figure 18.1. These deviations require understanding of the biological literature around the specific target and mathematically representing this knowledge.

If the target antigen is a receptor, then therapeutic mAb may have a shorter half-life due to receptor-mediated internalization. For brevity, the set of differential equations for this case are not mentioned here. Figure 18.2 explores the effect of different receptor levels and half-lives on the therapeutic mAb dosing.

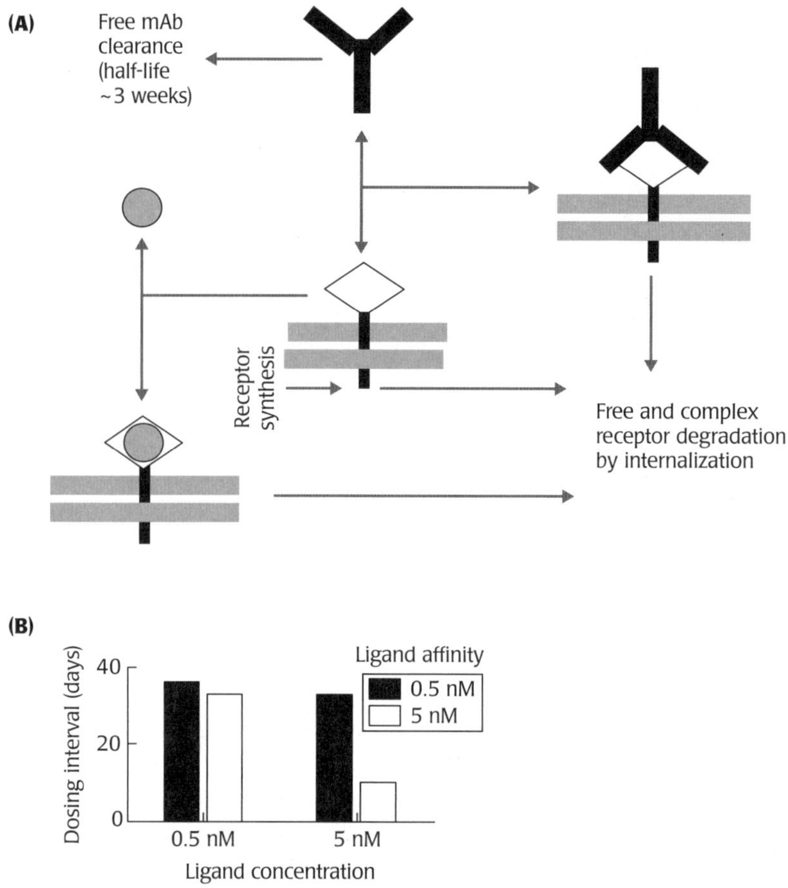

Figure 18-3: Effect of competition with ligand to bind to the target receptor on dosing interval. Dosing interval is defined as the duration for which the target is knocked down at least 90% of its pre-mAb dose level. **(A)** Representation of mAb and endogenous ligand interactions with target receptor. **(B)** The receptor is assumed to have a concentration of 0.1 n*M* and degradation half-life is 60 min. The mAb has an affinity of 1 n*M* for the target receptor and is injected intravenously at a dose of 1mg/kg in a human model. The dosing intervals are calculated for two receptor–ligand affinities (K_d): 0.5 n*M* and 5 n*M*, and two ligand concentrations: 0.5 n*M* and 5 n*M*. Competition with higher concentration of higher affinity ligand reduces dosing interval.

The model recaptures the understanding that a faster degrading high-level receptor will require more frequent dosing. In fact, it is possible that faster mAb loss caused by a high rate of receptor degradation can make mAb impractical for treating a disease condition. And, these cases can be predicted using mechanistic mathematical modeling in early discovery phases that can lead to significant savings in discovery and development costs.[23]

Further complexity can be added by the presence of an endogenous ligand, assuming that the target receptor has an endogenous ligand and that this receptor–ligand complex leads to undesired signaling. Therapeutic mAb might compete with the ligand for the same receptor epitope to avoid complex formation. Figure 18.3 shows that competition with a high-concentration ligand with tight receptor binding can cause more frequent dosing. Figures 18.1–18.3 emphasize that it can be challenging to design mAb drug properties, even in simple and intuitive cases, using mental or descriptive models of biological processes due to the dependence on many biological parameters. Mechanistic mathematical modeling is a systematic tool for integrating biological knowledge so that it results in an improved therapeutic mAb affinity and dose design.

18.4 MATHEMATICAL MODELING FOR PREDICTING TOXICITY

18.4.1 Antibody–antigen complex

Increase in the total level of target antigen in the form of antibody–antigen complex can occur after mAb dosing. Binding to mAb can protect the target antigen from clearing by its endogenous pathway. This is particularly true for small proteins that get cleared by kidney filtration only when they are not bound to mAb. If the mAb is targeted to the receptor-binding epitope of a ligand, it will prevent receptor binding and receptor-mediated clearance. The antibody–antigen complex accumulation has been reported for several cytokines including IL-3, IL-4, IL-6, and IL-7.[24] Injection of anti-IL6 mAb in a patient with multiple myeloma with *Escherichia coli* sepsis led to 1,000-fold increased levels of IL-6 in the form of IL-6-mAb complex.[25] The complex accumulation may have implications for the clinical outcome of a mAb treatment.

Despite strong biological evidence in favor of targeting IL-6 in cancer and autoimmune and inflammatory diseases, mAbs to IL-6 have not yielded expected clinical outcome.[26] Accumulation of antibody-IL-6 complex has been hypothesized as one of the reasons for incomplete neutralization of IL-6 activity.[26] Another example of a negative impact on a clinical trial due to accumulation of antibody–antigen complex formation was presented by anti-CCL2/monocyte chemotactic protein 1 (MCP-1) mAb.[27] The anti-CCL2 mAb in patients with rheumatoid arthritis caused up to 2,000-fold buildup of the antibody–antigen complex. The antibody–antigen complex could have been the reason for ineffectiveness and worsening of rheumatoid arthritis in patients in the clinical trial.

A high level of a complex formation can be a safety concern for three main reasons: (a) prolongation of short-lived target antigen activity, (b) residual activity of the targeted epitope in the antibody–antigen complex, and (c) residual activity of the nontargeted epitope in the antibody–antigen complex, which can lead to unintended biological effect. The prolongation effect of the antigen due to antibody–antigen complex has been reported for IL-3[28] and IL-6[29] in mice. The antibody spreads the acute activity of a short-lived cytokine over a longer duration. A positive feedback effect of antibody–antigen complex on increasing the antigen production has also been suggested to contribute to the prolongation of cytokine activity.[30]

The residual activity of antibody–antigen complex can arise due to a very small activity of the target antigen retained by the antibody–antigen complex as a result of less than 100% neutralization of the targeted epitope by the mAb.

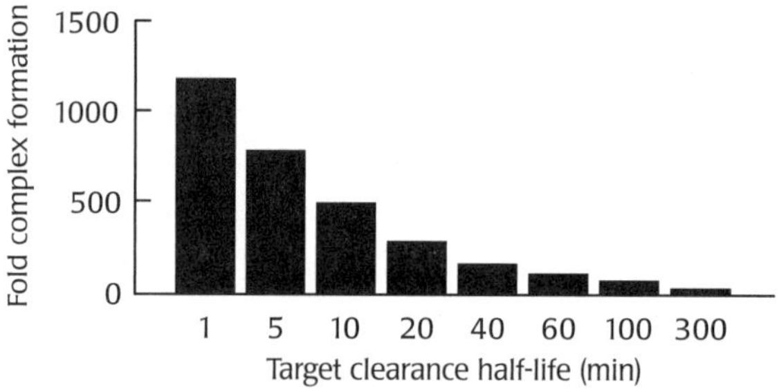

Figure 18-4: Mathematically calculated mAb-target complex formation for targets with half-lives varying over 1–300 min. The fold complex formation has been defined as the ratio of mAb-target complex concentration at the end of first week after mAb dosing and predose level of target. The predose target concentration is 50 p*M* and a dose of 10 mg/kg of 1 n*M* mAb is given in a human model.

The small residual activity can contribute significantly to the overall activity of the antigen at high level of antibody–antigen complex. For example, a 1,000-fold higher level of antibody-antigen complex, as compared to pretreated free antigen level, with 1% residual activity is equivalent to a 10-fold elevation of activity of the target antigen. This can actually lead to worsening of the diseased condition after therapeutic mAb treatment.

The target antigen may also show multiple activities exerted by distinct sites on the antigen molecule all of which may not be blocked by the mAb. These activities may contribute to off-target effects at high antibody–antigen complex accumulation. IL-6-anti-IL-6 autoantibody complex has been reported to have over 60% residual IL-6 activity that may be due to two distinct epitopes on IL-6 molecule: one recognized by IL-6 autoantibodies and the other the binding site of IL-6 to its receptors.[31]

The extent of target-mAb formation can be predicted using mechanistic mathematical modeling, which can help in determining optimal drug dosage prescription. Figure 18.4 shows the predicted levels of complex formation in a week for antigens clearing at different rates. As expected, short-lived antigens lead to more complex formation as is found with short-lived cytokines (5–20 min) in serum.

18.4.2 Uptake of the mAb by nontarget cells and tissues

The target antigen can be expressed in nontarget tissues which can lead to unintended effects. An example is the cardiac toxicity observed in some patients treated with trastuzumab for HER2-overexpressing metastatic breast cancer.[32] The mechanism of cardiac toxicity has not been fully elucidated, but it may be related to the protective role of HER2 in cardiac function.[33,34]

Inhibition of the biological function of the target antigen is a general safety concern and mechanistic mathematical modeling can help in optimally designing dosage and affinity of the therapeutic mAb. A mechanistic mathematical model can be written using ordinary differential equations, similar to Equation 1, to describe the transient concentrations of target, mAb and mAb-target complex in target and nontarget tissues. The local concentrations of target in different tissues and transport rates of target and mAb between plasma and tissues are important factors in predicting the uptake of mAb in target and nontarget tissues. It should be mentioned that different molecular weights of target and mAb may influence the transport properties, and these differences must be considered in the model.

The issue of uptake by nontarget cells plays a central role in cytotoxic antibody drug conjugates (ADCs) used for treating cancer. Although there is only one ADC in clinical use, Gemtuzumab Ozogamicin (marketed as Mylotarg), several ADCs in preclinical and clinical phases emphasize the need for understanding and predicting the clinical safety profile.[35] A cytotoxic compound (e.g., diphtheria toxin or doxorubicin) is conjugated to a mAb that targets an antigen highly expressed in cancer (e.g., HER2). The target antigen is chosen to be highly selective in differentiating cancer versus normal cells to avoid normal cell killing. However, finding a target antigen that is completely absent from all cells except cancer cells is idealistic. Therefore, an important question for an ADC drug discovery project is linking the target expression profile to selectivity in terms of normal versus cancer cell killing. Moreover, there is a risk of killing endothelial cells due to nonspecific uptake by fluid phase endocytosis. A high affinity ADC may reduce selectivity advantage by binding in normal tissues with low target expression. Similarly, a high dose of ADC can lead to substantial nonspecific uptake by endothelial cells leading to vascular toxicity. Furthermore, the selectivity will be influenced by the transport rates between plasma and the tissue. Considering the additional complexity, designing an optimal dosage and affinity of ADC to deliver maximal efficacy in target tissues with minimal toxicity in nontarget tissues can be helped by mechanistic mathematical modeling.

18.4.3 Immunogenicity

Immunogenicity is a general concern with the therapeutic use of proteins.[36] The clinical implications of immunogenicity can range from reduction in efficacy to life-threatening allergic or anaphylactic response.[37,38] The immunogenicity is influenced by a number of factors related to variations from human protein, route of administration, dose, length of treatment, contaminants and process-related impurities, formulation, storage and patient characteristics (e.g., weakened immune system in cancer).[39] It has also been suggested that mAb targeting cell-bound antigens tend to induce more antibody formation than those targeting circulating antigen.[40]

The extent of difference between the exogenous and endogenous protein should be the main source of immunogenicity. Proteins from an animal source, including murine mAbs, carry a great risk of a human immunogenic response. Therefore, humanized mAbs held the promise for solving immunogenicity issues. The humanization reduces the risk of immunogenicity but it does not completely eliminate it. In a clinical trial with fully humanized mAb natalizumab, 7% of the patients developed antibodies.[41] In fact, the administration of any protein, including fully human proteins, can lead to the development of antibodies. In a clinical trial with 100 diabetic patients, recombinant human insulin led to the development of antibodies in 44% of the patients over 12 months.[42]

The first-generation murine-derived mAbs triggered a classical vaccine-type immune response. However, the immune response by humanized mAbs is thought to be based on breaking of B cell tolerance. The process is not completely understood but takes up to a year of chronic treatment. This results in antibodies, which can lead to neutralization of the target antigen, reducing efficacy and even can neutralize endogenous protein causing safety concerns.[40] In addition to the role of B cell tolerance, T cell tolerance also plays an important role in immunogenicity. It has been hypothesized that therapeutic mAbs have not been produced in a human where selection against self reactivity has been eliminated by thymus surveillance. Production mAbs are manufactured under conditions that, even if in the case of fully humanized mAb, have not been counterselected. It is not clear what the magnitude of this effect is.

Current literature does not provide any example of predictive mathematical modeling for immunogenicity by humanized mAbs mainly due to poorly understood underlying biological mechanism. Mathematical modeling has been applied to the immune system since 1960s, but the field is still in its infancy due to underlying biological complexities and lack of mechanistic details.[43,44] Many of the past efforts have been directed toward viral dynamics and infection (e.g., HIV, HCV, and HBV) and antiviral immune response including T cell dynamics. Attempts have also been made to mathematically describe intracellular signaling events following immune receptor activation.[45] However, experimental measurements of intracellular milieu are tedious. Modeling of immunogenicity will require mathematical representations of more complex immunological processes involved in B cell and T cell tolerance. In addition to the limited mechanistic depth, the mathematical modeling in this area is restricted by the lack of quantitative experimental measurements.

18.4.4 Infusion reactions

Infusion reactions are the most common safety issue with mAbs. Typical infusion reactions are injection-site reactions such as itching, rash, redness, swelling, and pain.[46] These reactions have been reported for all the generally used administration routes: intravenous, subcutaneous, and intramuscular. As may be expected, subcutaneous administration has been associated more with injection-site reactions. The mechanisms underlying injection-site reactions are not well understood, making mechanism-based modeling an impossible task. However, it should be mentioned that mathematical models have been developed to represent the absorption kinetics after therapeutic administration.[47,48]

In addition to injection-site reactions, other mild to moderate reactions include fever, dizziness, sweating, and nausea. Low incidences of severe infusion reactions (e.g., hypotension, cardiac dysfunction, anaphylaxis, and bronchospasms) have also been reported with Rituximab, Cetuximab, and even with humanized mAb Trastuzumab.[46] Once again, the underlying mechanisms are poorly understood, limiting the application of mechanistic mathematical modeling for predicting infusion site reactions.

18.5 CONCLUSION

Mechanistic mathematical modeling can be applied from early discovery to clinical phases. As discussed in this chapter, a mechanistic model can be very powerful in early phases of drug discovery when the mAb affinity needs to be designed. Mechanistic mathematical models can be used to test whether a target antigen can be altered to a desired level using reasonable mAb properties including affinity, dose, and dosing frequency. The reasonable range depends on the disease indication and requires input from clinical groups. For example, in chronic diseases such as rheumatoid arthritis and diabetes, frequent administration of mAb may not be desirable. However, that may not be an issue in those types of cancers where alternative treatments are much less effective.

First-in-human (FIH) dose predications can be made using mechanism-based scaling. In moving from the preclinical to the clinical phase, a mechanistic mathematical model can be validated using animal data. The validated animal model can be scaled to the human model by changing each parameter's value based on mechanism from animal to human. The recently introduced approach of the minimal anticipated biological effect level (MABEL) for dose selection can be perceived as an important step by regulatory authorities toward using mechanism-based scaling. The MABEL standard suggests calculating first-in-human dose based on target receptor occupancy model.[49] The concept of MABEL was initiated as a result of the severe adverse reactions in phase 1 clinical trial of TGN1412.[50,51] The first-in-human dose of TGN1412 corresponded to saturating receptor occupancy of the target receptor.[51]

In conclusion, mechanistic mathematical modeling can help testing the feasibility of a mAb approach to treat a disease and picking the mAb properties for optimal therapeutic index. As a result, the use of mechanistic mathematical models in drug discovery will lead to reduction in clinical attrition by increasing the chance of producing a safe and effective drug.

REFERENCES

1. Maggon K. Global pharmaceutical market review & world top ten/twenty drugs 2008. http://knol.google.com/k/krishan-maggon/global-pharmaceutical-market-review/3fy5eowy8suq3/6# Accessed March 28, 2009.
2. Aggarwal S. What's fueling the biotech engine? *Nat Biotech.* 2007;25(10):1097–1104.
3. Derendorf H, Meibohm B. Modeling of pharmacokinetic/pharmacodynamic (PK/PD) relationships: Concepts and perspectives. *Pharma Res.* 1999;16(2):176–185.
4. Gibaldi M, Perrier D. *Pharmacokinetics.* 2nd ed.New York, NY: Informa HealthCare; 1982.

5. Rowland M, Tozer TN. *Clinical Pharmacokinetics: Concepts and Applications.* 3rd ed.Philadelphia, PA: Lippincott Williams & Wilkins; 1995.
6. West GB, Brown JH, Enquist BJ. A general model for the origin of allometric scaling laws in biology. *Science.* 1997;276(5309):122–126.
7. Mager DE. Quantitative structure–pharmacokinetic/pharmacodynamic relationships. *Adv Drug Deliv Rev.* 2006;58(12–13):1326–1356.
8. Wang W, Wang EQ, Balthasar JP. Monoclonal antibody pharmacokinetics and pharmacodynamics. *Clin Pharmacol Ther.* 2008;84(5):548–558.
9. Garg A, Balthasar J. Physiologically-based pharmacokinetic (PBPK) model to predict IgG tissue kinetics in wild-type and FcRn-knockout mice. *J Pharmacokinet Pharmacodynam.* 2007;34(5):687–709.
10. Davda JP, Jain M, Batra SK, Gwilt PR, Robinson DH. A physiologically based pharmacokinetic (PBPK) model to characterize and predict the disposition of monoclonal antibody CC49 and its single chain Fv constructs. *Int Immunopharmacol.* 2008;8(3):401–413.
11. Lammerts van Bueren JJ, Bleeker WK, Bogh HO, et al. Effect of target dynamics on pharmacokinetics of a novel therapeutic antibody against the epidermal growth factor receptor: Implications for the mechanisms of action. *Cancer Res.* 2006;66(15):7630–7638.
12. Tabrizi MA, Tseng C-ML, Roskos LK. Elimination mechanisms of therapeutic monoclonal antibodies. *Drug Discov Today.* 2006;11(1–2):81–88.
13. Klee EW, Carlson DF, Fahrenkrug SC, Ekker SC, Ellis LBM. Identifying secretomes in people, pufferfish and pigs. *Nucleic Acids Res.* 2004;32(4):1414–1421.
14. Grimmond SM, Miranda KC, Yuan Z, et al. The mouse secretome: Functional classification of the proteins secreted into the extracellular environment. *Genome Res.* 2003;13:1350–1359.
15. Strachan RT, Ferrara G, Roth BL. Screening the receptorome: An efficient approach for drug discovery and target validation. *Drug Discov Today.* 2006;11(15–16):708–716.
16. Oda K, Matsuoka Y, Funahashi A, Kitano H. A comprehensive pathway map of epidermal growth factor receptor signaling. *Mol Syst Biol.* 2005;1–17.
17. Hendriks BS, Hua F, Chabot JR. Analysis of mechanistic pathway models in drug discovery: p38 pathway. *Biotechnol Progr.* 2008;24(1):96–109.
18. Wiley HS, Shvartsman SY, Lauffenburger DA. Computational modeling of the EGF-receptor system: A paradigm for systems biology. *Trends Cell Biol.* 2003;13(1): 43–50.
19. Levenspiel O. *Chemical Reaction Engineering.* 3rd ed.Hoboken, NJ: Wiley; 1998.
20. Deen WM. *Analysis of Transport Phenomena.*New York, NY: Oxford University Press; 1998.
21. Dickman S. Tough mining. *Plos Biol.* 2003;1(2):144.
22. Roopenian DC, Akilesh S. FcRn: The neonatal Fc receptor comes of age. *Nat Rev Immunol.* 2007;7:715–725.
23. Bueren JJLv, Bleeker WK, Bøgh HO, et al. Effect of target dynamics on pharmacokinetics of a novel therapeutic antibody against the epidermal growth factor receptor: Implications for the mechanisms of action. *Cancer Res.* 2006;66:7630–7638.
24. Finkelman FD, Madden KB, Morris SC, et al. Anti-cytokine antibodies as carrier proteins. Prolongation of in vivo effects of exogenous cytokines by injection of cytokine-anti-cytokine antibody complexes. *J Immunol.* 1993;151(3):1235–1244.
25. Lu Z-Y, Brailly H, Rossi J-F, Wijdenes J, Bataille R, Klein B. Overall interleukin-6 production exceeds 7 mg/day in multiple myeloma complicated by sepsis. *Cytokine.* 1993;5(6):578–582.
26. Kishimoto T. Interleukin-6: Discovery of a pleiotropic cytokine. *Arthritis Res. Ther.* 2006;8(Suppl 2):S2.
27. Haringman JJ, Gerlag DM, Smeets TJM, et al. A randomized controlled trial with an anti-CCL2 (anti-monocyte chemotactic protein 1) monoclonal antibody in patients with rheumatoid arthritis. *Arthritis & Rheumatism.* 2006;54(8):2387–2392.

28. Jones AT, Ziltener HJ. Enhancement of the biologic effects of interleukin-3 in vivo by anti- interleukin-3 antibodies. *Blood.* 1993;82(4):1133–1141.
29. Mihara M, Koishihara Y, Fukui H, Yasukawa K, Ohsugi Y. Murine anti-human IL-6 monoclonal antibody prolongs the half-life in circulating blood and thus prolongs the bioactivity of human IL-6 in mice. *Immunology.* 1991;74(1):55–59.
30. Slifka MK, Whitton JL. Clinical implications of dysregulated cytokine production. *J Molec Med.* 2000;78(2):74–80.
31. Suzuki H, Takemura H, Yoshizaki K, et al. IL-6-anti-IL-6 autoantibody complexes with IL-6 activity in sera from some patients with systemic sclerosis. *J Immunol.* 1994;152(2):935–942.
32. Ewer SM, Ewer MS. Cardiotoxicity profile of trastuzumab. *Drug Saf.* 2008;31(6): 459–467.
33. Perez EA. Cardiac toxicity of ErbB2-targeted therapies: what do we know? *Clin Breast Cancer.* 2008;8:S114-S120.
34. Suter TM, Cook-Brunsb, Bartonc C. Cardiotoxicity associated with trastuzumab (Herceptin) therapy in the treatment of metastatic breast cancer. *The Breast.* 2004;13(3):173–183.
35. Kovtun YV, Goldmacher VS. Cell killing by antibody–drug conjugates. *Cancer Lett.* 2007;255(2):232–240.
36. Schellekens H. Immunogenicity of therapeutic proteins: Clinical implications and future prospects. *Clin Therapeut.* 2002;24(11):1720–1740.
37. Pendley C, Schantz A, Wagner C. Immunogenicity of therapeutic monoclonal antibodies. *Curr Opin Molec Therapeut.* 2003;5:172–179.
38. Kessler M, Goldsmith D, Schellekens H. Immunogenicity of biopharmaceuticals. *Nephrology Dialysis Transplantation.* 2006;21:v9–v12.
39. Schellekens H. Bioequivalence and the immunogenicity of biopharmaceuticals. *Nat Rev Drug Discov.* 2002;1(6):457–462.
40. Crommelin DJA, Sindelar RD, Meibohm B, eds. *Pharmaceutical Biotechnology: Fundamentals and Applications.* 3rd ed.Philadelphia, PA: Informa HealthCare; 2007.
41. Ghosh S, Goldin E, Gordon FH, et al. Natalizumab for active Crohn's disease. *N Engl J Med.* 2003;348(1):24–32.
42. Fineberg SE, Galloway JA, Fineberg NS, Rathbun MJ, Hufferd S. Immunogenicity of recombinant DNA human insulin. *Diabetologia.* 1983;25(6):465–469.
43. Perelson AS. Modelling viral and immune system dynamics. *Nat Rev Immunol.* 2002;2(1):28–36.
44. Chakraborty AK, Dustin ML, Shaw AS. In silico models for cellular and molecular immunology: successes, promises and challenges. *Nat Immunol.* 2003;4(10):933–936.
45. Goldstein B, Faeder JR, Hlavacek WS. Mathematical and computational models of immune-receptor signalling. *Nat Rev Immunol.* 2004;4(6):445–456.
46. Lenz H-J. Management and preparedness for infusion and hypersensitivity reactions. *The Oncologist.* 2007;12(5):601–609.
47. Mosekilde E, Jensen KS, Binder C, Pramming S, Thorsteinsson B. Modeling absorption kinetics of subcutaneous injected soluble insulin *J Pharmacokinet Pharmacodynam.* 1989;17(1):67–87.
48. Wach P, Trajanoski Z, Kotanko P, Skrabal F. Numerical approximation of mathematical model for absorption of subcutaneously injected insulin. *Med Biol Eng Comput.* 1995;33(1):18–23.
49. Muller PY, Brennan FR. Safety assessment and dose selection for first-in-human clinical trials with immunomodulatory monoclonal antibodies. *Clin Pharmacol Ther.* 2009;85(3):247–258.
50. Suntharalingam G, Perry MR, Ward S, et al. Cytokine storm in a phase 1 trial of the anti-CD28 monoclonal antibody TGN1412. *N Engl J Med.* 2006;355(10):1018–1028.
51. Duff GW. *Expert Group on Phase One Clinical Trials.*Norwich, UK: Department of Health (UK); 2006.

19 **Vaccine toxicology**

Nonclinical predictive strategies

Sarah Gould and Raymond Oomen

19.1 INTRODUCTION

Vaccines are one of the safest and most effective preventative treatments against infectious diseases. The first vaccine was against smallpox, and developed by Edward Jenner (1796) as a simple preparation of crude vaccinia. Today's vaccines are composed of a diverse range of products, which may include live attenuated or inactivated bacteria, virus or parasites, living irradiated cells, crude fractions or purified parts of microorganisms, polysaccharides, toxoids, recombinant proteins/polypeptides, and vector-based and DNA vaccines. Formulations may include novel adjuvants, excipients, and multiple antigen combinations and be delivered by novel routes via viral vectors or new delivery systems.[1–3] Vaccines also offer wider possibilities with the promise of therapeutic benefit against various disorders such as cancer, prevention or treatment of immune-mediated diseases, and antismoking therapy.[4]

Vaccines have an exemplary safety record, with a benefit that is immeasurable. With today's risk-averse society and heightened awareness, vaccine safety attracts intense scrutiny, particularly in the case of preventative vaccines, which are given to healthy adults, infants, and children. The safety benefit ratio is skewed heavily toward safety and as many infectious diseases are not prevalent today, many people may not perceive the benefit. In fact, in recent years, there has been a shift toward a risk benefit for the individual, and as a result of certain alleged safety issues, there has been a reduction in vaccinations, (e.g., Japan and DTP vaccines, MMR in UK, polio in African regions); this will ultimately lead to decreased herd immunity, and the prevalence of certain diseases may return. Thus, the need to ensure safety is of utmost importance. It should be noted that the risk benefit may differ slightly for therapeutic vaccines. However, the emphasis on safety remains.

For successful development of any medicine, including vaccines, potential safety alerts should be identified as early as possible; this will reduce potential safety issues in the clinic and stop development early where needed. When considering predictive strategies, an understanding of alleged safety issues can provide key guidance. Vaccines may be associated with transient reactogenicity-type symptoms, as a result of stimulating the immune system and may include reddening of the injection site, headache, and fever; such reactions – considering the risk benefit – are acceptable. However, specific safety concerns, which require further consideration, have been raised. For example, in the 1960s, vaccines against respiratory syncytial virus (RSV) and chlamydia were alleged to be associated with exacerbated disease symptoms following exposure to the infectious agent[5–7] (see Section 19.5). In the 1970s, clinical reports noted an association between the whole cell pertussis vaccine and adverse clinical reactions, including convulsions, continuous screaming, and collapses, with and without apnea.[8] More recently, a vaccine against simian human reassortant rotavirus was reported to cause intussusception (blockage of the intestine) and mortality in vaccinated infants.[9] Other associated adverse events following vaccination are discussed in reviews by O'Hagan and Rappuoli[10] and Bonhoeffer and Heininger.[11]

This chapter considers some predictive strategies, which may identify potential safety alerts, augment our understanding of mechanisms of action, and contribute to the safety of vaccines.

19.2 PREDICTIVE STRATEGIES

The principle of a safety evaluation for vaccines, for traditional pharmaceuticals and biopharmaceutical products, is to screen, identify, and characterize any potential toxicity and target organs. The initial safety evaluation is to support a phase I first-in-human (FIH) clinical trial, in which ultimately human safety will be evaluated. The earlier that potential safety issues are identified, the better. A step-by-step approach is advisable, with special attention to potential pharmacological effects associated with the immune system (e.g., severe local or systemic reactions, immunotoxicology) (see Section 19.5). Following a phase I trial, additional assessments may be required dependent upon changes in manufacturing process, route of administration, and addition of a different adjuvant or if any safety concerns arose during the clinical trial and if a particular patient population needs to be considered (e.g., women of child-bearing potential).[12]

In predicting safety, several factors need to be considered including the intrinsic toxicity of the antigen and/or components of the vaccine, as well as the pharmacodynamic and biological activities, which may trigger either direct or indirect effects.[2,13] To date, *in vivo* animal models represent the best model for predicting potential adverse events prior to dosing in human. There are *in vitro* and/or *in silico* models that may be considered, particularly in early development. It should be acknowledged that there will always be limitations in accurately predicting human safety,[14] and rare toxicities and potential effects on specific subpopulations may only ever be addressed in humans.

A safety assessment needs to be tailored to each individual investigational vaccine (case-by-case) and will need to consider the type of vaccine, its components (e.g., presence of a novel adjuvant), the clinical dose, and the schedule and route of administration. There are three key guidelines concerned with the safety of vaccine:

1. European Medicines Evaluation Agency (EMEA) notes for guidance on preclinical pharmacological and toxicological testing of vaccines[15]
2. World Health Organization (WHO) guidelines on nonclinical evaluation of vaccines[16]
3. FDA CBER draft guidance for industry: considerations for reproductive toxicity studies for preventative vaccines for infectious disease indications[17]

Other guidelines exist, are more specific (e.g., for influenza, smallpox vaccines), or cover specific topics (e.g., adjuvants). Brennan and Dougan[2] and Dempster and Howarth[3] present a list of the most relevant guidelines. Also of note is the fact that guidelines may differ between countries; for example, Japan considers a DNA/plasmid vaccine a gene therapy product. All pivotal studies should be conducted in compliance with Good Laboratory Practice (GLP).[18]

An environmental risk assessment may also be required, particularly for Genetically Modified Organism (GMO) medicinal products. The following should be considered: genetic structure and stability, the possibility to disseminate and survive in the environment, the ability of the vaccine to transfer potential pathogenicity or virulent factors to other microorganisms, and its ability to stably convert to a toxicogenic phenotype.[19,20]

19.2.1 *In vivo* toxicological evaluation

Typical predictive *in vivo* studies conducted to evaluate vaccine safety include general toxicity studies (either single or repeat dose), local tolerance, and developmental studies. Other studies that may be considered depending on the vaccine and/or adjuvant include safety pharmacology, biodistribution, integration, and neurovirulence studies. Carcinogenicity and genotoxicity studies are not generally relevant for vaccines as these are large macromolecules, with limited ability to cross the cell membrane and integrate into the DNA. However, genotoxicity testing may be considered for certain adjuvants, process residues and/or excipients present in the vaccine formulation.[15,16]

19.2.2 General toxicology

The aim of a general toxicity study is to identify potential systemic toxicity effects by the timely evaluation of various endpoints, including life observations, body weight, food consumption, local reactions, clinical pathology (hematology, biochemistry, and coagulation), ophthalmology, organ weights, and histopathology (for more details see References 2, 4, 15, 16). The study is designed to attain a no adverse effect level (NOAEL). The maximum tolerated dose is not normally evaluated, although there may be some exceptions (e.g., for a novel adjuvant, or toxin). Single acute studies are generally not required,[15,16] but there are examples in the literature where acute studies have been conducted, for instance, as part of the development of a recombinant plasmid DNA antirabies vaccine.[21] However, the necessity for such a study could be argued.

19.2.3 Design of toxicology studies

The design of a nonclinical safety study should use the most appropriate species and take into account the clinical route of administration, the dose, and the dosing schedule. In the clinic, the dosing schedule is usually episodic, either weeks or months apart. In the animal studies, this dosing period can be reduced to approximately 2 to 3 weekly intervals (see Sections 19.2.4 and 19.2.5).

The number of doses will normally depend on the vaccine and the proposed clinical dosing schedule. In most cases, a $N + 1$ approach is used (one dose more than the clinical schedule[22]), which should provide an overage in the safety margin. However, in certain cases, only a single dose is needed. For example, for a Japanese encephalitis vaccine, to assess the effect of a viremia, only one dose was given to support a clinical regimen of one dose; the viremia was only evident after one dose (unpublished data).

In an animal study, the human clinical dose is usually the only dose level required to be assessed and, if possible, is given in the human dose volume: 0.5 mL is the standard intramuscular (IM) volume. A single human dose is given with the assumption that this dose will be NOAEL. Such a dose should provide an adequate safety margin over the human dose. However, this concept was challenged at a DIA meeting in 2006, as the consequence of this rule is that the safety margin depends largely on the size of the animal model selected.[23] For a pediatric population, depending on the species selected, there may therefore be no safety margin. Assessing other dose levels may be more appropriate in certain cases, and administering multiple doses, including above the human dose or testing the most immunogenic dose level,[2] may provide more meaningful information.

The size of the groups usually depends on the animal model selected. For small animals (e.g., rodents), approximately 10 animals per sex per group per sacrifice time should be studied. For larger animals, the number is reduced: approximately four to five per group per sex per sacrifice time for rabbits and between two and three per group per sex for primates.[16,17]

The study should include a period of time in which either reversibility and/or a delayed effect may be evaluated and is normally a period of between 14 and 28 days.

19.2.4 Species selection

It is critical that the most appropriate or relevant model is selected. For vaccines, like other biopharmaceuticals, this criterion is normally based on pharmacological activity.[2,24] The main criteria are as follows:

1. The development of a humoral immune response[15,16,25]
2. The susceptibility of the species to the targeted pathology; applicable to live or attenuated vaccines and/or toxin-based vaccines[16,25] (see following discussion of *S. typhi*)
3. Availability of a reasonable amount of background and historical data for the species

4. The size of the muscle mass, particularly if administering a human dose at 0.5 mL via intramuscular administration (For smaller species, the amount injected will need to be adjusted. For mice, the dose may be reduced to a 1/10th of the dose, and for the rat the dose may be given at 250 μL x 2.)

Another consideration in species selection is the cell-mediated immune response. However, this area is less well considered or understood at present and should be considered carefully, case by case (see Section 19.2.5).

In general, vaccine safety assessment programs use a single species, with rodent and rabbit being the most common.[22,15,16] Other species may be considered including the nonhuman primate and mini-pig, although, if possible, for ethical reasons, primates should be avoided. Hamster,[26] ferret, and guinea pig are sometimes used, but usually for more specific investigations. In certain cases, two species may be appropriate.[15,16]

A preliminary exploratory study may provide valuable information and help to confirm the relevance of the animal species regarding its ability to induce an immune response, or to understand the timing of certain responses, such as viremia.

In cases where a relevant species has not been identified, a multifaceted approach may be taken. This was the case for *S. typhi*, a human-restricted strain vaccine, which used a combination of *in vitro* and *in vivo* studies and a weight of evidence approach. Also, by changing the formulation to include hog mucin and the route of administration from subcutaneous to intraperitoneal, the mouse, which was previously not sensitive, became sensitive to the pathogen, which enabled levels of attenuation to be assessed. The vaccine entered into a phase I clinical trial with no reported safety issues.[27]

For some vaccines, particularly, therapeutic vaccines, the target may be a specific human self antigen target, or involve a vector that expresses a human-specific antigen (e.g., a human cytokine). In these cases, a homologous animal gene may be generated or a model adapted to be responsive to the specific encoded gene.[3] Trovax, a viral vector vaccine, developed to induce responses against cells bearing the human tumor-associated antigen 5T4 in the treatment of various solid tumors, required a mouse-specific antigen vaccine to be developed alongside the human vaccine. The reason being was to enable an appropriate reprotoxicity evaluation, as the protein 5T4 is expressed in the placenta and therefore the risk of any potential effects during pregnancy were assessed by ensuring the appropriate antigen/antibody interactions were tested.[28]

Other selection criteria may be considered. The mini-pig is a good model for studying intracutaneous or topical vaccines.[29] For a mucosal vaccine, Glueck[30] used the baboon to investigate a novel adjuvant for intranasal immunization, based on the physiological and pharmacology similarity with man. However, other species should be considered first, and certainly rats, mice, and rabbits have been used. For further discussion, see safety evaluation of toxin adjuvants delivered intranasally by Lang.[31]

19.2.5 Immunogenicity evaluation

The toxicology study should include an evaluation of the immune response, which will provide evidence that the vaccine was dosed, show that the species is responsive to the vaccine, and might allow the correlation between a toxic effect and the immune response induced. For further details, see References 4, 15, 16, 22.

At present, the aim is to ensure that a humoral response is generated. For mucosal vaccines, IgA may be more appropriate.[2,15,16] T cell–mediated responses may also be considered, and advances in knowledge and the development of different types of vaccines and/or adjuvants suggest that cell-mediated responses may be just as or more important than the humoral response, when considering the selection of species. Adjuvants can selectively switch the T helper cell response, which may influence a protection or pathology dependent response (see Section 19.2.5). However, the current understanding and interpretation of such data are limited in terms of predicitivity, and there are also limitations in the immunoassays developed for species routinely used in nonclinical testing. This is a key area where further development is required.

19.2.6 Local tolerance

Reactogenicity or local tolerance is an important safety endpoint for vaccines and may be evaluated as part of the general toxicity study or in a separate study. For such a study, an appropriate scoring system should be used (e.g., the adapted Draize scale and the appropriate dose volume to muscle ratio given). Rabbit is often the preferred model for IM injection, as a typical human dose of 0.5 mL can be given. Other species may be considered. For example, the mini-pig has an epidermis similar to that of humans and may be the most appropriate model for assessing intradermal or patch dosing. There are some limitations in certain models, in particular rodents, where administration of dose volume is limited and the choice of muscle is important. It is also important to consider the histopathological changes that can arise simply by the procedure, as both in rats and rabbits, histopathological reactogenicity are seen as a result of dosing sodium chloride.[32]

19.2.7 Reproductive and developmental studies

The target population for vaccines may include women of child-bearing potential who may become pregnant during the vaccination period or just after, or the vaccine may be specifically designed for maternal immunization to prevent infectious diseases in the neonate by the passive transfer of antibodies (e.g., the vaccine against group B streptococcus, which can be life threatening during the neonatal period).[33]

Assessment of potential adverse effects on reproduction and development of fetuses and pups must therefore be considered.[34] As with general toxicology, any

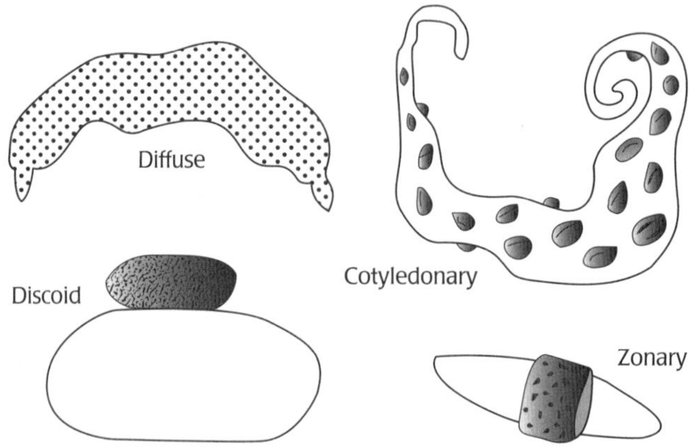

Figure 19-1: Classification of placenta shape. *Discoid/hemichorial*: a single placenta is formed, discoid in shape (e.g., primates, rabbits, rodents, humans). Attachment of the primate placenta is bidiscoid and rats and mice have three trophoblastic layers between the maternal and fetal environment. *Diffuse/epitheliochorial*: almost entire surface of the allantochorion is involved in formation of the placenta (e.g., horses, pigs). *Zonary/endotheliocorial*: placenta has complete or incomplete bands of tissue surrounding the fetus (e.g., dogs, cats, seals, bears, and elephants). *Cotyledonary*: multiple discrete areas of attachment called cotyledons are formed by interaction of patches of allantochorion with endometrium. This type of placentation is observed in ruminants.

potential adverse effects of the inherent biological activity of the vaccine antigen and the constituents of the vaccine, including adjuvant, should be assessed. There are exceptions, and certain vaccines may automatically be contraindicated to pregnant women or to those planning to become pregnant. For example, the smallpox vaccine, which is contraindicated for women who are pregnant and women who plan to become pregnant within 4 weeks after vaccination. Furthermore, pregnant women are advised to avoid close contact with persons recently vaccinated, as in the case of rubella.[35]

The selection of species, dose, and dosing schedule should be considered in the study design, and previous or preliminary nonclinical data may be supportive. The FDA[17] guidance for conducting developmental studies for both preventative vaccines and therapeutic vaccines provide clear guidance. A single species is usually considered adequate and should develop an immune response to the antigen (as discussed in Section 19.2.5). In addition, the fetus should be exposed to maternal antibodies. The temporal passage of antibodies between the species may vary and is likely to be a consequence of physiological and anatomical differences between species. Figure 19.1 shows different placental shapes between species and the table below (Table 19.1) provides information regarding IgG transfer, possibly as a consequence of these differences.

The majority of human vaccines tend to be immunogenic in rodents and rabbits. Rabbits have the added advantage that their antibody transfer is similar to man, and they are a well understood reproductive model. For more practical reasons, rats are also commonly used, although the transfer of antibodies mainly occurs postnatally, which means the assessment of the antibody on the fetus is limited; this factor could be a key concern particularly for some therapeutic

Table 19-1. IgG transfer varies between species

Species	IgG transfer
Human	Starts second trimester and reaches maternal levels by birth (100%)[103]
Primate and rabbits	Similar to humans – 100% prenatal transfer[104,105]
Rat, mice	10% before birth; 90% Ab transferred postnatally in milk, [106,107]
Pig, cow, goat, horse, sheep	After birth

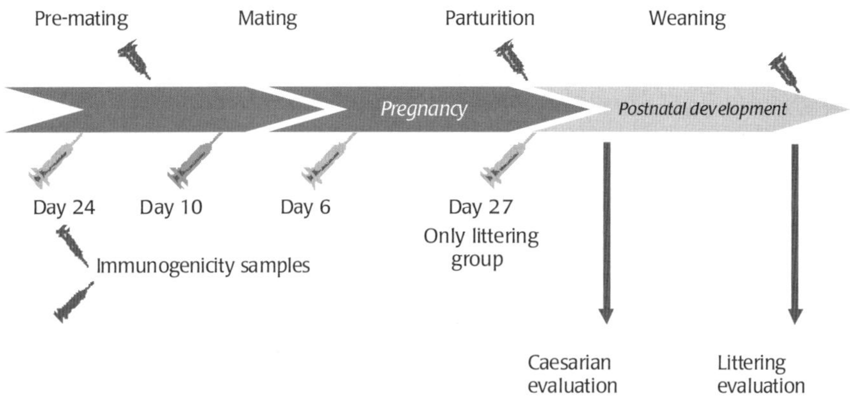

Figure 19-2: An example and schematic representation of a dosing schedule used in a DART study.

vaccines, such as those targeted against a fetally expressed self antigen. In some cases, the nonhuman primate is the only suitable species, although there are technical and logistical difficulties associated with timing and numbers of offsprings, particularly if a postnatal examination is considered (see review by Weinbauer et al.[36]).

The study design and dosing schedule should reflect the clinical route of administration and dose level and should ensure the fetus is exposed to peak maternal antibodies at key periods (e.g., during organogenesis and postnatal weaning period). The frequency of dosing may depend on the (a) type of vaccine, (b) individual species, (c) Ab response/kinetic profile. Premating priming doses may be required to reach a peak antibody response during organogenesis. For a postnatal examination, another dose may be required just prior to littering. Episodic dosing is usually the most appropriate dosing schedule (see Figure 19.2), and overexposure to the vaccine could result in immune tolerance.

The endpoints measured in the developmental and reproductive toxicity (DART) study are consistent with studies conducted on small molecules and biotherapeutics. For further information, see FDA and International Conference on Harmonization (ICH) guidelines. Organs essential to the normal functioning of the immune system are not typically assessed in DART studies, and revisiting this should be considered as suggested by Holsapple et al.[37]

For males, the only assessment of the reproductive tract is in the general toxicology study. Fertility studies in males are not conducted unless there is a particular cause for concern.[17]

19.2.8 Safety pharmacology

Safety pharmacology studies investigate potential undesirable pharmacodynamic effects on physiological functions and are recommended for small molecules.[38] For vaccines, the guidance is slightly contradictory. The EMEA suggests measuring certain hemodynamic endpoints (e.g., blood pressure and heart rate) as a consequence of findings from the pertussis and *Haemophilus influenza* vaccines.[23] However, it can be generally argued that safety pharmacology studies are not required for vaccines unless there is a finding in the general toxicology study, or a specific case, (e.g., development of a toxoid vaccine and/or use of a novel adjuvant).[15,16,23]

The assessment for potential prolongation of QT interval for vaccines is not considered relevant as these are macromolecules, which are unlikely to bind with internal KCNH2/hERG channel receptors. However, as Turner et al.[39] point out, KCNH2/hERG is a transmembrane protein and has an external pore region, and therefore raises the theory that it would be possible for a biological to bind and was reported for the scorpion toxin BeKm-1. Could this be relevant therefore to vaccines, the answer is likely to depend upon the nature and target of the vaccine and should not be dismissed completely without due consideration.

19.2.9 Biodistribution studies

Biodistribution studies are conducted to evaluate the dissemination and persistence of nucleic acid/DNA and viral vector-based vaccines. Vector persistence should be examined at more than one time point up to at least 21 days or more after the last injection;[22] unpublished data) and the biodistribution and persistence of a plasmid is usually dependent upon the route of administration.[20] These studies can be combined with a general toxicology study or may be conducted separately. In most cases, the DNA is extracted from the selected tissues and assessed by quantitative Polymerase Chain Reaction (qPCR).[15,16]

19.2.10 Integration studies

Integration studies are normally considered for DNA vaccines, which deliver antigen genes via a DNA expression vector[20] and where integration into the genome could ultimately lead to unwanted effects such as oncogenesis via activation of oncogenes or inactivation of tumor suppressor genes. Integration studies are also needed if a biodistribution study showed persistence of plasmid in tissues at levels exceeding 30,000 copies per microgram of host DNA at termination of the study.[20,40]

To determine the risk of integration, genomic DNA is isolated and compared with appropriate negative and positive controls to determine the presence of potential integrated vaccine plasmid DNA.[41] Most DNA vaccines are delivered intramuscularly (IM), and to date, integration studies have shown no concerns. However, Wang et al.[42] showed how electroporation can increase the levels of plasmid uptake, which could increase the risk.

19.2.11 Juvenile or elderly populations

Toxicology studies conducted specifically to support juvenile or elderly populations are not evident in the published literature. The general practice is to support such populations with standard nonclinical safety studies (as discussed previously) and clinical data generated in adults.

Neonatal vaccination may offer a better way of protecting against certain pathogens, such as HIV, *B. pertussis* and *H. influenzae B*,[43] and neonate and juvenile models have been developed to evaluate efficacy.[44] One of the key safety issues for a neonatal vaccine is the induction of immune tolerance.[43,45] Studies conducted in neonatal mice have shown that tolerance can be antigen specific and that vaccination at an early age induced no immune response and that mice remained unresponsive as adults, in terms of antibody response when exposed to the antigen.[45] There is some evidence of this in humans with certain vaccines, which Siegrist[43] suggests may be circumnavigated in the future by priming the immune system in a specific way, such that it alters the T and B cell response in neonates. There is no doubt that the safety of vaccines in neonate, juvenile and elderly population needs further consideration, particularly with the development of novel adjuvants, therapeutic vaccines, and neonatal vaccines.

19.3 IMMUNOLOGY MEETS TOXICOLOGY (IMMUNOPHARMACOTOXICOLOGY)

Potential safety issues should be predicted as early as possible. For vaccines, adverse events are often the result of pharmacological activity, and may include, for example, cross-reactivity of induced antibodies with innate antigens, allergy, autoimmunity, local reactogenicity, and disease exacerbation. Early identification of potential safety issues will allow vaccine developers to engineer antigens that do not have these safety issues while retaining efficacy.

19.3.1 Autoimmunity risk and vaccination

The question regarding autoimmunity and a link with vaccine administration has been a common topic of debate for some years. Autoimmunity may be described as an inappropriate response of the immune system to self antigens that can lead to organ or tissue damage.[47] The cause, although unknown, is likely to be multifactorial and may include hormonal, immunological, genetic, and environmental factors.[47,48] In the past few years, there have been several reports of potential links between various vaccines (e.g., hepatitis B, tetanus toxoid, measles, polio) and certain autoimmune type diseases (e.g., multiple sclerosis, Guillain-Barré syndrome, systemic lupus erythematosus, diabetes mellitus).[49–51] It is encouraging to note that, although the potential appears to exist at a theoretical level, epidemiology studies have so far failed to show a link between autoimmunity and vaccination[51–55] and perhaps provide some reassurance that the theoretical risk has not been confirmed. However, although these links may be disputed, they cannot be completely ignored, and questions of the potential risk must be considered during the development of any new product. This also applies to the development of new adjuvants that may invoke stronger, not always fully understood, immune responses (see review by Wraith et al.[55]).

The next section considers further how the risk of autoimmunity may be addressed.

19.3.2 Predicting autoimmunity

To predict the onset or potential development of autoimmune diseases is a challenge. First, the response is rare; second, the etiology is unknown; and third, the cause is likely to be multifactorial.

There are two key factors to be considered in the development of autoimmunity:

1. Induction of a *de novo* autoimmune disease
2. Exacerbation of existing autoimmune disorders

Bioinformatics and animal models may offer some predictive value in determining the potential for autoimmune reactions (see Section 19.3.3).

One key hypothesis regarding the etiology of autoimmunity is that of molecular mimicry, where a microbial antigen may contain epitopes that are sufficiently similar to human molecular determinants, and for which the immune system cannot discriminate between.[47,56] The degree to which epitope mimicry occurs, under what conditions, and its pathological significance remains controversial.[56] Criteria by which to demonstrate molecular mimicry-induced autoimmunity are outlined in a review by Ang et al.[58]

One of the first cases of possible molecular mimicry was that of rheumatic fever, in which the symptoms were caused by antigens that mimic cardiac myosin.[56,59] A simple rabbit study demonstrated how the administration of the key antigen induced strong inflammatory and myocardial changes as a result of host immune response to self antigens.[59]

More recently, studies on *Campylobacter jejuni* have demonstrated how specific bacterial carbohydrate antigens can mimic the fine structure of human cell surface glycolipid structures and elicit autoimmune reactivity. Yuki et al.[61] first identified that the lipooligosaccharide (LOS) of *C. jejuni* mimicked human G(M)1 ganglioside and subsequently extended these studies to demonstrate that specific single amino acid variants of the *C. jejuni* Cst-II sialyltransferase protein are responsible for the synthesis of LOS variants that in turn, mimic different human ganglioside variants, leading to clinically distinct neuropathological syndromes.[62]

In contrast to the modification of carbohydrate structures linking *C. jejuni* infection to autoimmune disease, molecular mimicry of protein-derived B or T cell epitopes is not always easily demonstrated as the sole causative factor of autoimmune disease in humans. For example, although streptococcal M protein was considered at one time to be a prime potential causative factor for rheumatic fever (see previous discussion), evidence has also been presented that molecular mimicry is not the mechanism and that, instead, it is the complex formed between bacterial M proteins and human collagen IV that presents an autoimmunogenic epitope against which antibodies are induced.[63,64] Another example can be taken from the apparent molecular mimicry between the OspA protein from *Borrelia burgdorferi*, the causative pathogen for Lyme disease, and human LFA-1.[65] This apparent molecular mimicry was identified as possibly leading to the development of antibiotic treatment-resistant Lyme arthritis in genetically susceptible individuals who had been administered an OspA vaccine. In fact, these individuals were already predisposed to arthritogenesis on the basis of their HLA types, but the potential link contributed to the withdrawal of an OspA-containing vaccine from the market.[66] However, despite many compelling *in vitro* experiments, a clear causative role for OspA-mediated molecular mimicry in the development of treatment-resistant Lyme arthritis in genetically susceptible individuals is lacking.[67]

Nevertheless, the potential for autoimmune disease would clearly exist if one considers the polyspecificity of immune recognition molecules such as B cell receptors, antibodies, T cell receptors and MHC molecules. Further, the polyspecificity of immune receptors is also able to transcend the biochemically defined classes of biomolecules. For instance, the monoclonal antibody SYA/J6 has been demonstrated to have a dual specificity, binding a specific carbohydrate or a specific peptide with comparable affinity.[68] Detailed analysis of the interatomic interactions between the antibody combining site and either the carbohydrate or the peptide antigens demonstrated that functional mimicry is possible without exact structural mimicry. This example underlines the case that it is not possible to predict with certainty whether the molecular surfaces of all potentially cross-reactive epitopes, whether of foreign or self molecules, will, or will not, be able to bind to a specific antibody.

DNA vaccines have also been associated with the induction of autoimmunity, particularly in that the presence of unmethylated CpG motifs in the plasmid backbone. These motifs can lead to anti-DNA antibodies, which were believed to accelerate the development of autoimmune disease.[69–71]

19.3.3 Autoimmunity and bioinformatics

Bioinformatics can play a key role and provide information regarding the potential risk of inducing an autoimmune reaction, within the limits of current knowledge and keeping in mind some skepticism regarding molecular mimicry, especially that of B or T cell epitopes derived from protein antigens, which have not been unequivocally demonstrated as a causative factor of autoimmune disease in humans.

Currently no regulations or guidelines exist regarding acceptable levels of sequence similarity between pathogen vaccine antigens and human proteins, and assessments are made on a case-by-case basis. In the food industry, where allergenicity of foodstuffs could be a health hazard, the potential for introducing genetically-modified organisms, or their proteins, that may be cross-reactive with allergen-specific IgE antibodies is a concern. Consequently, guidelines have been developed over time by the Food and Agriculture Organization and the World Health Organization[72,73] to reduce the risk of introducing potentially allergenic proteins into the food supply as a consequence of genetic modification of foodstuffs. Since the variable domain repertoire for IgE is the same as for other immunoglobulin classes, and the same principles of antigen–antibody interaction apply to allergens, it might be useful to consider how these guidelines may inform prediction of cross-reactive antigens in vaccine formulations.

The FAO/WHO Codex Alimentarius recommends that cross-reactivity be considered a concern when either of two conditions is satisfied: (a) when amino acid sequence identity between an introduced protein and a known allergen is greater than 35% over a window of 80 residues, or (b) when there are more than six identical contiguous residues. First, when the sequences of protein allergens is examined, it has been observed that in most cases, cross-reactivity requires at least 70% identity, and that cross-reactivity is considered rare when identity is under 50% identity.[73] Under these criteria, 35% identity is a very conservative threshold. Although a sliding window of 80 residues may be considered a way to focus on the modular domain structure of proteins, this window size is a somewhat arbitrary measure, and leads to a higher rate of false positives than a straightforward implementation of the FASTA sequence comparison algorithm would provide.[75] Second, in the case of short sequence matches of eight contiguous residues or less, it has been shown that the likelihood of finding such matches is extremely high, and that six-residue matches are highly predicted on the basis of chance alone.[76] Essentially, such short-sequence matches are in themselves unlikely to provide useful information about the potential for cross-reactivity between an antigen and self proteins. Ultimately, although neither of these criteria seem to have a solid scientific foundation,[77] they nevertheless represent public points of reference that must be addressed.

In the absence of reliable predictive methods for assessing potential immunological cross-reactivity, a comparative sequence analysis approach can be used to identify whether or not known epitopes from human proteins exist in a candidate vaccine antigen. The Immune Epitope Database (IEDB) provides a comprehensive reference data set for known epitopes.[78] When screening potential vaccine candidates, the presence of known human-derived epitopes can be ruled out by comparison against the IEDB (www.iedb.org).

19.3.4 Autoimmunity and animal models

Animal models may provide further understanding of the pathology or etiology of autoimmune disease. However, they should be considered with caution as they do not perfectly mimic the human situation, and the models developed to date are manipulated to have a susceptibility to developing autoimmune disease (see review by Taneja and David[79]). In 1996, Classen[80] showed an increase in spontaneously developed Insulin Dependent Diabetes Mellitus (IDDM) in Nonobese Diabetic (NOD) mice exposed to the pertussis or *Haemophilus influenza B* (Hib) vaccine. However, this finding has been disputed within the scientific community. A repeat study in NOD mice with a Hib vaccine showed no such evidence (unpublished data), and subsequent publication by Ravel et al.[81] showed no increase in autoimmunity in NOD mouse when treated with multivalent diphtheria, tetanus, pertussis, poliomyelitis, and hemophilus vaccines, and therefore it is difficult to draw conclusions. Another model that was tested used mercuric chloride (believed to induce autoimmunity) to determine when coadministered with hepatitis B vaccine would predispose a genetically susceptible species to develop autoimmunity. The study showed an increase in anti-double-stranded (ds) DNA and antinuclear antibodies in vaccine treated groups, compared to mercuric chloride alone, and indicated that both genetic disposition and environment may increase the risk of developing autoimmunity following vaccination.[82] However, the authors were reluctant to draw firm conclusions, and there was neither a direct comparison with the vaccine alone and the presence of anti-ds DNA and antinuclear antibodies.

19.4 ALLERGY/HYPERSENSITIVITY

Vaccines have been associated with allergic reactions, which can present via a number of different forms, including skin rash, anaphylaxis reactions, and vasculitis.[83] Anaphylaxis is possibly the most life threatening, and serious hypersensitivity reaction that can be evoked. However, it is considered extremely rare, with a risk of approximately 0.65 cases per million doses that resulted in death.[84] Predicting potential allergic reactions in animal models has proven to be a challenge, and today there are no good models for assessing hypersensitivity. The best proposed method is to use the conventional endpoints in a general toxicology study even though the limited animal numbers and lack of genetic variability, compared to the human population, limits the power in these current preclinical studies.[3]

Inducing a strong immune response following vaccination is essential for providing protection. However, instead of protection, some experimental vaccines have led to disease exacerbation, following postvaccine exposure to the pathogen. The examples are not numerous, and often the confirmatory studies or studies designed to elucidate the nature of the observed phenomena are lacking. Examples are measles,[85] chlamydia trachoma,[7] and RSV vaccine.[5] The mechanism for such phenomena remains poorly understood.[86,87] In the case of chlamydia, no further investigations were conducted, and the data are questionable as to whether the phenomenom exists. Studies with RSV and the cotton tail rat have suggested that the induction of the immunopathological effect of RSV may be related to a Th_2-biased immune response,[88,89] which may be triggered by formalin, and specifically related to the carbonyl groups on formaldehyde.[90] Studies have shown that if Th_2 cytokines (e.g., interleukin-4 (IL-4) and IL-10) are depleted, there is a reduction in the severity of enhanced disease.[90] Dosing regime, schedule, and age may all be other critical components to the induction of protection or pathology,[92,93] as well as the hypothesis that a strong unbalanced T cell response, producing Th_2 IL13 and Il5 may increase the risk.[94]

The potential link of formaldehyde-inactivated vaccines adjuvanted with aluminium and observed with the RSV prototype vaccines raised concerns that the *influenza* H5N1 pandemic formaldehyde-inactivated adjuvanted vaccine could cause an immunopathological effect. As a result, a challenge study in macaque monkeys was conducted; it measured both humoral and cell-mediated immune responses and evaluated lung histopathology as an endpoint. The study concluded that there was no disease enhancement.[95]

A recent case concerning an HIV vaccine, which used a replication defective adenovirus type 5 (Ad5) vector, was stopped after a clinical trial showed an increase in HIV infections postvaccination. A followup investigation by Perreau et al.,[96] using *ex vivo* modeling with dendritic cells, showed how the formation of Ad5 immune complexes, a consequence of previous adenovirus exposure, can lead to specific CD4 and 8 T cell responses, which are targeted more toward the adenovirus than the HIV antigen, and as a consequence are less protective.

The mechanisms behind this enhanced disease phenomena are far from understood and are likely to be multifactorial. To investigate exacerbated reactions usually requires the development of an appropriate model, and that itself may be a challenge. A review by Byrd and Prince[97] lists some points to consider in terms of developing an animal model for RSV, and are relevant for other vaccines, and the authors highlight the challenge regarding the ability to predict such a phenomena.

19.5 OTHER SAFETY CONSIDERATIONS

19.5.1 DNA vaccines

When developing DNA vaccines, there are some specific issues to consider in terms of theoretical safety risks. One key factor relates to the sequence design: Certain genes and sequences (e.g., those involved with integration, transposition, or replication promoter or enhancer sequences), which could alter oncogenes[96] or sequences that are homologous with the host DNA, should be avoided (see review by Schalk et al.[20]).

Other safety concerns include

1. Fate of the plasmid in the vaccinated animals
2. Risk of DNA integration into host genome
3. Induction of autoimmunity

At one time, the risk of inducing anti-DNA antibodies was recognized as an issue but this no longer considered the case.[98] However, the long-term expression of foreign antigens and the use of costimulatory molecules such as cytokines may modulate a deviated reaction, and therefore an accurate assessment of additional risks should always be considered.

19.5.2 Toxins

Many antigens currently marketed would be inherently toxic except for the fact they have been stringently detoxified. Some of the most successful and durable vaccines today include toxoided forms of tetanus, pertussis, and diphtheria toxins. During the manufacturing process, these toxoids undergo significant chemical modifications, and their toxic properties are effectively eliminated. The safety is assured with every batch release and defined within safety characterization/quality control tests, which are not discussed in this chapter.

Bacteria produce a wide variety of proteins with toxic effects, and it is possible to detect the potential for such biological activities by sequence homology to known molecules, or by the identification of specific amino acid motifs that are diagnostic for a particular activity (e.g., proteolysis or membranolysis). In these cases, it is often possible to introduce specific mutations by genetic engineering to render the protein nontoxic. Careful selection of the mutations, especially if done in the context of available structural information, such as an atomic-resolution model of the antigen, can produce a fully detoxified molecule that retains the antigenic properties that make it attractive as a vaccine candidate.

Many pathogens have evolved mechanisms to sabotage the host immune system by provoking or initiating irrelevant or counterproductive immune responses. Although not classically grouped as toxins, the potential exists to alter the binding sites or effector regions of these molecules to render them inactive in the same manner as described earlier.

19.5.3 Adjuvants

Many vaccines require additional help to stimulate the immune system to achieve an efficacious immune response. For many years, aluminum has been the gold standard with a good safety record, although there have been concerns regarding macrophagic myofasciitis,[99] and the role alum plays in shifting the immune system toward a Th_2 bias. Today, new adjuvants that aim to provide a more specific immune modulation, with improved efficacy and safety, are being developed. This brings new challenges in the development of such products, and the safety of adjuvants needs to be considered carefully, particularly as they may stimulate the immune system via mechanisms not clearly understood. The assessment of the adjuvant should be considered case by case and may be classified as a synthetic rather than biological, which may therefore require additional safety testing to those normally considered for a vaccine alone (see EMEA adjuvant guidelines[99]).

19.5.4 Biomarkers/genomics/proteomics

In predicting safety issues, there are a range of biomarkers that may be considered, many of which are those standard biomarkers currently used in toxicology studies (e.g., hematology and blood chemistry parameters) plus newly identified specialized markers.

The evaluation of certain immunological parameters such as cytokines may also be included. Although, there are currently a limited number of validated assays and understanding regarding the interpretation of this data. Some immune-related biological markers are not necessarily linked to pathological consequences. For example, it is possible to measure autoantibodies.[100] However, there is no clear relationship between serum autoantibodies and the risk of autoimmune disease,[101] and in the absence of conclusive data, autoantibodies should not be considered a predictive tool.[100]

The increasing amount of genome-scale data being generated offers the possibility of a much wider range of biomarkers becoming available in the future. For example, as libraries of tissue-specific patterns of gene expression become increasingly well-defined and the critical parameters surrounding the definition of healthy and pathological states of gene expression are clarified, reference patterns for specific tissues should become available. However, caution is required in understanding results and how levels of gene expression can be considered in relation to safety and current safety margin principles.

19.6 PREDICTIVE *IN VITRO* SYSTEMS

In vitro systems can offer a number of advantages: saving animals and providing a quick, easy screening method, which may be particularly useful in early development. Various *in vitro* models were reviewed by Brennan and Dougan[2] and will not be rediscussed in this chapter.

One fairly new system is the Modular Immune *in vitro* Construct technology system (MIMIC), which can measure innate and adaptive immune responses and evaluate cytokines, antibodies, and chemokines *in vitro*. The system is based on a multidimensional interrogation of quiescent primary human cells mainly of blood origin that can reproduce immune responses in a cell-based high-throughput screen and rapidly capture the effect of an immunoresponsive agent (e.g.,

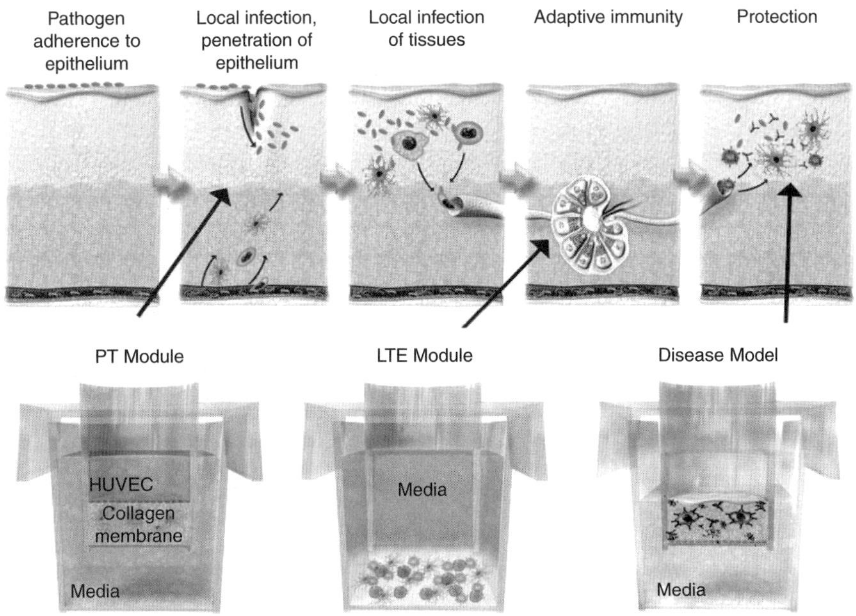

Figure 19-3: Graphical representation of an immune response and how it is modeled via the PTE, LTE, and disease model (functional assay) modules of the MIMIC system. *See color plates.*

a vaccine or immunotherapeutic) on human population subgroups defined by genetic diversity (e.g., HLA haplotypes) as well as differences due to age and gender.

There are three components in the MIMIC system, which can act independently as described (see Figure 19.3):

- Peripheral Tissue Equivalent (PTE) module: a three-dimensional construct that recapitulates the innate arm of the immune system
- Lymphoid Tissue Equivalent (LTE) module: an artificial lymph node, where generated antigen-presenting cells (APCs) efficiently interact with T and B lymphocytes to initiate antigen-specific immune responses
- Functional assays that assess neutralizing Ab, hemagglutinin inhibition, cytotoxic T cell, and other effector functions

The PTE module reproduces the human *in vivo* immune-physiology of peripheral tissues, such as the skin, and can recreate the natural immune-reactogenicity. The system is able to simultaneously generate autonomous monocyte-derived dendritic cells (DCs) and macrophages and intrinsic signals can be measured.[102] When stimulated by vaccines, the PTE module mimics the *in vivo* state, and the inflammatory reaction can be determined by measuring cytokine (e.g., TNF, interleukins, PGE2) levels. Figure 19.4 shows the general innate reactogenicity of the vaccines DTaP, Fluzone, and Recombivax, assessed by measuring proinflammatory cytokines. Figure 19.5 demonstrates how the PTE system using CD33+ selected monocytes can be used to analyze for prostaglandin production using standard Enzyme-Linked Immunosorbent Assay (ELISA) methods.

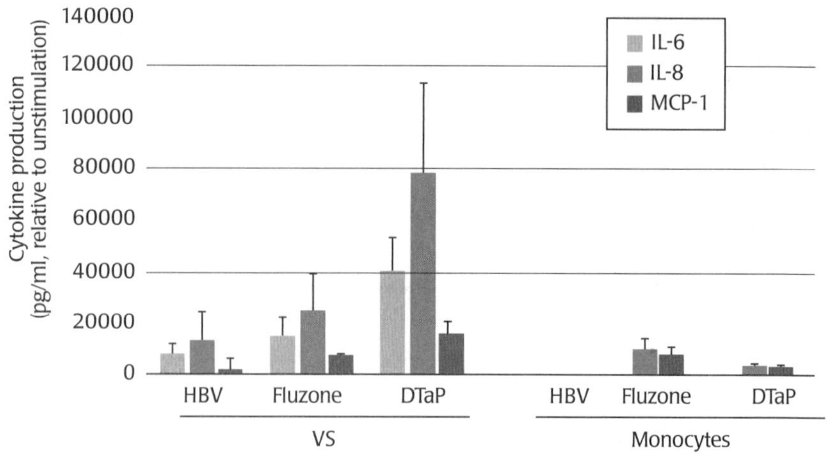

Figure 19-4: Reactogenicity of commercial vaccines in the PTE module and by monocytes alone. Vaccines hepatitis B virus (HBV 1:200), influenza virus vaccine (Fluzone 1:400), and tetanus toxoid vaccine (DTaP 1:200) were used in the study. PTE is the peripheral tissue equivalent module containing CD33+ positively selected cells (left). CD33+ monocytes alone do not produce any appreciable cytokines nor chemokines when stimulated with the vaccines (right).

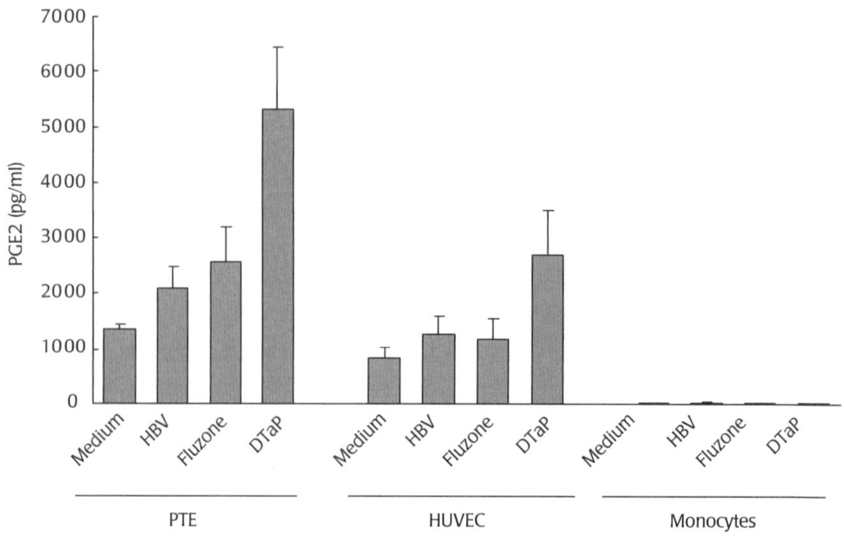

Figure 19-5: Prostaglandin E2 production induced by the vaccines hepatitis B virus (HBV 1:200), influenza virus vaccine (Fluzone 1:400), and Tetanus toxoid vaccine (DTaP 1:200). PTE is the peripheral tissue equivalent module containing CD33+ positively selected cells (left). HUVEC (center) is the empty PTE and also produces PGE2 when stimulated. CD33+ monocytes alone do not produce PGE2 when stimulated with vaccines (right).

To evaluate the immunopotency of toll-like receptor (TLR) agonists in the *in vitro* PTE module, TLR-induced cytokine can be measured. TLR agonists often induce higher levels of cytokines in the PTE module than in conventional PBMC cultures and may be considered more sensitive. For example, Poly I:C and CpG 2006 both induced proinflammatory cytokines IL-1 a/b in the PTE module, but neither of these were observed in PBMC cultures. Poly I:C also triggered the

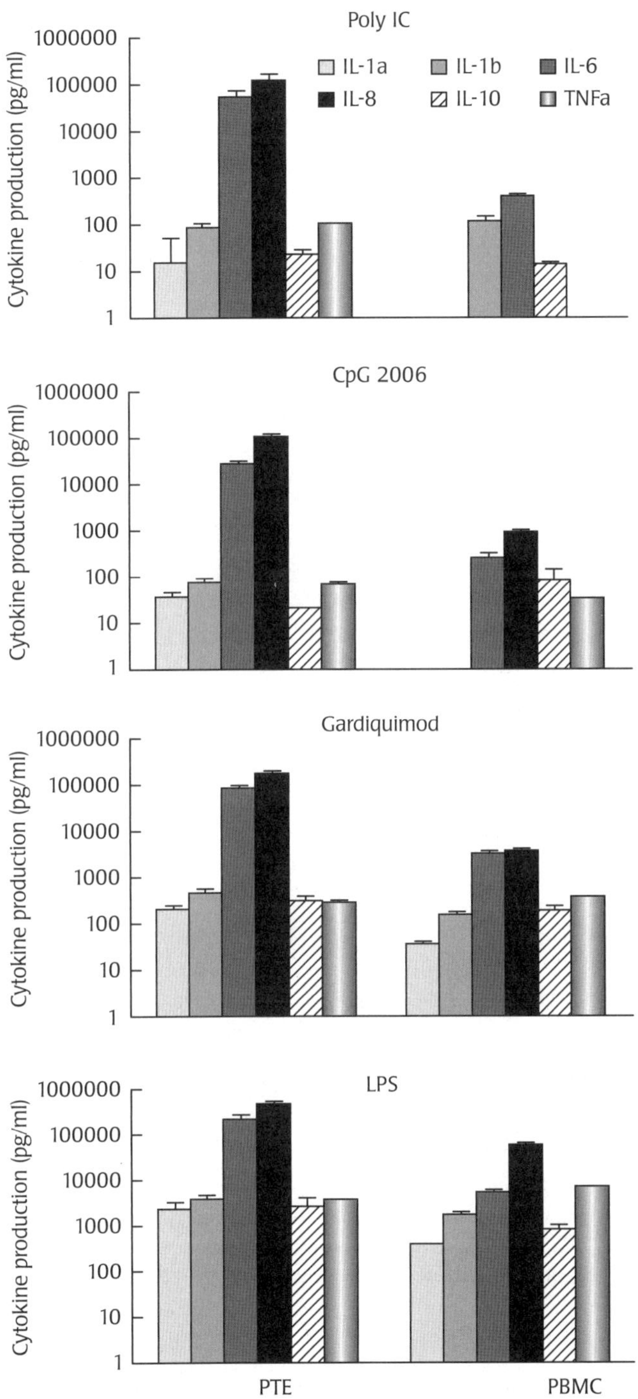

Figure 19-6: TLR agonists induce cytokine production in the PTE module. The culture supernatants were collected after 24-h incubation, the cytokine levels in supernatants were analyzed by Q-plex cytokine array. The data shown in the figure are the relative cytokine production for each treatment after subtraction of the basal production in unstimulated PTE modules. The numbers shown in the bar graphs represent the mean ± SE of three or four different donors.

production TNFalpha only in the PTE culture (Figure 19.3). Moreover, Poly I:C and CpG 2006 treatments elicited approximately 100- to 1,000-fold greater levels of IL-6 and IL-8 in the PTE module than in PBMC culture. Although Gardiquimod and LPS dramatically induced IL-1 a/b, IL-6, IL-8, IL-10, and TNFalpha both in the PTE module and in the PBMC culture, the PTE module produced approximately three- to sixfold more IL-1 a/b and IL-10, and 10- to 50-fold more IL-6 and IL-8 than PBMC culture (Figure 19.6).

19.7 CONCLUSIONS

Vaccines are one of the greatest success stories of modern medicine. At the turn of the twentieth century, catching pneumonia could be a death sentence. Today, society is protected against a number of highly infectious and often deadly diseases. Ensuring safety of vaccines is of utmost importance, as they are given to millions of healthy individuals, including, infants, children, and adults. There are a number of well-used methods for detecting potential safety issues, these are mainly *in vivo*, but also *in vitro* and *in silico* methods exist, and can be considered, particularly prior to the first dose in humans. There is always room for improvement, better understanding, and predictivity, even rare events, particularly as vaccines increase their target and with the development of new adjuvants.

ACKNOWLEDGMENTS

We would like to acknowledge the following who have either directly contributed to the writing of this chapter or who have volunteered to provide time and feedback, including Caroline Ruat, Guillaume Ravel and Artur Pedyczak. We would like to thank VaxDesign who provided the information regarding *in vitro* systems and Richard Bown of Colorado State University for the use of his placenta diagram.

REFERENCES

1. Bonnet MC, Targaglia J, Verdier F, Kourilsky P, Lindberg A, Klein M, Moingeon P. Recombinant viruses as a tool for therapeutic vaccination against human cancers. *Immunol Lett.* 2000;74:11–25.
2. Brennan FR, Dougan D. Non-clinical safety evaluation of novel vaccines and adjuvants: New products, new strategies. *Vaccine.* 2005;23:3210–3222.
3. Dempster AM, Haworth R. Pre-clinical safety evaluation of viral vaccines. In: Cavagnaro JA, ed. Preclinical Safety Evaluation of Biopharmaceuticals. *John Wiley & Sons Inc. Hoboken, New Jersey.* 2008;31:683–712.
4. Sela M. and Hilleman MR. Therapeutic vaccines: Realities of today and hopes for tomorrow. *PNAS*, 2004;101(2):14559.
5. Chin J, Magoffin RL, Shearer LA, Schieble JH, Lenette EH. Field evaluation of a respiratory syncytial virus vaccine and a trivalent parainfluenza virus vaccine in a pediatric population. *Am J Epidemiol.* 1969;89:449–463.

6. Kim HW, Canchola JG, Brandt CD, Pyles G, Chanock R, Jensen K, Parrott RH. Respiratory syncytial virus disease in infants despite prior administration of antigenic inactivated vaccine. *Am J Epidemiol.* 1969;89(4):422–434.
7. Grayston JT, Foy HM, Kenny ER. The epidemiology of mycoplasma infections of the human respiratory tract. In: Hayflick L, ed. *The Mycoplasmatales and the L-Phase of Bacteria Amsterdam, The Netherlands: Appelton-Century-Crofts* 1969: 651.
8. Stewart GT. Toxicity of pertussis vaccine: Frequency and probability of reactions. *J Epidemiol Community Health.* 1979;33:150–156.
9. Murphy TV, Gargiullo PM, Massoudi MS, Nelson DB, Jumaan AO, Okoro C, Zanardi LR, Setia S, Fair E, LeBaron CW, Wharton M, Livingood J. Intussusception among infacts given an oral rotavirus vaccine. For the rotavirus intussuception investigation team. *N Eng J Med.* 2001;344(8):564–572.
10. O'Hagan DT, Rappuoli R. Novel approaches to vaccine delivery. *Pharma Res.* 2004;21(9):1519–1530.
11. Bonhoeffer J, Heininger U. Adverse events following immunization: perception and evidence. *Curr Opin Infect.* 2007;20;237–246.
12. Sutkowski EM, Gruber MF. Non Clinical safety evaluation of preventative vaccines-regulatory considerations, Business briefing. *Future Drug Discov. 3rd edition.* 2003;34–37.
13. Verdier F. Non-clinical vaccine safety assessment. *Toxicology.* 2002:174;37–43.
14. Olsen, H, Betton G, Robinson D, Thomas K, Monro A, Kolaja G, Lilly P, Sanders J, Sipes G, Bracken W, Dorato M, Van Duen K, Smith P, Berger B, Heller A. Concordance of the toxicity of pharmaceuticals in humans and in animals. *Regul Toxicol Pharmacol.* 2000;32:56–67.
15. EMEA. Note for guidance on preclinical pharmacological and toxicological testing of vaccines. CPMP/SWP/465/95. 1997.
16. WHO. Guidelines on nonclinical evaluation vaccines. Technical report series No. 927. 2005.
17. FDA CBER. Guidance for industry: considerations for reproductive toxicity studies for preventative vaccines for infectious disease indications. Draft guidance. 2006.
18. OECD. Principles on Good Laboratory Practice (as revised in 1997).
19. Viret JF, Favre GD. Biosafety aspects of the recombinant live oral *Vibrio cholerae* vaccine strain CVD 103-HgR. *Vaccine.* 2004;22:2457–2469.
20. Schalk J, Mooi FR, Berbers G, Van Aerts L, Ovelgonne H, Kimman TG. Preclinical and clinical safety studies on DNA vaccines. *Human Vaccines.* 2006;2(2):45–53.
21. Kumar PU, Kumar D, Annapurnav V, Kirshna P, Kalyansundaram S, Suresh P, Harishankar N, Jagadeesan V, Hariahran S, Naidu N, Krishnaswamy K, Rangarajan PN, Srinivasan VA, Reddy GS, Sesikeran B. Nonclinical toxicology study of recombinant – Plasmid DNA anti-rabies vaccines. *Vaccine.* 2006;24:2790–2798.
22. Lebron JA, Wolf JJ, Kaplanski CV, Ledwith BJ. Ensuring the quality, potency and safety of vaccines during preclinical development. *Vaccine.* 2005;4(6): 855–866.
23. Van der Laan JW, Forstor R, Ledwith B, Gruber M, Gould S, Penninks A. Non clinical testing of vaccines: Report from a workshop. *Drug Inf J.* 2009;43:75–85.
24. Subramanyam M, Rinaldi N, Mertssching E, Hutto D. Selection of relevant species. (In: Cavagnaro JA, ed. Preclinical Safety Evaluation of Biopharmaceuticals. *John Wiley & Sons Inc. Hoboken, New Jersey.*; 2008;9:181–206.
25. Kantor J, Irvine K, Abrams S, Snoy P, Olsen R, Greiner J, Kaufman H, Eggensperger D, Schlom J. (1992). Immunogenicity and safety of a recombinant vaccinia virus vaccine expressing the carcinoembryonic antigen gene in a nonhuman primate. *Cancer Res.* 1992;52:6917–6925.
26. Tang RS, Spaete RR, Thompson MW, MacPhail M, Guzzetta JM, Ryan PC, Reisinger K, Chandler P, Hilty M, Walker RE, Gomez MM, Losonsky GA. Development of a PIV-vectored RSV vaccine: Preclinical evaluation of safety, toxicity and enhanced disease and initial clinical testing in healthy adults. *Vaccine.* 2008;26: 373–6382.

27. Pasetti MF, Levine MM, Sztein MB. Animal models paving the way for clinical trials of attenuated Salmonella enterica serovar Typhi live oral vaccines and live vectors. *Vaccine*. 2003;21:401–418.
28. Woods AM, Wang WW, Shaw DM, Ward CM, Carroll MW, Rees B, Stern PI. Characterization of the murine 5T4 oncofoetal antigen: A target for immunotherapy in cancer. *Biochem. J.* 2002;366:353–365.
29. Gerdts V, Littel-van den Hurk S, Drunen, Griebel PJ, Babiuk LA. Use of animal models in the development of human vaccine s *Future Microbiol.* 2007;2(6): 667–675.
30. Glueck R. Pre-clinical and clinical investigation of the safety of a novel adjuvant for intranasal immunization. *Vaccine*. 2002;20:S42–244.
31. Lang D. Safety evaluation of toxin adjuvants delivered intranasally. Meeting notes. National Institute of Allergy and Infectious Diseases. 2001.
32. Thuilliez C, Dorso L, Howroyd P, Gould S, Chanut F, Burnett R. (2008). Histopathological lesions following intramuscular administration of saline in laboratory rodents and rabbits. *Exp Toxicol Pathol*. 2008;61:13–21.
33. Gruber MF. Maternal immunization: US FDA regulatory considerations. *Vaccine*. 2003;21:3487–3491.
34. Verdier F, Barrow P, Burge J. Reproductive toxicity testing of vaccines. *Toxicology*. 2003;85:213–219.
35. Amstey MS, Gall SA. Smallpox vaccine and pregnancy. *Obstet Gynecol*. 2002;100:87–93.
36. Weinbauer GF, Frings W, Fuchs A, Niehaus M, Osterburg I. Reproductive/development toxicity assessment of biopharmaceuticals in non human primates In: Cavagnaro JA, ed. Preclinical Safety Evaluation of Biopharmaceuticals. *John Wiley & Sons Inc. Hoboken, New Jersey*. 2008;18:379–397.
37. Holsapple MP, West LJ, Landreth KS. Species comparison of anatomical and functional immune system development. *Birth Defects Res. (Part B)*. 2003;68:321–334.
38. ICH7A. Harmonised tripartite guideline on safety pharmacology studies for human pharmaceuticals. *S7A*, Step 4. 2000.
39. Turner JR, Durham TA. Nonclinical Development Integrated Cardiac Safety: Assessment Methodologies for Non-cardiac Drugs in Discovery, Development, and Postmarketing Surveillance. *John Wiley & Sons Inc. Hoboken, New Jersey*. 2009:111–134.
40. FDA CBER. Draft guidance for industry: Considerations for plasmid DNA vaccines for infectious disease indications. 2007.
41. Ledwith BJ, Manam S, Troilo PJ, Barnum AB, Pauley CJ, Griffiths TG, Harper LB, Schock HB, Zhang H, Faris JE, Way PA, Beare CM, Bagdon WJ, Nichols WW. Plasmid DNA vaccines: Assay for integration into host genomic DNA. *Dev Biol (Basel)*. 2000;104:33–43.
42. Wang Z, Troilo PJ, Griffiths II TG Pacchione SJ, Barnum AB, Harper LB, Pauley CJ, Nui Z, Denisova L, Follmer TT, Rizzuto G, Ciliberto G, Fattori E, Monica NL, Manam S, Ledwith BJ. Detection of integration of plasmid DNA into host genomic DNA following intramuscular and electroporation. *Gene Therapy*. 2004;11: 711–721.
43. Siegrist CA. Neonatal and early life vaccinology. *Vaccine*. 2001;19:3331–3346.
44. Marthas M, Rompay KV, Earl P, Tartaglia J. Conference on Retroviruses and Opportunistic Infections. Program Abstr Conf Retrovir Oppor Infect 11th 2004 San Franc Calif. 2004 Feb 8–11; 11: abstract no. 271.
45. Silverstein AM, Segal S. The ontogeny of antigen-specific T cells. *J Exp Med*. 1975;142(3):802–804.
46. Mor G, Yamshchikov G, Sedegah M. Induction of neonatal tolerance by plasmid DNA vaccination of mice. *J. Clin.Invest*. 1996;98:2700–2705.
47. Samarkos M, Vaiopoulos G. The role of infections in the pathogenesis of autoimmune diseases. *Inflammation and allergy*. 2005;4:99–103.

48. Deodhar SD. Autoimmune diseases: overview and current concepts of pathogenesis. *Clin Biochem.* 1992;25(3):181–185.
49. Marshall E. A shadow falls on hepatitis B vaccination effort. *Science.* 1998; 281(5377):630–631.
50. Dickman S. (Possible cause found for Lyme arthritis. *Science.* 1998;281(5377): 631–632.
51. Shoenfeld Y, Aron-Maor A. Vaccination and autoimmunity – "vaccinosis" A dangerous liaison? *J Autoimmun.* 2000;14:1–10.
52. Monteyne P, André FE. Is there a causal link between hepatitis B vaccination and multiple sclerosis? *Vaccine.* 2000;18:1994–2001.
53. Brickman CM, Shoenfeld Y. The mosaic of autoimmunity. *Scand J Clin Lab Invest Suppl.* 2001;235:3–15.
54. Chen RT, Pless R, Destefano F. Epidemiology of autoimmune reactions induced by vaccination. *J. Autoimmun.* 2001;16:309–318.
55. Wraith DC, Goldman M, Lambert PH. Vaccination and autoimmune disease: what is the evidence? *Lancet.* 2003;362 (9396): 1659–1666.
56. Tsuchiya N, Williams RC. Molecular mimicry- hypothesis or reality? *West J Med.* 1992;157:133–138.
57. Christen U, von Herrath MG Infections and autoimmunity – good or bad? *J. Immunol.* 2005;174(12):7481–7486.
58. Ang CW, Jacobs BC, Laman JD. The Guillain-Barré syndrome: A true case of molecular mimicry. *Trends Immunol.* 2004;25(2):61–66.
59. Guilherme L, Oshiro SE, Fae KC, Cunha-Neto E, Renesto G, Goldberg AC, Tanaka AC, Pomerantzeff PM, Kiss MH, Silva C, Guzman F, Patarroyo ME, Southwood S, Sette A, Kalil J. T-cell reactivity against streptococcal antigens in the periphery mirrors reactivity of heart-infiltrating T lymphocytes in rheumatic heart disease patients. *Infect Immun.* 2001;69:5345–5351.
60. Burova LA, Nagornev VA, Pigarevky PV, Gladilina MM, Gavrilova EA, Seliverstova VG, Totolian AA, Thern A, Shalen C. Myocardial tissue damage in rabbits injected with group A streptococci, types M1 and M22. Role of bacterial immunoglobulin G-binding surface proteins. *Acta Pathol Microbiol Immunol Scand.* 2004;113(1):21–30.
61. Yuki N, Susuki K, Koga M, Nishimoto Y, Odaka M, Hirata K, Taguchi K, Miyatake T, Furukawa K, Kobata T, Yamada M. Carbohydrate mimicry between human ganglioside GM1 and Campylobacter jejuni lipooligosaccharide causes Guillain-Barre syndrome. *Proc Natl Acad Sci USA.* 2004;101(31):11404–11409. Epub 2004 Jul 26.
62. Yuki N. Campylobacter sialyltransferase gene polymorphism directs clinical features of Guillain-Barré syndrome. *J Neurochem.* 2007;103(Suppl 1):150–158.
63. Dinkla K, Nitsche-Schmitz DP, Barroso V, Reissmann S, Johansson HM, Frick IM, Rohde M, Chhatwal GS. Identification of a streptococcal octapeptide motif involved in acute rheumatic fever. *J Biol Chem.* 2007;282(26):18686–18693. Epub Apr 23.
64. Dinkla K, Talay SR, Mörgelin M, Graham RM, Rohde M, Nitsche-Schmitz DP, Chhatwal GS. Crucial role of the CB3-region of collagen IV in PARF-induced acute rheumatic fever. *PLoS One.* 2009;4(3):e4666. Epub Mar 2.
65. Gross DM, Forsthuber T, Tary-Lehmann M, Etling C, Ito K, Nagy ZA, Field JA, Steere AC, Huber BT. Identification of LFA-1 as a candidate autoantigen in treatment-resistant Lyme arthritis. *Science.* 1998;281(5377):703–706.
66. Abbott A. Lyme disease: Uphill struggle. *Nature.* 2006;439 (7076):524–525.
67. Ball R, Shadomy SV, Meyer A, Huber BT, Leffell MS, Zachary A, Belotto M, Hilton E, Bryant-Genevier M, Schriefer ME, Miller FW, Braun MM. HLA type and immune response to *Borrelia burgdorferi* outer surface protein a in people in whom arthritis developed after Lyme disease vaccination. *Arthritis Rheum.* 2009;60(4):1179–1186.
68. Vyas NK, Vyas MN, Chervenak MC, Bundle DR, Pinto BM, Quiocho FA. Structural basis of peptide-carbohydrate mimicry in an antibody-combining site. *Proc Natl Acad Sci USA.* 2003;100(25):15023–15028.

69. Donnelly JJ, Ulmer JB, Shiver JW, Liu MA. DNA vaccines. *Annu Rev Immunol.* 1997;15:617–648.
70. Gurunathan S, Klinman DM, Seder RA. DNA vaccines: Immunology, application and optimization. *Annu Rev Immunol.* 2000;18:927–974.
71. Krieg AM. CpG motifs in bacterial DNA and their immune effects. *Annu Rev Immunol.* 2002;20:709–760.
72. FAO/WHO. Evaluation of allergenicity of genetically modified foods. Report of a joint FAO/WHO expert consultation on allergenicity of foods derived from biotechnology. (Food and Agriculture Organization of the United Nations (FAO), Rome, 2001. http://www.who.int/foodsafety/publications/biotech/en/ec_jan2001.pdf. 2001.
73. FAO/WHO. Codex Alimentarius Commission. Alinorm 03/34: Joint FAO/WHO Food Standard Programme, Codex Alimentarius Commission, Twenty-Fifth Session, Rome, 30 June–5 July, 2003. Appendix III, Guideline for the conduct of food safety assessment of foods derived from recombinant-DNA plants and Appendix IV, Annex on the assessment of possible allergenicity, 2003:47–60.
74. Aalberse RC. Structural biology of allergens. *J Allergy Clin Immunol.* 2000;106(2):228–238.
75. Ladics GS, Bannon GA, Silvanovich A, Cressman RF. Comparison of conventional FASTA identity searches with the 80 amino acid sliding window FASTA search for the elucidation of potential identities to known allergens. *Mol Nutr Food Res.* 2007;51(8):985–998.
76. Silvanovich A, Nemeth MA, Song P, Herman R, Tagliani L, Bannon GA. The value of short amino acid sequence matches for prediction of protein allergenicity. *Toxicol Sci.* 2006;90(1):252–258.
77. Goodman RE, Vieths S, Sampson HA, Hill D, Ebisawa M, Taylor SL, van Ree R. Allergenicity assessment of genetically modified crops – What makes sense? *Nat Biotechnol.* 2008;26(1):73–81.
78. Zhang Q, Wang P, Kim Y, Haste-Andersen P, Beaver J, Bourne PE, Bui HH, Buus S, Frankild S, Greenbaum J, Lund O, Lundegaard C, Nielsen M, Ponomarenko J, Sette A, Zhu Z, Peters B. Immune epitope database analysis resource (IEDB-AR). *Nucleic Acids Res.* 2008;36:W513–W518. Epub 2008 May 31.
79. Taneja V, David CS. Lessons from animal models for human autoimmune diseases. *Nat Immunol.* 2001;2(9),781–784.
80. Classen JB. The timing of immunization affects the development of diabetes in rodents. *Autoimmunity.* 1996;24(3):137–145.
81. Ravel G, Christ M, Liberge P, Burnett R, Descotes J. Effects of two pediatric vaccines on autoimmune diabetes in NOD female mice. *Toxicol Lett.* 2003;146:93–100.
82. Ravel G, Christ M, Howard F, Descotes J. Autoimmunity, environmental exposure and vaccination; Is there a link? *Toxicology.* 2004;196:211–216.
83. Descotes J, Ravel G, Ruat C. Vaccines: Predicting the risk of allergy and autoimmunity. *Toxicology.* 2002;174:45–51.
84. Bohlke K, Davis RL, Marcy SM, Braun MM. Risk of anaphylaxis after vaccination of children and adolescents. *Pediatrics.* 2003;112:815–820.
85. Fulginiti VA, Eller JJ, Downie AW, Kempe CH. Altered reactivity to measles virus. Atypical measles in children previously immunized with inactivated measles virus vaccine. *J Am Med Assoc.* 1967;202 (12):1075–1080.
86. Graham BS, Henderson GS, Tang YW, Lu X, Neuzil KM, Colley DG. Priming immunization determines T helper cytokine mRNA expression patterns in lungs of mice challenged with respiratory syncytial virus. *J Immunol.* 1993;151(4):2032–2040.
87. Waris ME, Tsou C, Erdman DD, Zaki SR,Anderson LJ. Respiratory syncytial virus infection in BALB/c mice previously immunized with formalin-inactivated virus induces enhanced pulmonary inflammatory response with a predominant Th2-like cytokine pattern. *J Virol.* 1996;70(5):2852–2860.

88. Prince GA, Jenson AB, Hemming VG, Murphy BR, Walsh EE, Horswood RL, Chanock R. Enhancement of respiratory syncytial virus pulmonary pathology in cotton rats by prior intramuscular inoculation of formalin inactivated virus. *J Virol.* 1986;57(3):721–728.
89. Prince GA, Curtis SJ, Yim KC, Porter DD. Vaccine-enhanced respiratory syncytial virus disease in cotton rats following immunization with Lot 100 or a newly prepared reference vaccine. *J Gen Virol.* 2001;82:2881–2888.
90. Moghaddam A, Olszewska W, Wang B, Tregoning JS, Helson R, Sattentau QJ, Openshaw PJ. A potential molecular mechanism for hypersensitivity caused by formalin-inactivated vaccines. *Nat Med.* 2006;12(8):905–907.
91. Igietseme JU, Ananaba GA, Bolie J, Bowers S, Moore T, Belay T, Eko FO,Lyn D, Black CM. Suppression of endogenous IL-10 gene expression in dendritic cells enhances antigen presentation for specific Th1 induction: potential for cellular vaccine development. *J Immunol.* 2000;164:4212–4219.
92. Openshaw P, Culley FJ, Olszewska W. Immunopathogenesis vaccine-enhanced RSV disease. *Vaccine.* 2001;20:S27–S31.
93. Opensahw PJ, Tregoning JS. Immune responses and disease enhancement during respiratory syncytial virus infection. *Clin Microbiol Rev.* 2005;18(3):541–555.
94. De Swart LT, Kuiken T, Timmerman HH, van Amerongen G, Van den Hoogen B, Vos HW, Neijens HJ, Andeweg AC, Osterhaus A. Immunization of macaques with formalin-inactivated respiratory syncytial virus (RSV) induces interleukin-13 associated hypersensitivity to subsequent RSV infection. *J Virol.* 2002;76(22):11561–11569.
95. Ruat C, Caillet C, Bidaut A, Simon J, Osterhaus A. Vaccination of macaques with adjuvanted formalin – invactivated influenza A virus (HRN1) vaccines: Protection against HRN1 challenge without disease enhancement. *J Virol.* 2008;82(5):2565–2569.
96. Perreau M, Pantaleo G, Kremer EJ. Activation of a dendritic cell-T cell axis by Ad5 immune complexes creates an improved environment for replication of HIV in T cells. *J Exp Med.* 2008;12:2717–2725.
97. Byrd LG, Prince GA. Animal models of respiratory syncytial virus infection. *Clin Infect Dis.* 1997;25:1363–1368.
98. Medjitna T, Stadier C, Bruckner L, Griot C, Ottiger HP. DNA vaccines: Safety aspect assessment and regulation. *Dev Biol.* 2006;126 (Discussion 327):261–270.
99. Verdier F, Burnett R, Michelet-Habchi C, Moretto P, Fievet-Groyne F, Sauzeat E. Aluminium assay and evaluation of the local reaction at several time points after intramuscular administration of aluminium containing vaccines in the Cynomolgus monkey. *Vaccine.* 2005;23:1359–1367.
100. EMEA. Guideline on adjuvants in vaccines for human use. EMEA/CHMP/VEG/134716/2004. 2005.
101. Verdier F, Patriarca C, Descotes J. Autoantibodies in conventional toxicity testing. *Toxicology.* 1997;119(1):51–58.
102. Shoenfeld Y, Isenberg D. The mosaic of autoimmunity. In: Turk JL, ed. *Research Monographs in Immunology.* Amsterdam: Elsevier; 1989: 1–52.
103. Randolph GJ, Beaulieu S, Lebecque S, Steinman RM, Muller WA. Differentiation of monocytes into dendritic cells in a model of transendothelial trafficking. *Science.* 1998;282: 480–483.
104. Simister N. Placental transport of immunoglobulin G. *Vaccine.* 2003;24: 3365–3369.
105. Fujimoto K, Terao K, Cho F, Honjo S. The placental transfer of IgG in the cynomologus monkey. *Jpn J Med Sci Biol.* 1993;36:171–176.
106. Rojas R, Apodaca G. Immunoglobulin transport across polarized epithelial cells. *Nat Rev Mol Cell Biol.* 2002;3:1–12.
107. Appleby P, Catty D. Transmission of immunoglobulin to foetal and neonatal mice. *J Reproductive Immunol.* 1983;5:203–213.

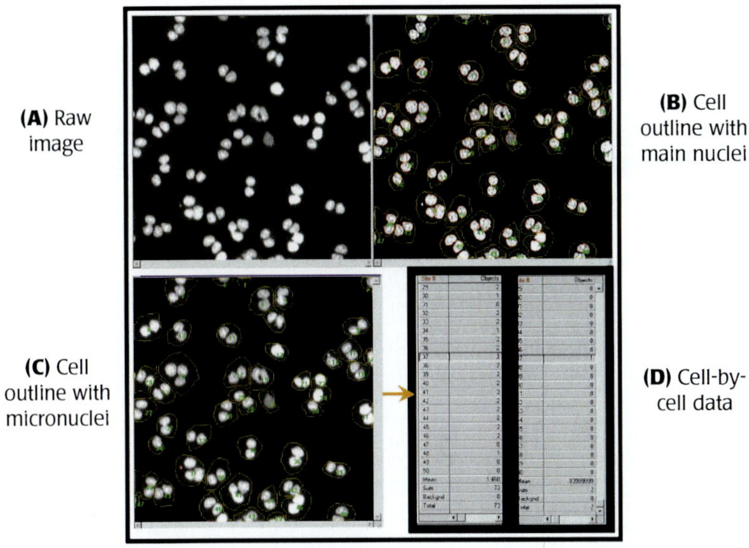

Figure 2-4: Automated image analysis of the *in vitro* micronucleus assay.

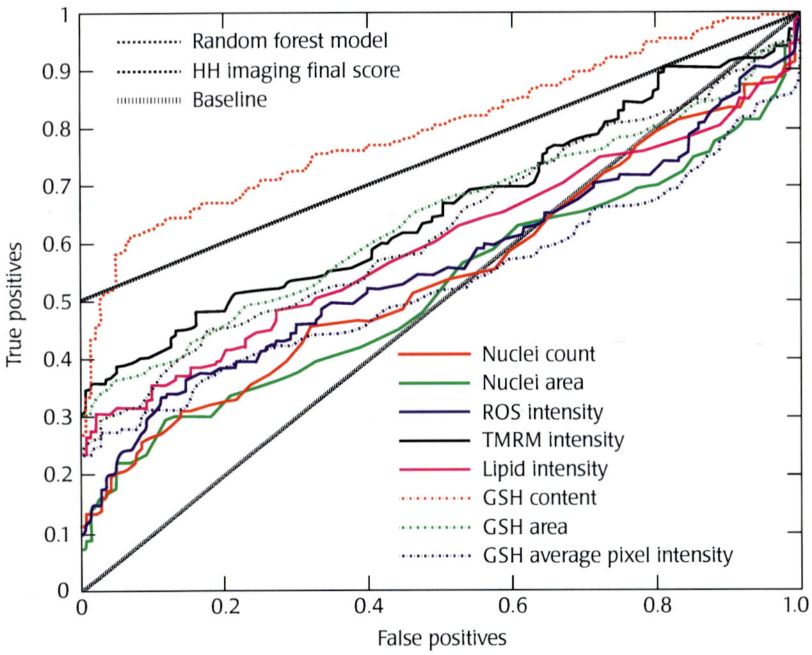

Figure 4-2: Receiver operator characteristic (ROC) curve showing the fractions of both true positives and false positives at any given threshold of HIAT imaging parameters. Automated image analysis and standard machine learning algorithms were applied to generate the ROC curves, for both individual imaging readout and various combined readouts. The best threshold yielded data point toward the top left of the curve (i.e., high true positive rate and low false positive rate). The combined human hepatocytes imaging score and random forest model produced the best balance of true positive (50–60 percent) and false positive rates (0–5 percent). Reprinted with permission from Xu et al.[108]

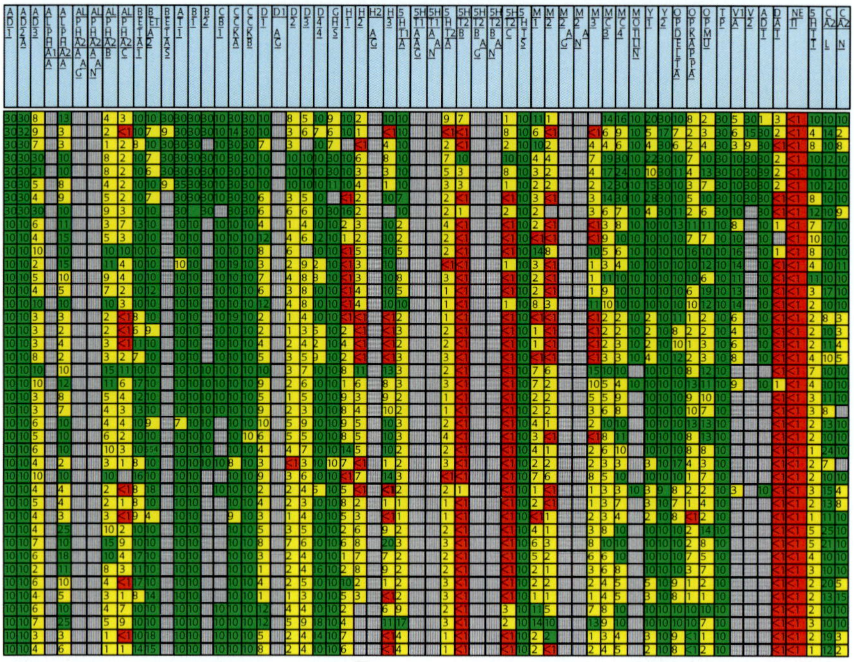

Figure 10-2: Heatmap of compounds submitted by a drug discovery project for off-target profiling. Each row represents a compound and columns are assigned to off-targets. This particular project has a serious problem with pharmacological promiscuity as compounds hit several targets at submicromolar potency. Red squares represent IC_{50} <1 μ*M*, yellow 1–10 μ*M*, and green >10 μ*M*. AG: agonist activity; AN: antagonist activity measured in functional assays.

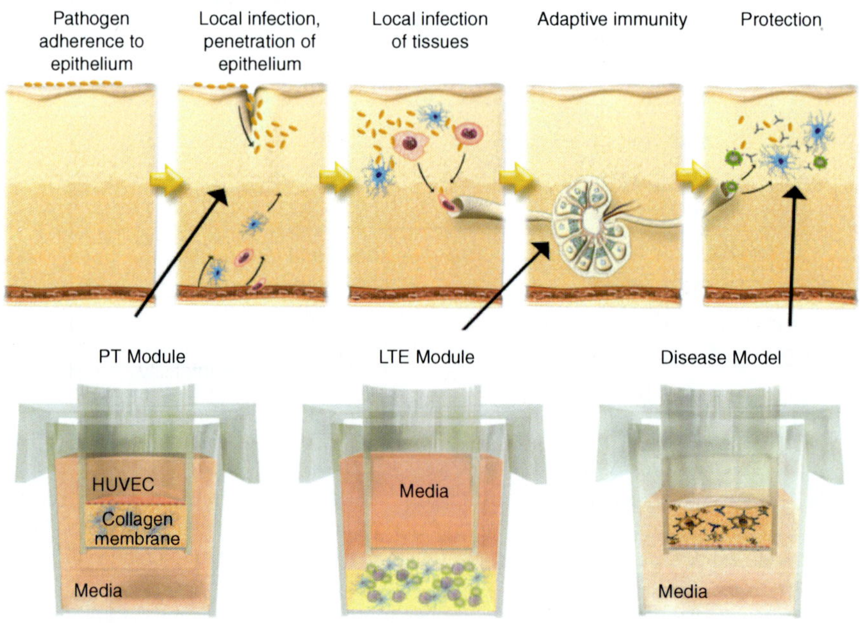

Figure 19-3: Graphical representation of an immune response and how it is modeled via the PTE, LTE, and disease model (functional assay) modules of the MIMIC system.

Epilogue

"to travel hopefully is a better thing than to arrive"

Robert Louis Stevenson

A year ago and hundreds of pages earlier, Jim and I have embraced a journey with fellow toxicologists to navigate the treacherous road through safety assessment to destination "SUCCESSFUL DRUGS." This book is the result – a roadmap – of this effort. Our traveling companion co-authors share their experiences and provide plenty of good advice, but this safety travel guide also raises important questions about the present status regarding the safety assessment of future medicines: It is a bumpy road.

We asked our colleagues to focus on integrated safety assessment models within their expert area of preclinical toxicology with an open eye on advances predicted by novel scientific discoveries and innovative experimental design. The content of this book reveals the richness of the landscape of preclinical safety, which is increasingly enhanced by ideas and methodologies offered by genomics, metabolomics, and proteomics. We are confident that readers using this book will find their topic of interest in preclinical toxicology and will be provided with an updated account of the field. All or most chapters combine theoretical and technological information and give guidance on data interpretation. We realize that today everyone is swamped with information, which does not always generate knowledge. Ever more pharmaceutical and biotechnology companies and academic institutions realize that the use of smart information technology and *in silico* tools is necessary to correlate and interpret data.

At the end of this book, we would like to supply some food for thoughts and highlight two major elements of modern preclinical toxicology. We start with the concept of early integrated risk assessment. The combination of *in vitro* and *in vivo* data with the knowledge of the possible modifying effects of some diseases provides a new power for safety assessment. A recent clinical candidate with a low micromolar hERG IC_{50} in functional, cellular assays is an excellent case to support this approach. Nonrodent telemetry data of this compound predicted a therapeutic index of >30, and the early clinical phase trials showed no sign of LQT or arrhythmia. However, once the compound was tried for the selected indication restricted to diabetic patients, LQT and arrhythmia developed. In a conventional scenario of safety support, one would rely overwhelmingly on the *in vivo* data, yet it has to be considered that "latent" off-target activity could manifest during a pathological condition. In the case at hand, the correct decision could be either to use an *in vivo* model of relevant pathology (e.g., diabetes) or to consider the off-target data early and then design the *in vivo* telemetry with such high doses that it will be able to support an increased therapeutic window. Alternatively, the compound should be abandoned. Termination would have saved millions of dollars as well.

However, if the safety assessment data and their correct interpretation are available early during drug development, there is a better way to go. This brings us to the second concept, namely mitigation of predicted liabilities during lead optimization. Signals of a certain off-target activity or organ-specific toxicity often can be associated with structural features within a chemical series, and chemists could use SAR to mitigate liabilities. An increasing number of off-targets are associated with clinical adverse drug reactions and increasingly *in vitro* assays or a combination of assays can support SAR in a cost-effective and predictive manner. They allow rapid testing of a relatively large number of compounds and their prioritization by improved side effect prediction. An additional benefit comes from the generation of large pools of data, which could serve as training sets for developing *in silico* tools. The power of this approach is that it makes possible mitigating safety issues during early drug discovery at relatively low cost and could prevent or improve late, expensive attrition during clinical trials.

As most new *in vitro* toxicology tests and assays use human cells, tissues, and proteins expressed in various cells, species specificity can also be investigated fairly early. When animal experiments signal unexpected toxic effects, one can sift through the extensive *in vitro* data and determine if the expected target molecule shares homology between the human and animal species.

It is most appropriate to sign off this book by highlighting the major aim of every safety assessment, which is to ensure the safety and well-being of the patient. Predicting clinical performance, toxic effects, and adverse reactions is by far not perfect, not just during drug discovery but within the more rigorous testing regimen of the preclinical development phase. While on average only one in hundreds of compounds in drug discovery will achieve the status of a clinical candidate, it is critically important to keep a watchful eye not just on the drug's potency but also on its drug-like behaviors and toxic effects. Early attrition is now well managed within ADME (absorption, distribution, metabolism, and excretion) with excellent predictive power for clinical performance. Interestingly, *in silico* and *in vitro* methods led the way to achieve this. Introduction of more detailed and sophisticated pharmacokinetics during lead optimization further improved the process.

Unfortunately, safety-related attrition is still high partly because of less awareness of early signals for toxic effects and partly because more complex and less understood biological processes can culminate in unwanted conditions. This book makes an effort to provide a single tome to help drug discovery scientists use the best tools available and make better decisions based on integrated risk assessments for drug safety.

If there is a single message we would like to deliver before you close these pages, it is: Always think about how to use the best knowledge and scientific power to discover and develop medicines that cure and "do no harm" (επι δηλησει δε και αδικιηι ειρξειν) to the patient.

Laszlo Urban and Jinghai J. Xu
November 1, 2009

Index